FIX-IT and FORGET-IT
Diabetic Cookbook

"Each of the hundreds of recipes for appetizers, main courses, soups, vegetables, breakfast dishes, and snacks comes with a nutritional analysis, and timely healthy tips are scattered among the recipes. Good also includes a week of sample menus (with nutritional breakdowns), answers the '10 Most Asked Questions about Diabetes' and gives a brief reading list."

—Publishers Weekly

Other slow cooker cookbooks in this series—

Fix-It and Forget-It Cookbook
Fix-It and Forget-It Lightly
Fix-It and Forget-It 5-Ingredient Favorites
Fix-It and Forget-It Recipes for Entertaining
More than 7.5 million copies of these cookbooks already sold!

FIX-IT and FORGET-IT

Diabetic Cookbook

Slow Cooker Favorites—
To Include Everyone!

New York Times bestselling author
Phyllis Pellman Good
with **American Diabetes Association**

RODALE

Exclusive direct mail edition published in June 2012 by Rodale Inc.
Reprinted by arrangement with Good Books, Intercourse, PA 17534.

© 2005 by Good Books

Illustrations by Cheryl Benner
Photographs by Mitch Mandel/Rodale Images
Book design by Christina Gaugler

Library of Congress Cataloging-in-Publication Data

Good, Phyllis Pellman.
    Fix-it and forget-it diabetic cookbook : slow cooker favorites, to include everyone / Phyllis Pellman Good ; with American Diabetes Association.
        p.   cm.
    Includes index.
    ISBN 978-1-60961-834-6 hardcover
    1. Diabetes—Diet therapy—Recipes.   2. Electric cooking, Slow.   I. American Diabetes Association.   II. Title.
    RC662.G66   2012
    641.5'6314—dc23   2012004828

Distributed to the trade by Macmillan
2   4   6   8   10   9   7   5   3   1   hardcover

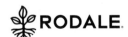

RODALE.

We inspire and enable people to improve their lives and the world around them.
For more of our products visit rodalestore.com or call 800-848-4735

Contents

The Main Courses

The Extras

About *Fix-It and Forget-It Diabetic Cookbook*

The recipes in this collection are for everyone! No more isolating persons with diabetes at mealtime. In fact, these delicious recipes offer both great taste and nutritional value—and easy preparation—the Fix-It and Forget-It trademark.

The American Diabetes Association joined us in this cookbook, using their know-how to adapt the recipes and analyze them so they fit into meal plans. Each recipe is followed by its Exchange List Values and its Basic Nutritional Values. Persons with diabetes need this information so they can manage their calories, and their carb, fat, and sodium counts.

Do You Wish You Knew More about Diabetes?

Don't miss the basic information given in our introduction, A Few Thoughts about Eating and Cooking When You Have Diabetes (pages ix–x), and after the recipes, 10 Most Asked Questions about Diabetes (pages 387–389). If you want to learn more, see the Recommended Reading List on page 390.

Would you like a little more help to manage your own or your loved one's eating? The American Diabetes Association provides a Week of Menus on pages 371–386, using one or two recipes from this cookbook each day.

Calculating the Nutritional Analyses

If the number of servings is given as a range, we used the higher number to do the nutritional analyses calculations.

The nutritional analysis for each recipe includes all ingredients except those labeled "optional," those listed as "to taste," or those calling for a "dash." If an ingredient is listed with a second choice, the first choice was used in the analysis. If a range is given for the amount of an ingredient, the first number was used. Foods listed as "serve with" at the end of a recipe, or accompanying foods listed without an amount, were not included in the recipe's analysis. In recipes calling for cooked rice, pasta, or other grains, the analysis is based on the starch being prepared without added salt or fat, unless indicated otherwise in the recipe.

The analyses were done assuming that meats were trimmed of all visible fat, and that skin was removed from poultry, before being placed in the slow cooker.

Relax and Enjoy These Recipes!

Mealtimes should be refreshing. Now you can relax and enjoy these recipes because you know the content of what you're preparing and how that will affect a meal plan.

These easy-to-prepare recipes take so little time and attention, they'll help you stick to your food goals.

Diabetes need not keep us from all gathering around the table together, eating tasty, wholesome food.

After all, a diet that's healthy for persons with diabetes is healthy for everyone. And everyone can eat and enjoy it when you use recipes from *Fix-It and Forget-It Diabetic Cookbook: Slow Cooker Favorites—To Include Everyone!*

—Phyllis Pellman Good

A Few Thoughts about Eating and Cooking When You Have Diabetes

No matter what the latest diet fad is, people with diabetes must always focus on carbohydrates, because carbohydrates raise blood sugar. Choosing the right foods, exercising every day (such as walking), and taking diabetes medications are the three things these people do to balance their blood sugar levels and stay healthy. (Actually, the first two are what we all should do to stay healthy!)

What Exactly Is a Carbohydrate?

Now, you may have been cooking all your life and still not be sure what a carbohydrate (carb) is. Our mothers and grandmothers showed us how to design a meal, and this is still pretty much the way we fill a plate:

Meat	
Starch (rice, pasta, potato, squash, corn, peas, beans)	carb
Vegetable	
Salad	
Bread	carb
Milk, water, tea	carb
Dessert (fruit, cake, ice cream, etc.)	carb

You see carbohydrates (carbs) in the starches (rice, pasta, potato, squash, corn, peas, or beans), in the bread and milk, the sugar in your tea, and the dessert (including fruit). These are foods we all like to eat, and none of us can—or should—go for more than about two weeks without carbohydrates in our meals. We need the nutrients that come in carbohydrate foods, which are our body's favorite fuel. The trick is in choosing which ones, because today we have so many choices that our grandmothers didn't have.

Why Vegetables Work for You

Leafy green, red, and orange vegetables do contain some carbohydrates, but—unlike starchy potatoes, squash, corn, peas, and beans—they don't have much. So these types of vegetables will have a smaller impact on your blood glucose. Don't forget that vegetables are also a powerhouse of vitamins and minerals—and that's great for your health.

Vegetables also have fiber, which slows down digestion of your food, which in turn slows down the rise in your blood sugar. (Can you see that vegetables really are the stars of the dinner plate?) Eating foods with fiber keeps your body working well. Simply put, these are the qualities within carbs that your body prefers, whether it is a whole grain, fruit, or vegetable. These foods come to you straight from the farmer's field, so they contain lots of vitamins, minerals, and fiber. Some whole grains to look for are slow-cooking oats (sometimes called "rolled oats"), whole wheat flour, stone-ground cornmeal, and brown rice.

Watch Out for These!

Other carbs are part of the bread, starch, drink, or dessert categories, but they have traveled far from the farmer's field before getting to you. Processed grains, such as white flour and white rice, have had their germ, bran, and fiber removed. That takes out a lot of their natural vitamins and minerals, so the food manufacturer puts some artificial vitamins back in. You can read the names of these artificial vitamins on the food labels attached to the packages containing breads, cookies, and other products. Because they don't have fiber, these carbs are digested quickly, raising blood sugar more quickly, too.

Chips, cookies, and desserts are carb foods that also contain fat. Fat slows down digestion, so it helps balance the blood sugar spike caused by white flour and white sugar. But some fats are better for you than others. Most processed foods contain fats called "trans fats" that are found in the "hydrogenated veg-etable oil" listed on the ingredients label. We are learning that trans fats may be the worst of the saturated fats, so food processors are starting to use other fats in their products.

Good Fats

Research shows that we all need to eat some fat every day. Our bodies just don't work right without fats. So which fats are best for your health? You probably have heard that you shouldn't eat a lot of solid fats, such as margarine, butter, marbled meat, or cheese. Vegetable oils are better, and olive oil and canola oil are the best oils because they contain balanced amounts of omega-6 and omega-3 fats. These fats are important for your heart and blood vessels (which is why you should eat more fish and freshly ground flaxseeds).

Processed foods contain a lot of omega-6 fats, but almost no omega-3 fats. You need balance. You find balance and good fats in nuts; avocados; olives; nut butters; olive and canola oils; and sesame, pumpkin, flax, and sunflower seeds. In fact, you might try a handful or two of raw almonds as a part of your daily "bread."

Remember:

- Good carb choices: whole grains, fruits, and vegetables
- Good fat choices: olive oil, avocados, fish, nuts, and seeds

—*American Diabetes Association*

Serving Sizes for Recipes in
Fix-It and Forget-It Diabetic Cookbook

Serving sizes are based approximately on these measurements, portion sizes which are consistent with healthy-eating guidelines.

Appetizer dips: 1–2 Tbsp.

Beans and legumes, cooked: ½ cup

Beverages: 1 cup

Desserts: ½ cup, ⅛ pie

Fruit: ½ cup

Frozen desserts: ½ cup

Grains and pasta side dishes: ½ cup

Main-dish sauces (for pasta, potato toppings, etc.): ½ cup

Meat, poultry, and seafood, cooked: ⅓–½ cup

One-dish meals (meat, poultry, seafood, meatless), cooked: 1–1½ cups

Salad dressing, barbecue sauce: 2 Tbsp.

Salads: ½ cup vegetable, fruit, and grain salads; 1–2 cups lettuce

Sauces: 2 Tbsp.

Soup: ¾–1 cup (as a side dish or appetizer); 1–1½ cups (as a main dish)

Vegetables, cooked: ½ cup

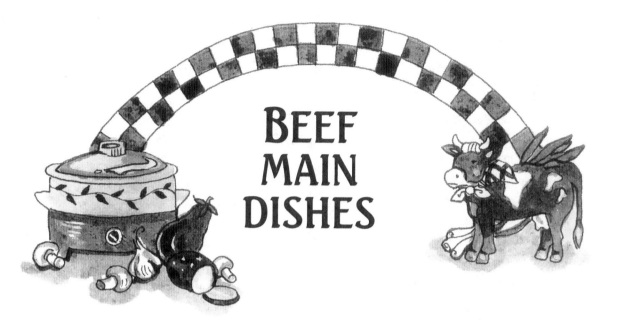

BEEF MAIN DISHES

Beef Stew

Wanda S. Curtin • Bradenton, FL / Paula King • Harrisonburg, VA / Miriam Nolt • New Holland, PA / Jean Shaner • York, PA / Mary W. Stauffer • Ephrata, PA / Alma Z. Weaver • Ephrata, PA

Makes 6 servings (Ideal slow cooker size: 4-quart)

2 lbs. beef chuck, cubed, trimmed of fat

¼–½ cup flour

¾ tsp. salt

½ tsp. pepper

1 tsp. paprika

1 tsp. Worcestershire sauce

1½ cups beef broth

half clove garlic, minced

1 bay leaf

4 medium carrots, sliced

2 medium onions, chopped

1 rib celery, sliced

3 medium potatoes, diced, unpeeled

1. Place meat in slow cooker.

2. Combine flour, salt, pepper, and paprika. Stir into meat until coated thoroughly.

3. Add remaining ingredients. Mix well.

4. Cover. Cook on Low 10–12 hours, or High 4–6 hours.

Exchange List Values: Starch 1.5, Vegetable 2.0, Meat, lean 2.0

Basic Nutritional Values: Calories 278 (Calories from Fat 55), Total Fat 6 gm (Saturated Fat 1.9 gm, Polyunsat Fat 0.5 gm, Monounsat Fat 2.8 gm, Cholesterol 75 mg), Sodium 598 mg, Total Carbohydrate 28 gm, Dietary Fiber 4 gm, Sugars 7 gm, Protein 28 gm

If someone you love has diabetes, you can help by learning about the disease, talking about your feelings (because diabetes affects you, too!), offering practical help, and getting help if needed.

Bavarian Beef

Naomi E. Fast • Hesston, KS

Makes 8 servings (Ideal slow cooker size: 4–5-quart)

3-lb. boneless beef chuck roast, trimmed of fat

1 Tbsp. canola oil

3 cups sliced carrots

3 cups sliced onions

2 large kosher dill pickles, chopped

1 cup sliced celery

$\frac{1}{2}$ cup dry red wine or beef broth

$\frac{1}{3}$ cup German-style mustard

2 tsp. coarsely ground black pepper

2 bay leaves

$\frac{1}{4}$ tsp. ground cloves

1 cup water

$\frac{1}{3}$ cup flour

1. Brown roast on both sides in oil in skillet. Transfer to slow cooker.

2. Add remaining ingredients except flour.

3. Cover. Cook on Low 6–7 hours.

4. Remove meat and vegetables to large platter. Cover to keep warm.

5. Mix flour with 1 cup of cooking broth until smooth. Return to cooker. Turn on High and stir, cooking until broth is smooth and thickened.

6. Serve over noodles or spaetzle.

Exchange List Values: Starch 0.5, Vegetable 2.0, Meat, lean 3.0

Basic Nutritional Values: Calories 251 (Calories from Fat 76), Total Fat 8 gm (Saturated Fat 2.4 gm, Polyunsat Fat 0.9 gm, Monounsat Fat 3.8 gm, Cholesterol 73 mg), Sodium 525 mg, Total Carbohydrate 17 gm, Dietary Fiber 4 gm, Sugars 7 gm, Protein 26 gm

Beef Stew with Shiitake Mushrooms

Kathy Hertzler • Lancaster, PA

Makes 4–6 servings (Ideal slow cooker size: 4–5-quart)

12 new potatoes, cut into quarters

$\frac{1}{2}$ cup chopped onions

8-oz. pkg. baby carrots

3.4-oz. pkg. fresh shiitake mushrooms, sliced, or 2 cups regular white mushrooms, sliced

16-oz. can whole tomatoes

$14\frac{1}{2}$-oz. can beef broth

$\frac{1}{2}$ cup flour

1 Tbsp. Worcestershire sauce

1 tsp. sugar

1 tsp. dried marjoram leaves

$\frac{1}{4}$ tsp. pepper

1 lb. beef stewing meat, cubed, trimmed of fat

1. Combine all ingredients except beef in slow cooker. Add beef.

2. Cover. Cook on Low 8–9 hours. Stir well before serving.

Exchange List Values: Starch 2.0, Vegetable 2.0, Meat, lean 1.0

Basic Nutritional Values: Calories 254 (Calories from Fat 29), Total Fat 3 gm (Saturated Fat 0.9 gm, Polyunsat Fat 0.4 gm, Monounsat Fat 1.4 gm, Cholesterol 38 mg), Sodium 534 mg, Total Carbohydrate 39 gm, Dietary Fiber 5 gm, Sugars 8 gm, Protein 18 gm

Dawn's Mushroom Beef Stew

Dawn Day • Westminster, CA

Makes 8–10 servings (Ideal slow cooker size: 4–5-quart)

1 lb. sirloin, cubed, trimmed of fat

2 Tbsp. flour

1 Tbsp. canola oil

1 large onion, chopped

2 cloves garlic, minced

½ lb. button mushrooms, sliced

2 ribs celery, sliced

3 large carrots, sliced

3–4 large potatoes, cubed

2 tsp. seasoning salt

14½-oz. can beef stock, or 2 bouillon cubes dissolved in 1⅔ cups water

½–1 cup good red wine

1. Dredge sirloin in flour and brown in oil in skillet. Reserve drippings. Place meat in slow cooker.

2. Saute onion, garlic, and mushrooms in drippings just until soft. Add to meat.

3. Add all remaining ingredients.

4. Cover. Cook on Low 6 hours. Test to see if vegetables are tender. If not, continue cooking on Low for another 1–1½ hours.

5. Serve with crusty bread.

Exchange List Values: Starch 1.5, Vegetable 2.0, Meat, lean 1.0, Fat 0.5

Basic Nutritional Values: Calories 247 (Calories from Fat 49), Total Fat 5 gm (Saturated Fat 1.1 gm, Polyunsat Fat 1.0 gm, Monounsat Fat 2.8 gm, Cholesterol 38 mg), Sodium 572 mg, Total Carbohydrate 33 gm, Dietary Fiber 5 gm, Sugars 7 gm, Protein 17 gm

Hungarian Barley Stew

Naomi E. Fast • Hesston, KS

Makes 8 servings (Ideal slow cooker size: 4-quart)

1½ lbs. beef cubes, trimmed of fat

2 Tbsp. canola oil

2 large onions, diced

1 medium-sized green pepper, chopped

28-oz. can whole tomatoes

½ cup ketchup

⅔ cup dry small pearl barley

½ tsp. salt

½ tsp. pepper

1 Tbsp. paprika

10-oz. pkg. frozen baby lima beans

3 cups water

1 cup fat-free sour cream

1. Brown beef cubes in oil in skillet. Add onions and green peppers. Saute. Pour into slow cooker.

2. Add remaining ingredients except sour cream.

3. Cover. Cook on High 5 hours.

4. Stir in sour cream before serving.

5. Serve with your favorite cabbage slaw.

Exchange List Values: Starch 1.5, Vegetable 2.0, Meat, lean 2.0

Basic Nutritional Values: Calories 286 (Calories from Fat 67), Total Fat 7 gm (Saturated Fat 1.3 gm, Polyunsat Fat 1.5 gm, Monounsat Fat 3.6 gm, Cholesterol 44 mg), Sodium 558 mg, Total Carbohydrate 36 gm, Dietary Fiber 6 gm, Sugars 11 gm, Protein 20 gm

Beef Burgundy and Bacon

Joyce Kaut • Rochester, NY

Makes 6 servings (Ideal slow cooker size: 3–4-quart)

1 slice bacon, cut in squares

2 lbs. sirloin tip or round steak, cubed, trimmed of fat

1/4 cup flour

1 tsp. canola oil

1/8 tsp. salt

1/2 tsp. seasoning salt

1/4 tsp. dried marjoram

1/4 tsp. dried thyme

1/4 tsp. pepper

1 clove garlic, minced

1 beef bouillon cube, crushed

1 cup burgundy wine

1/4 lb. fresh mushrooms, sliced

2 Tbsp. cornstarch

2 Tbsp. cold water

1. Cook bacon in skillet until browned. Remove bacon.

2. Coat beef with flour and brown on all sides in canola oil.

3. Combine steak, bacon drippings, bacon, seasonings, garlic, bouillon, and wine in slow cooker.

4. Cover. Cook on Low 6–8 hours.

5. Add mushrooms.

6. Dissolve cornstarch in water. Add to slow cooker.

7. Cover. Cook on High 15 minutes.

8. Serve over noodles.

Exchange List Values: Starch 0.5, Meat, lean 3.0

Basic Nutritional Values: Calories 202 (Calories from Fat 63), Total Fat 7 gm (Saturated Fat 2.0 gm, Polyunsat Fat 0.6 gm, Monounsat Fat 3.5 gm, Cholesterol 76 mg), Sodium 389 mg, Total Carbohydrate 8 gm, Dietary Fiber 0 gm, Sugars 1 gm, Protein 25 gm

Wash-Day Stew

Naomi E. Fast • Hesston, KS

Makes 14 servings (Ideal slow cooker size: 4–5-quart)

1 1/2–2 lbs. lean lamb or beef, cubed, trimmed of fat

2 15-oz. cans garbanzo beans, drained

2 15-oz. cans white beans, drained

2 medium onions, peeled and quartered

1 qt. water

1/2 tsp. salt

1 tomato, peeled and quartered

1 tsp. turmeric

3 Tbsp. fresh lemon juice

8–10 pita bread pockets

1. Combine all ingredients except pitas in slow cooker.

2. Cover. Cook on High 6–7 hours.

3. Lift stew from cooker with a strainer spoon and stuff into pita bread pockets.

Exchange List Values: Starch 3.0, Meat, lean 1.0

Basic Nutritional Values: Calories 287 (Calories from Fat 38), Total Fat 4 gm (Saturated Fat 1.1 gm, Polyunsat Fat 0.9 gm, Monounsat Fat 1.3 gm, Cholesterol 31 mg), Sodium 440 mg, Total Carbohydrate 42 gm, Dietary Fiber 7 gm, Sugars 5 gm, Protein 20 gm

Note: I learned to prepare this nutritious meal from a student from Iran, who was attending graduate school at the University of Nebraska. Fatimeh explained to me that her family prepared this dish every wash day. Very early in the morning, they made a fire in a large rock-lined pit outside. Then they placed a large covered kettle, filled with the ingredients from the opposite page, over the coals to cook slowly all day. At the end of a day of doing laundry, the food was ready with a minimum of preparation. Of course, they started with dry beans and dry garbanzos, presoaked the night before. They served this Wash-Day Stew spooned into pita bread and ate it with their hands.

Forget about your "ideal" weight, or how much you weighed in high school. Shoot for losing 10 pounds over 3–6 months and keeping it off!

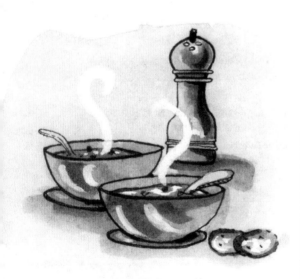

Tempting Beef Stew

Patricia Howard • Albuquerque, NM

Makes 10 servings (Ideal slow cooker size: 4–5-quart)

2 lbs. beef stewing meat, trimmed of fat

3 carrots, sliced thin

1-lb. pkg. frozen green peas with onions

1-lb. pkg. frozen green beans

16-oz. can whole or stewed tomatoes

$\frac{1}{2}$ cup beef broth

$\frac{1}{2}$ cup white wine

$\frac{1}{4}$ cup brown sugar

4 Tbsp. tapioca

$\frac{1}{2}$ cup bread crumbs

$1\frac{1}{2}$ tsp. salt

1 bay leaf

pepper to taste

1. Combine all ingredients in slow cooker.

2. Cover. Cook on Low 10–12 hours.

3. Serve over noodles, rice, couscous, or biscuits.

Exchange List Values: Starch 1.0, Vegetable 2.0, Meat, lean 1.0

Basic Nutritional Values: Calories 203 (Calories from Fat 36), Total Fat 4 gm (Saturated Fat 1.1 gm, Polyunsat Fat 0.4 gm, Monounsat Fat 1.8 gm, Cholesterol 45 mg), Sodium 588 mg, Total Carbohydrate 24 gm, Dietary Fiber 4 gm, Sugars 12 gm, Protein 18 gm

VARIATION: In place of the tapioca, thicken stew with $\frac{1}{4}$ cup flour dissolved in $\frac{1}{3}$-$\frac{1}{2}$ cup water. Mix in and turn cooker to High. Cover and cook for 15–20 minutes.

Note: Prepare this Tempting Beef Stew before your guests arrive. Give yourself time to relax instead of panicking in a last-minute rush.

1-2-3-4 Casserole

Betty K. Drescher • Quakertown, PA

Makes 8 servings (Ideal slow cooker size: 4-quart)

1 lb. 90%-lean ground beef

2 onions, sliced

3 carrots, thinly sliced

½ tsp. salt

⅛ tsp. pepper

½ tsp. cream of tartar

1 cup cold water

4 potatoes, thinly sliced, unpeeled

10¾-oz. can 98%-fat-free, reduced-sodium cream of mushroom soup

¼ cup fat-free milk

½ tsp. salt

⅛ tsp. pepper

1. Layer in greased slow cooker: ground beef, onions, carrots, ½ tsp. salt, and ⅛ tsp. pepper.

2. Dissolve cream of tartar in water in bowl. Toss sliced potatoes with water. Drain.

3. Combine soup and milk. Toss with potatoes. Add remaining salt and pepper. Arrange potatoes in slow cooker.

4. Cover. Cook on Low 7–9 hours.

Exchange List Values: Starch 1.5, Vegetable 1.0, Meat, lean 1.0, Fat 0.5

Basic Nutritional Values: Calories 216 (Calories from Fat 59), Total Fat 7 gm (Saturated Fat 2.6 gm, Polyunsat Fat 0.5 gm, Monounsat Fat 2.6 gm, Cholesterol 37 mg), Sodium 503 mg, Total Carbohydrate 24 gm, Dietary Fiber 3 gm, Sugars 6 gm, Protein 15 gm

VARIATIONS:

1. Substitute sour cream for the milk.

2. Top potatoes with ½ cup shredded cheese.

Herbed Beef Stew

Carol Findling • Princeton, IL

Makes 6–8 servings (Ideal slow cooker size: 4-quart)

1 lb. beef round, cubed, trimmed of fat

4 Tbsp. seasoned flour*

1½ cups beef broth

1 tsp. Worcestershire sauce

1 clove garlic

1 bay leaf

4 medium carrots, sliced

3 medium potatoes, cubed, unpeeled

2 medium onions, diced

1 rounded tsp. fresh thyme, or ½ tsp. dried thyme

1 rounded tsp. chopped fresh basil, or ½ tsp. dried basil

1 Tbsp. fresh parsley, or 1 tsp. dried parsley

1 rounded tsp. fresh marjoram, or 1 tsp. dried marjoram

1. Put meat in slow cooker. Add seasoned flour. Toss with meat. Stir in remaining ingredients. Mix well.

2. Cover. Cook on High 4–6 hours, or Low 10–12 hours.

Exchange List Values: Starch 1.5, Vegetable 2.0, Meat, lean 1.0

Basic Nutritional Values: Calories 220 (Calories from Fat 33), Total Fat 4 gm (Saturated Fat 1.2 gm, Polyunsat Fat 0.3 gm, Monounsat Fat 1.5 gm, Cholesterol 43 mg), Sodium 445 mg, Total Carbohydrate 28 gm, Dietary Fiber 4 gm, Sugars 7 gm, Protein 18 gm

*SEASONED FLOUR:

1 cup flour

1 tsp. salt

1 tsp. paprika

¼ tsp. pepper

Audrey's Beef Stew

Audrey Romonosky • Austin, TX

Makes 4–6 servings (Ideal slow cooker size: 4-quart)

3 medium carrots, sliced

3 medium potatoes, cubed, unpeeled

2 lbs. beef chuck, cubed, trimmed of fat

2 cups water

2 beef bouillon cubes

1 tsp. Worcestershire sauce

½ tsp. garlic powder

1 bay leaf

¼ tsp. salt

½ tsp. pepper

1 tsp. paprika

3 onions, chopped

1 rib celery, sliced

¼ cup flour

⅓ cup cold water

1. Combine all ingredients except flour and ⅓ cup cold water in slow cooker. Mix well.

2. Cover. Cook on Low 8 hours.

3. Dissolve flour in ⅓ cup water. Stir into meat mixture. Cook on High until thickened, about 10 minutes.

Exchange List Values: Starch 1.5, Vegetable 2.0, Meat, lean 2.0

Basic Nutritional Values: Calories 287 (Calories from Fat 54), Total Fat 6 gm (Saturated Fat 1.8 gm, Polyunsat Fat 0.5 gm, Monounsat Fat 2.8 gm, Cholesterol 75 mg), Sodium 501 mg, Total Carbohydrate 30 gm, Dietary Fiber 5 gm, Sugars 9 gm, Protein 28 gm

Pot Roast

Carole Whaling • New Tripoli, PA

Makes 8 servings (Ideal slow cooker size: 4-quart)

4 medium potatoes, cubed

4 medium carrots, sliced

1 medium onion, sliced

3–4-lb. rump roast, or pot roast, bone removed, trimmed of fat, and cut into serving-size pieces

1 tsp. salt

½ tsp. pepper

1 bouillon cube

½ cup boiling water

1. Put vegetables and meat in slow cooker. Stir in salt and pepper.

2. Dissolve bouillon cube in water, then pour over other ingredients.

3. Cover. Cook on Low 10–12 hours.

Exchange List Values: Starch 1.0, Vegetable 1.0, Meat, lean 3.0

Basic Nutritional Values: Calories 246 (Calories from Fat 56), Total Fat 6 gm (Saturated Fat 2.2 gm, Polyunsat Fat 0.3 gm, Monounsat Fat 2.5 gm, Cholesterol 73 mg), Sodium 485 mg, Total Carbohydrate 20 gm, Dietary Fiber 3 gm, Sugars 4 gm, Protein 27 gm

When flying, keep your medications and glucose meter with you in your carry-on luggage so there's no chance of things being lost.

Swiss Steak

Marilyn Mowry • Irving, TX

Makes 4–6 servings (Ideal slow cooker size: 4-quart)

3–4 Tbsp. flour

½ tsp. salt

¼ tsp. pepper

1½ tsp. dry mustard

1½–2 lbs. round steak, trimmed of fat

1 Tbsp. canola oil

1 cup sliced onions

1 lb. carrots, sliced

14½-oz. can whole tomatoes

1 Tbsp. brown sugar

1½ Tbsp. Worcestershire sauce

1. Combine flour, salt, pepper, and dry mustard.

2. Cut steak in serving pieces. Dredge in flour mixture. Brown on both sides in oil in saucepan. Place in slow cooker.

3. Add onions and carrots.

4. Combine tomatoes, brown sugar, and Worcestershire sauce. Pour into slow cooker.

5. Cover. Cook on Low 8–10 hours, or High 3–5 hours.

Exchange List Values: Vegetable 3.0, Meat, lean 3.0

Basic Nutritional Values: Calories 236 (Calories from Fat 71), Total Fat 8 gm (Saturated Fat 1.9 gm, Polyunsat Fat 1.0 gm, Monounsat Fat 3.6 gm, Cholesterol 64 mg), Sodium 426 mg, Total Carbohydrate 18 gm, Dietary Fiber 3 gm, Sugars 9 gm, Protein 23 gm

Hearty Beef Stew

Charlotte Shaffer • East Earl, PA

Makes 4–5 servings (Ideal slow cooker size: 4-quart)

2 lbs. stewing beef, cubed, trimmed of fat

5 medium carrots, sliced

1 large onion, cut in chunks

3 ribs celery, sliced

22-oz. can stewed tomatoes

½ tsp. ground cloves

2 bay leaves

¼ tsp. salt

¼–½ tsp. pepper

1. Combine all ingredients in slow cooker.

2. Cover. Cook on High 5–6 hours.

Exchange List Values: Vegetable 4.0, Meat, lean 3.0

Basic Nutritional Values: Calories 270 (Calories from Fat 66), Total Fat 7 gm (Saturated Fat 2.2 gm, Polyunsat Fat 0.5 gm, Monounsat Fat 3.4 gm, Cholesterol 90 mg), Sodium 575 mg, Total Carbohydrate 21 gm, Dietary Fiber 5 gm, Sugars 10 gm, Protein 31 gm

VARIATIONS:

1. Substitute 1 whole clove for ½ tsp. ground cloves. Remove before serving.

2. Use venison instead of beef.

3. Cut back the salt and use 1 tsp. soy sauce.

Judy's Beef Stew

Judy Koczo • Plano, IL

Makes 4–6 servings (Ideal slow cooker size: 4-quart)

2 lbs. stewing meat, cubed, trimmed of fat

5 medium carrots, sliced

1 medium onion, diced

3 ribs celery, diced

5 medium potatoes, cubed

28-oz. can tomatoes

⅓–½ cup quick-cooking tapioca

½ tsp. salt

½ tsp. pepper

1. Combine all ingredients in slow cooker.

2. Cover. Cook on Low 10–12 hours, or High 5–6 hours.

Exchange List Values: Starch 2.0, Vegetable 3.0, Meat, lean 2.0

Basic Nutritional Values: Calories 357 (Calories from Fat 55), Total Fat 6 gm (Saturated Fat 1.8 gm, Polyunsat Fat 0.6 gm, Monounsat Fat 2.8 gm, Cholesterol 75 mg), Sodium 518 mg, Total Carbohydrate 47 gm, Dietary Fiber 7 gm, Sugars 10 gm, Protein 29 gm

VARIATION: Add 1 whole clove and 2 bay leaves to stew before cooking.

Slow Cooker Stew

Trudy Kutter • Corfu, NY

Makes 6–8 servings (Ideal slow cooker size: 4-quart)

2 lbs. boneless beef, cubed, trimmed of fat

4–6 ribs celery, sliced

6–8 medium carrots, sliced

6 medium potatoes, cubed, unpeeled

2 medium onions, sliced

28-oz. can tomatoes

¼ cup minute tapioca

1 tsp. salt

¼ tsp. pepper

½ tsp. dried basil, or oregano

1 garlic clove, pressed or minced

1. Combine all ingredients in slow cooker.

2. Cover. Cook on Low 8–10 hours.

Exchange List Values: Starch 2.0, Vegetable 3.0, Meat, lean 1.0

Basic Nutritional Values: Calories 299 (Calories from Fat 42), Total Fat 5 gm (Saturated Fat 1.4 gm, Polyunsat Fat 0.5 gm, Monounsat Fat 2.1 gm, Cholesterol 56 mg), Sodium 549 mg, Total Carbohydrate 42 gm, Dietary Fiber 7 gm, Sugars 11 gm, Protein 23 gm

Italian Stew

Ann Gouinlock • Alexander, NY

Makes 6 servings (Ideal slow cooker size: 4-quart)

1½ lbs. beef cubes

2-3 carrots, cut in 1" chunks

3-4 ribs celery, cut in ¾-1" pieces

1-1½ cups coarsely chopped onions

14½-oz. can stewed, or diced, tomatoes

⅓ cup minute tapioca

1½ tsp. salt

¼ tsp. pepper

¼ tsp. Worcestershire sauce

½ tsp. Italian seasoning

1. Combine all ingredients in slow cooker.

2. Cover. Cook on Low 8–10 hours.

Exchange List Values: Starch 0.5, Vegetable 2.0, Meat, lean 2.0

Basic Nutritional Values: Calories 188 (Calories from Fat 41), Total Fat 5 gm (Saturated Fat 1.4 gm, Polyunsat Fat 0.3 gm, Monounsat Fat 2.1 gm, Cholesterol 56 mg), Sodium 508 mg, Total Carbohydrate 18 gm, Dietary Fiber 3 gm, Sugars 6 gm, Protein 19 gm

Anything that raises your pulse and makes you breathe harder—swimming, walking, jogging, dancing, or biking—is aerobic. Find something you enjoy and do it for 30 minutes, three or four times a week.

Venison or Beef Stew

Frances B. Musser • Newmanstown, PA

Makes 6 servings (Ideal slow cooker size: 4-quart)

1½ lbs. venison or beef cubes

2 Tbsp. canola oil

1 medium onion, chopped

4 medium carrots, peeled and cut into 1" pieces

1 rib celery, cut into 1" pieces

4 medium potatoes, peeled and quartered

12-oz. can whole tomatoes, undrained

10½-oz. can beef broth

1 Tbsp. Worcestershire sauce

1 Tbsp. parsley flakes

1 bay leaf

¼ tsp. salt

¼ tsp. pepper

2 Tbsp. quick-cooking tapioca

1. Brown meat cubes in skillet in oil over medium heat. Transfer to slow cooker.

2. Add remaining ingredients. Mix well.

3. Cover. Cook on Low 8–9 hours.

Exchange List Values: Starch 1.5, Vegetable 2.0, Meat, very lean 3.0, Fat 1.0

Basic Nutritional Values: Calories 313 (Calories from Fat 70), Total Fat 8 gm (Saturated Fat 1.5 gm, Polyunsat Fat 2.1 gm, Monounsat Fat 3.5 gm, Cholesterol 102 mg), Sodium 552 mg, Total Carbohydrate 29 gm, Dietary Fiber 4 gm, Sugars 7 gm, Protein 31 gm

VARIATION: For added color and flavor, add 1 cup frozen peas 5 minutes before end of cooking time.

Venison Swiss Steak

Dede Peterson • Rapid City, SD

Makes 6 servings (Ideal slow cooker size: 4-quart)

1/4 cup flour

2 tsp. salt

1/2 tsp. pepper

2 lbs. venison round steak

1 Tbsp. canola oil

2 medium onions, sliced

2 ribs celery, diced

1 cup carrots, diced

2 cups fresh, or stewed, tomatoes

1 Tbsp. Worcestershire sauce

1. Combine flour, salt, and pepper. Dredge steak in flour mixture. Brown in oil in skillet. Place in slow cooker.

2. Add remaining ingredients.

3. Cover. Cook on Low 7 1/2–8 1/2 hours.

Exchange List Values: Starch 0.5, Vegetable 2.0, Meat, very lean 4.0, Fat 1.0

Basic Nutritional Values: Calories 277 (Calories from Fat 59), Total Fat 7 gm (Saturated Fat 1.7 gm, Polyunsat Fat 1.6 gm, Monounsat Fat 2.5 gm, Cholesterol 135 mg), Sodium 527 mg, Total Carbohydrate 14 gm, Dietary Fiber 3 gm, Sugars 6 gm, Protein 39 gm

Swiss Steak

Wanda S. Curtin • Bradenton, FL /
Jeanne Hertzog • Bethlehem, PA

Makes 6 servings (Ideal slow cooker size: 4-quart)

1 1/2 lbs. round steak, about 3/4" thick, trimmed of fat

2–4 tsp. flour

1/2–1 tsp. salt

1/4 tsp. pepper

1 medium onion, sliced

1 medium carrot, chopped

1 rib celery, chopped

14 1/2-oz. can diced tomatoes, or 15-oz. can tomato sauce

1. Cut steak into serving pieces.

2. Combine flour, salt, and pepper. Dredge meat in seasoned flour.

3. Place onions in bottom of slow cooker. Add meat. Top with carrots and celery and cover with tomatoes.

4. Cover. Cook on Low 8–10 hours, or High 3–5 hours.

5. Serve over noodles or rice.

Exchange List Values: Vegetable 2.0, Meat, lean 2.0

Basic Nutritional Values: Calories 172 (Calories from Fat 48), Total Fat 5 gm (Saturated Fat 1.7 gm, Polyunsat Fat 0.3 gm, Monounsat Fat 2.2 gm, Cholesterol 64 mg), Sodium 381 mg, Total Carbohydrate 8 gm, Dietary Fiber 2 gm, Sugars 4 gm, Protein 22 gm

Margaret's Swiss Steak

Margaret Rich • North Newton, KS

Makes 6 servings (Ideal slow cooker size: 4-quart)

1 cup chopped onions

½ cup chopped celery

2-lb., ½"-thick round steak, trimmed of fat

¼ cup flour

3 Tbsp. oil

1 tsp. salt

¼ tsp. pepper

16-oz. can diced tomatoes

¼ cup flour

½ cup water

1. Place onions and celery in bottom of slow cooker.

2. Cut steak in serving-size pieces. Dredge in ¼ cup flour. Brown on both sides in oil in saucepan. Place in slow cooker.

3. Sprinkle with salt and pepper. Pour on tomatoes.

4. Cover. Cook on Low 9 hours. Remove meat from cooker and keep warm.

5. Turn heat to High. Blend together ¼ cup flour and water. Stir into sauce in slow cooker. Cover and cook 15 minutes. Serve with steak.

Exchange List Values: Starch 0.5, Vegetable 1.0, Meat, lean 4.0, Fat 0.5

Basic Nutritional Values: Calories 305 (Calories from Fat 124), Total Fat 14 gm (Saturated Fat 2.8 gm, Polyunsat Fat 2.4 gm, Monounsat Fat 7.0 gm, Cholesterol 85 mg), Sodium 592 mg, Total Carbohydrate 14 gm, Dietary Fiber 2 gm, Sugars 4 gm, Protein 30 gm

Nadine & Hazel's Swiss Steak

Nadine Martinitz • Salina, KS / Hazel L. Propst • Oxford, PA

Makes 6-8 servings (Ideal slow cooker size: 4-quart)

3-lb. round steak, trimmed of fat

⅓ cup flour

1 tsp. salt

½ tsp. pepper

3 Tbsp. canola oil

1 large onion, or more, sliced

1 large bell pepper, or more, sliced

14½-oz. can stewed tomatoes, or 3-4 fresh tomatoes, chopped

water

1. Sprinkle meat with flour, salt, and pepper. Pound both sides. Cut into 6 or 8 pieces. Brown meat in canola oil over medium heat on top of stove, about 15 minutes. Transfer to slow cooker.

2. Brown onion and pepper. Add tomatoes and bring to boil. Pour over steak. Add water to completely cover steak.

3. Cover. Cook on Low 6-8 hours.

Exchange List Values: Vegetable 2.0, Meat, lean 4.0, Fat 0.5

Basic Nutritional Values: Calories 296 (Calories from Fat 116), Total Fat 13 gm (Saturated Fat 2.9 gm, Polyunsat Fat 1.9 gm, Monounsat Fat 6.4 gm, Cholesterol 96 mg), Sodium 547 mg, Total Carbohydrate 11 gm, Dietary Fiber 1 gm, Sugars 4 gm, Protein 33 gm

VARIATION: To add some flavor, stir in your favorite dried herbs when beginning to cook the steak, or add fresh herbs in the last hour of cooking.

Beef, Tomatoes, & Noodles

Janice Martins • Fairbank, IA

Makes 8 servings (Ideal slow cooker size: 4-quart)

1½ lbs. stewing beef, cubed, trimmed of fat

¼ cup flour

2 cups stewed tomatoes (if you like tomato chunks), or 2 cups crushed tomatoes (if you prefer a smoother gravy)

1 tsp. salt

¼-½ tsp. pepper

1 medium onion, chopped

water

12-oz. bag noodles

1. Combine meat and flour until cubes are coated. Place in slow cooker.

2. Add tomatoes, salt, pepper, and onion. Add water to cover.

3. Cover. Simmer on Low 6–8 hours.

4. Serve over cooked noodles.

Exchange List Values: Starch 2.0, Vegetable 1.0, Meat, lean 2.0

Basic Nutritional Values: Calories 286 (Calories from Fat 46), Total Fat 5 gm (Saturated Fat 1.8 gm, Polyunsat Fat 0.7 gm, Monounsat Fat 2.1 gm, Cholesterol 83 mg), Sodium 490 mg, Total Carbohydrate 39 gm, Dietary Fiber 2 gm, Sugars 4 gm, Protein 20 gm

Before and after working out, you should check your blood sugar levels. If you will be exercising for more than an hour, check your levels during the activity, too.

Big Beef Stew

Margaret H. Moffitt • Bartlett, TN

Makes 6–8 servings (Ideal slow cooker size: 4–5-quart)

3-lb. beef roast, cubed, trimmed of fat

1 large onion, sliced

1 tsp. dried parsley flakes

1 medium green pepper, sliced

3 ribs celery, sliced

4 medium carrots, sliced

28-oz. can tomatoes with juice, undrained

1 clove garlic, minced

2 cups water

1. Combine all ingredients.

2. Cover. Cook on High 1 hour. Reduce heat to Low and cook 8 hours.

3. Serve on rice or noodles.

Exchange List Values: Vegetable 3.0, Meat, lean 3.0

Basic Nutritional Values: Calories 224 (Calories from Fat 61), Total Fat 7 gm (Saturated Fat 2.1 gm, Polyunsat Fat 0.4 gm, Monounsat Fat 3.1 gm, Cholesterol 85 mg), Sodium 248 mg, Total Carbohydrate 12 gm, Dietary Fiber 3 gm, Sugars 7 gm, Protein 28 gm

Note: For additional zest, add ¾ tsp. black pepper.

Spanish Round Steak

Shari Jensen • Fountain, CO

Makes 4–6 servings (Ideal slow cooker size: 4-quart)

1 small onion, sliced

1 medium green pepper, sliced in rings

1 rib celery, chopped

2 lbs. round steak, trimmed of fat

2 Tbsp. chopped fresh parsley, or 2 tsp. dried parsley

1 Tbsp. Worcestershire sauce

1 Tbsp. dry mustard

1 Tbsp. chili powder

2 cups canned tomatoes

2 tsp. dry minced garlic

1/2 tsp. salt

1/4 tsp. pepper

1. Put half of onion, green pepper, and celery in slow cooker.

2. Cut steak into serving-size pieces. Place steak pieces in slow cooker.

3. Put remaining onion, green pepper, and celery over steak.

4. Combine remaining ingredients. Pour over meat.

5. Cover. Cook on Low 8 hours.

6. Serve over noodles or rice.

Exchange List Values: Vegetable 2.0, Meat, lean 3.0

Basic Nutritional Values: Calories 222 (Calories from Fat 67), Total Fat 7 gm (Saturated Fat 2.3 gm, Polyunsat Fat 0.5 gm, Monounsat Fat 3.0 gm, Cholesterol 85 mg), Sodium 414 mg, Total Carbohydrate 8 gm, Dietary Fiber 2 gm, Sugars 5 gm, Protein 30 gm

Slow-Cooked Pepper Steak

Carolyn Baer • Conrath, WI / Ann Driscoll • Albuquerque, NM

Makes 6–8 servings (Ideal slow cooker size: 4-quart)

1 1/2–2 lbs. beef round steak, trimmed of fat, cut in 3" x 1" strips

2 Tbsp. canola oil

1/4 cup soy sauce

1 clove garlic, minced

1 cup chopped onions

1 tsp. sugar

1/4 tsp. pepper

1/4 tsp. ground ginger

2 large green peppers, cut in strips

4 medium tomatoes cut in eighths, or 16-oz. can diced tomatoes

1/2 cup cold water

1 Tbsp. cornstarch

1. Brown beef in oil in saucepan. Transfer to slow cooker.

2. Combine soy sauce, garlic, onions, sugar, pepper, and ginger. Pour over meat.

3. Cover. Cook on Low 5–6 hours.

4. Add green peppers and tomatoes. Cook 1 hour longer.

5. Combine water and cornstarch to make paste. Stir into slow cooker. Cook on High until thickened, about 10 minutes.

6. Serve over rice or noodles.

Exchange List Values: Vegetable 2.0, Meat, lean 2.0

Basic Nutritional Values: Calories 174 (Calories from Fat 68), Total Fat 8 gm (Saturated Fat 1.5 gm, Polyunsat Fat 1.3 gm, Monounsat Fat 3.7 gm, Cholesterol 48 mg), Sodium 546 mg, Total Carbohydrate 10 gm, Dietary Fiber 2 gm, Sugars 6 gm, Protein 17 gm

Pepper Steak Oriental

Donna Lantgen • Rapid City, SD

Makes 6 servings (Ideal slow cooker size: 4-quart)

1-lb. round steak, trimmed of fat, sliced thin

3 Tbsp. light soy sauce

$\frac{1}{2}$ tsp. ground ginger

1 clove garlic, minced

1 medium green pepper, thinly sliced

4-oz. can mushrooms, drained, or 1 cup fresh mushrooms

1 medium onion, thinly sliced

$\frac{1}{2}$ tsp. crushed red pepper

1. Combine all ingredients in slow cooker.

2. Cover. Cook on Low 6–8 hours.

3. Serve as steak sandwiches topped with provolone cheese, or over rice.

Exchange List Values: Vegetable 1.0, Meat, lean 2.0

Basic Nutritional Values: Calories 122 (Calories from Fat 32), Total Fat 4 gm (Saturated Fat 1.2 gm, Polyunsat Fat 0.2 gm, Monounsat Fat 1.5 gm, Cholesterol 43 mg), Sodium 368 mg, Total Carbohydrate 6 gm, Dietary Fiber 2 gm, Sugars 3 gm, Protein 16 gm

Powerhouse Beef Roast with Tomatoes, Onions, and Peppers

Donna Treloar • Gaston, IN

Makes 5–6 servings (Ideal slow cooker size: 4–5-quart)

3-lb. boneless chuck roast, trimmed of fat

1 clove garlic, minced

1 Tbsp. canola oil

2–3 medium onions, sliced

2–3 green and red peppers, sliced

16-oz. jar salsa

2 14$\frac{1}{2}$-oz. cans Mexican-style stewed tomatoes

1. Brown roast and garlic in oil in skillet. Place in slow cooker.

2. Add onions and peppers.

3. Combine salsa and tomatoes and pour over ingredients in slow cooker.

4. Cover. Cook on Low 8–10 hours.

5. Slice meat to serve.

Exchange List Values: Vegetable 4.0, Meat, lean 4.0

Basic Nutritional Values: Calories 327 (Calories from Fat 97), Total Fat 11 gm (Saturated Fat 3.1 gm, Polyunsat Fat 1.3 gm, Monounsat Fat 4.7 gm, Cholesterol 106 mg), Sodium 565 mg, Total Carbohydrate 19 gm, Dietary Fiber 5 gm, Sugars 12 gm, Protein 38 gm

VARIATION: Make Beef Burritos with the leftovers. Shred the beef and heat with remaining peppers, onions, and $\frac{1}{2}$ cup of the broth. Add 1 Tbsp. chili powder, 2 tsp. cumin, and salt to taste. Heat thoroughly. Fill warm flour tortillas with mixture and serve with sour cream, salsa, and guacamole.

Steak San Morco

Susan Tjon • Austin, TX

Makes 4–6 servings (Ideal slow cooker size: 4-quart)

2 lbs. stewing meat, cubed, trimmed of fat

1 envelope sodium-free dry onion soup mix

29-oz. can peeled, or crushed, tomatoes

1 tsp. dried oregano

garlic powder to taste

2 Tbsp. canola oil

2 Tbsp. wine vinegar

1. Layer meat evenly in bottom of slow cooker.

2. Combine soup mix, tomatoes, spices, oil, and vinegar in bowl. Blend with spoon. Pour over meat.

3. Cover. Cook on High 6 hours, or Low 8–10 hours.

Exchange List Values: Carbohydrate 0.5, Vegetable 1.0, Meat, lean 3.0

Basic Nutritional Values: Calories 237 (Calories from Fat 94), Total Fat 10 gm (Saturated Fat 2.1 gm, Polyunsat Fat 1.7 gm, Monounsat Fat 5.5 gm, Cholesterol 75 mg), Sodium 252 mg, Total Carbohydrate 10 gm, Dietary Fiber 2 gm, Sugars 5 gm, Protein 25 gm

Pat's Meat Stew

Pat Bishop • Bedminster, PA

Makes 4–5 servings (Ideal slow cooker size: 4-quart)

1–2 lbs. beef roast, cubed, trimmed of fat

1 tsp. salt

1/4 tsp. pepper

2 cups water

2 small carrots, sliced

2 small onions, sliced

4–6 small potatoes, unpeeled, cut up in chunks, if desired

1/4 cup quick-cooking tapioca

1 bay leaf

10-oz. pkg. frozen peas, or mixed vegetables

1. Brown beef in nonstick saucepan. Place in slow cooker.

2. Sprinkle with salt and pepper. Add remaining ingredients except frozen vegetables. Mix well.

3. Cover. Cook on Low 8–10 hours, or on High 4–5 hours. Add vegetables during last 1–2 hours of cooking.

Exchange List Values: Starch 2.0, Vegetable 1.0, Meat, lean 1.0

Basic Nutritional Values: Calories 257 (Calories from Fat 33), Total Fat 4 gm (Saturated Fat 1.1 gm, Polyunsat Fat 0.3 gm, Monounsat Fat 1.7 gm, Cholesterol 45 mg), Sodium 567 mg, Total Carbohydrate 36 gm, Dietary Fiber 6 gm, Sugars 7 gm, Protein 20 gm

Ernestine's Beef Stew

Ernestine Schrepfer • Trenton, MO

Makes 5–6 servings (Ideal slow cooker size: 4-quart)

1½ lbs. stewing meat, cubed, trimmed of fat

2¼ cups no-salt-added tomato juice

10½-oz. can consommé

1 cup chopped celery

2 cups sliced carrots

4 Tbsp. quick-cooking tapioca

1 medium onion, chopped

¼ tsp. salt

¼ tsp. pepper

1. Combine all ingredients in slow cooker.

2. Cover. Cook on Low 7–8 hours. (Do not peek.)

Exchange List Values: Starch 0.5, Vegetable 2.0, Meat, lean 2.0

Basic Nutritional Values: Calories 193 (Calories from Fat 40), Total Fat 4 gm (Saturated Fat 1.4 gm, Polyunsat Fat 0.3 gm, Monounsat Fat 2.1 gm, Cholesterol 57 mg), Sodium 519 mg, Total Carbohydrate 17 gm, Dietary Fiber 3 gm, Sugars 7 gm, Protein 21 gm

Becky's Beef Stew

Becky Harder • Monument, CO

Makes 6–8 servings (Ideal slow cooker size: 4-5-quart)

1½ lbs. beef stewing meat, cubed, trimmed of fat

2 10-oz. pkgs. frozen vegetables—carrots, corn, peas

4 large potatoes, unpeeled, cubed

1 bay leaf

1 medium onion, chopped

15-oz. can stewing tomatoes of your choice— Italian, Mexican, or regular

8-oz. can tomato sauce

2 Tbsp. Worcestershire sauce

1 tsp. salt

¼ tsp. pepper

1. Put meat on bottom of slow cooker. Layer frozen vegetables and potatoes over meat.

2. Mix remaining ingredients together in large bowl and pour over other ingredients.

3. Cover. Cook on Low 6–8 hours.

Exchange List Values: Starch 2.0, Vegetable 2.0, Meat, lean 1.0

Basic Nutritional Values: Calories 259 (Calories from Fat 31), Total Fat 3 gm (Saturated Fat 1.0 gm, Polyunsat Fat 0.4 gm, Monounsat Fat 1.6 gm, Cholesterol 42 mg), Sodium 506 mg, Total Carbohydrate 39 gm, Dietary Fiber 6 gm, Sugars 9 gm, Protein 19 gm

Santa Fe Stew

Jeanne Allen • Rye, CO

Recipe photo appears in color section.

Makes 4–6 servings (Ideal slow cooker size: 4-quart)

2 lbs. sirloin, or stewing meat, trimmed
    of fat, cubed

1 large onion, diced

2 cloves garlic, minced

2 Tbsp. canola oil

1½ cups water

1 Tbsp. dried parsley flakes

1 beef bouillon cube

1 tsp. ground cumin

¼ tsp. salt

3 medium carrots, sliced

1-lb. pkg. frozen green beans

1-lb. pkg. frozen corn

4-oz. can diced green chilies

1. Brown meat, onion, and garlic in oil in saucepan until meat is no longer pink. Place in slow cooker.

2. Stir in remaining ingredients.

3. Cover. Cook on High 30 minutes. Reduce heat to Low and cook 4–6 hours.

Exchange List Values: Starch 1.0, Vegetable 3.0, Meat, lean 3.0

Basic Nutritional Values: Calories 322 (Calories from Fat 99), Total Fat 11 gm (Saturated Fat 2.2 gm, Polyunsat Fat 2.0 gm, Monounsat Fat 5.6 gm, Cholesterol 75 mg), Sodium 554 mg, Total Carbohydrate 30 gm, Dietary Fiber 7 gm, Sugars 10 gm, Protein 28 gm

Gone-All-Day Casserole

Beatrice Orgish • Richardson, TX

Recipe photo appears in color section.

Makes 8 servings (Ideal slow cooker size: 4–5-quart)

1 cup uncooked wild rice, rinsed and drained

1 cup chopped celery

1 cup chopped carrots

2 4-oz. cans mushrooms, stems and pieces, drained

1 large onion, chopped

1 clove garlic, minced

½ cup slivered almonds

2 beef bouillon cubes

1¼ tsp. seasoned salt

2 lbs. boneless round steak, trimmed of fat, cut into 1" cubes

3 cups water

1. Place ingredients in order listed in slow cooker.

2. Cover. Cook on Low 6–8 hours, or until rice is tender. Stir before serving.

Exchange List Values: Starch 1.0, Vegetable 1.0, Meat, lean 3.0

Basic Nutritional Values: Calories 264 (Calories from Fat 77), Total Fat 9 gm (Saturated Fat 1.7 gm, Polyunsat Fat 1.3 gm, Monounsat Fat 4.5 gm, Cholesterol 56 mg), Sodium 615 mg, Total Carbohydrate 23 gm, Dietary Fiber 4 gm, Sugars 4 gm, Protein 24 gm

Eat plenty of green leafy vegetables; red, orange, and yellow fruits and vegetables; citrus fruits; nuts and seeds; and meat and fish. They are good for your heart and help prevent cancer.

Full-Flavored Beef Stew

Stacy Petersheim • Mechanicsburg, PA

Makes 6 servings (Ideal slow cooker size: 4-quart)

2-lb. beef roast, trimmed of fat, cubed

2 cups sliced carrots

2 cups diced potatoes, unpeeled

1 medium onion, sliced

1½ cups frozen or fresh peas

2 tsp. quick-cooking tapioca

½ tsp. salt

½ tsp. pepper

8-oz. can tomato sauce

1 cup water

1 Tbsp. brown sugar

1. Combine beef and vegetables in slow cooker. Sprinkle with tapioca, salt, and pepper.

2. Combine tomato sauce and water. Pour over ingredients in slow cooker. Sprinkle with brown sugar.

3. Cover. Cook on Low 8 hours.

Exchange List Values: Starch 1.0, Vegetable 2.0, Meat, lean 3.0

Basic Nutritional Values: Calories 271 (Calories from Fat 54), Total Fat 6 gm (Saturated Fat 1.9 gm, Polyunsat Fat 0.4 gm, Monounsat Fat 2.8 gm, Cholesterol 75 mg), Sodium 539 mg, Total Carbohydrate 26 gm, Dietary Fiber 5 gm, Sugars 11 gm, Protein 28 gm

VARIATION: Add peas one hour before cooking time ends to keep their color and flavor.

Lazy Day Stew

Ruth Ann Gingrich • New Holland, PA

Makes 8 servings (Ideal slow cooker size: 4-quart)

2 lbs. stewing beef, trimmed of fat, cubed

2 cups diced carrots

2 cups diced potatoes, unpeeled

2 medium onions, chopped

1 cup chopped celery

10-oz. pkg. lima beans

2 tsp. quick-cooking tapioca

1 tsp. salt

½ tsp. pepper

8-oz. can tomato sauce

1 cup water

1 Tbsp. brown sugar

1. Place beef in bottom of slow cooker. Add vegetables.

2. Sprinkle tapioca, salt, and pepper over ingredients.

3. Mix together tomato sauce and water. Pour over top.

4. Sprinkle brown sugar over all.

5. Cover. Cook on Low 8 hours.

Exchange List Values: Starch 1.0, Vegetable 2.0, Meat, lean 2.0

Basic Nutritional Values: Calories 229 (Calories from Fat 41), Total Fat 5 gm (Saturated Fat 1.4 gm, Polyunsat Fat 0.4 gm, Monounsat Fat 2.1 gm, Cholesterol 56 mg), Sodium 558 mg, Total Carbohydrate 25 gm, Dietary Fiber 5 gm, Sugars 8 gm, Protein 22 gm

VARIATION: Instead of lima beans, use 1½ cups green beans.

Rose M. Hoffman • Schuylkill Haven, PA

Beef with Mushrooms

Doris Perkins • Mashpee, MA

Makes 4–6 servings (Ideal slow cooker size: 4-quart)

1½ lbs. stewing beef, trimmed of fat, cubed

4-oz. can mushroom pieces, drained (save liquid)

half a clove garlic, minced

¾ cup sliced onions

3 Tbsp. canola oil

1 beef bouillon cube

1 cup hot water

8-oz. can tomato sauce

2 tsp. sugar

2 tsp. Worcestershire sauce

1 tsp. dried basil

1 tsp. dried oregano

½ tsp. salt

⅛ tsp. pepper

1. Brown meat, mushrooms, garlic, and onions in oil in skillet.

2. Dissolve bouillon cube in hot water. Add to meat mixture.

3. Stir in mushroom liquid and rest of ingredients. Mix well. Pour into slow cooker.

4. Cover. Cook on High 3 hours, or until meat is tender.

5. Serve over cooked noodles, spaghetti, or rice.

Exchange List Values: Vegetable 2.0, Meat, lean 2.0, Fat 1.0

Basic Nutritional Values: Calories 210 (Calories from Fat 101), Total Fat 11 gm (Saturated Fat 1.8 gm, Polyunsat Fat 2.3 gm, Monounsat Fat 6.1 gm, Cholesterol 56 mg), Sodium 385 mg, Total Carbohydrate 8 gm, Dietary Fiber 2 gm, Sugars 5 gm, Protein 19 gm

Beef Pot Roast

Alexa Slonin • Harrisonburg, VA

Makes 8–10 servings (Ideal slow cooker size: 4–5-quart)

12-oz. can whole tiny new potatoes, or 2 medium potatoes, cubed, or 2 medium sweet potatoes, cubed

8 small carrots, cut in small chunks

2 small onions, cut in wedges

2 ribs celery, cut up

2½–3 lbs. beef chuck, or pot roast, trimmed of fat

2 Tbsp. canola oil

¾ cup water, dry wine, or tomato juice

1 Tbsp. Worcestershire sauce

1 tsp. instant beef bouillon granules

1 tsp. dried basil

1. Place vegetables in bottom of slow cooker.

2. Brown roast in oil in skillet. Place on top of vegetables.

3. Combine water, Worcestershire sauce, bouillon, and basil. Pour over meat and vegetables.

4. Cover. Cook on Low 10–12 hours.

Exchange List Values: Starch 0.5, Vegetable 2.0, Meat, lean 2.0, Fat 0.5

Basic Nutritional Values: Calories 233 (Calories from Fat 78), Total Fat 9 gm (Saturated Fat 2.1 gm, Polyunsat Fat 1.3 gm, Monounsat Fat 4.1 gm, Cholesterol 61 mg), Sodium 231 mg, Total Carbohydrate 16 gm, Dietary Fiber 3 gm, Sugars 5 gm, Protein 22 gm

Pot Roast

Janet L. Roggie • Linville, NY

Makes 6–8 servings (Ideal slow cooker size: 4-quart)

3 potatoes, thinly sliced

2 large carrots, thinly sliced

1 onion, thinly sliced

1 tsp. salt

½ tsp. pepper

3–4-lb. pot roast, trimmed of fat

½ cup water

1. Put vegetables in bottom of slow cooker. Stir in salt and pepper. Add roast. Pour in water.

2. Cover. Cook on Low 10–12 hours.

Exchange List Values: Starch 1.0, Vegetable 1.0, Meat, lean 3.0

Basic Nutritional Values: Calories 219 (Calories from Fat 55), Total Fat 6 gm (Saturated Fat 2.2 gm, Polyunsat Fat 0.3 gm, Monounsat Fat 2.5 gm, Cholesterol 73 mg), Sodium 361 mg, Total Carbohydrate 14 gm, Dietary Fiber 2 gm, Sugars 3 gm, Protein 26 gm

VARIATIONS:

1. Add ½ tsp. dried dill, a bay leaf, and ½ tsp. dried rosemary for more flavor.

2. Brown roast on all sides in saucepan in 2 Tbsp. oil before placing in cooker.

Debbie Zeida • Mashpee, MA

Did you know that one trip to the salad bar can add up to more than 1,000 calories? Watch out for side dishes like potato salad, pasta salad, and creamy soups; choose low-fat or fat-free dressing.

Easy Pot Roast and Veggies

Tina Houk • Clinton, MO / Arlene Wines • Newton, KS

Recipe photo appears in color section.

Makes 6 servings (Ideal slow cooker size: 4–5-quart)

3–4-lb. chuck roast, trimmed of fat

4 medium potatoes, cubed, unpeeled

4 medium carrots, sliced, or 1-lb. pkg. baby carrots

2 ribs celery, sliced thin, optional

1 envelope dry onion soup mix

3 cups water

1. Put roast, potatoes, carrots, and celery in slow cooker.

2. Add onion soup mix and water.

3. Cover. Cook on Low 6–8 hours.

Exchange List Values: Starch 1.5, Vegetable 1.0, Meat, lean 3.0

Basic Nutritional Values: Calories 325 (Calories from Fat 76), Total Fat 8 gm (Saturated Fat 2.9 gm, Polyunsat Fat 0.5 gm, Monounsat Fat 3.6 gm, Cholesterol 98 mg), Sodium 560 mg, Total Carbohydrate 26 gm, Dietary Fiber 4 gm, Sugars 6 gm, Protein 35 gm

VARIATIONS:

1. To add flavor to the broth, stir 1 tsp. kitchen bouquet, ½ tsp. salt, ½ tsp. black pepper, and ½ tsp. garlic powder into water before pouring over meat and vegetables.

Bonita Ensenberger • Albuquerque, NM

2. Before putting roast in cooker, sprinkle it with the dry soup mix, patting it on so it adheres.

Betty Lahman • Elkton, VA

Rump Roast and Vegetables

Kimberlee Greenawalt • Harrisonburg, VA

Makes 6–8 servings (Ideal slow cooker size: 4–5-quart)

1½ lbs. small potatoes (about 10), or medium potatoes (about 4), halved, unpeeled

2 medium carrots, cubed

1 small onion, sliced

10-oz. pkg. frozen lima beans

1 bay leaf

2 Tbsp. quick-cooking tapioca

2–2½-lb. boneless beef round rump, round tip, or pot roast, trimmed of fat

2 Tbsp. canola oil

10¾-oz. can condensed vegetable beef soup

¼ cup water

¼ tsp. pepper

1. Place potatoes, carrots, and onions in slow cooker. Add frozen beans and bay leaf. Sprinkle with tapioca.

2. Brown roast on all sides in oil in skillet. Place over vegetables in slow cooker.

3. Combine soup, water, and pepper. Pour over roast.

4. Cover. Cook on Low 10–12 hours, or High 5–6 hours.

5. Discard bay leaf before serving.

Exchange List Values: Starch 2.0, Vegetable 1.0, Meat, lean 2.0

Basic Nutritional Values: Calories 288 (Calories from Fat 71), Total Fat 8 gm (Saturated Fat 1.9 gm, Polyunsat Fat 1.3 gm, Monounsat Fat 3.7 gm, Cholesterol 50 mg), Sodium 349 mg, Total Carbohydrate 32 gm, Dietary Fiber 6 gm, Sugars 5 gm, Protein 22 gm

Hearty New England Dinner

Joette Droz • Kalona, IA

Makes 6–8 servings (Ideal slow cooker size: 4–5-quart)

2 medium carrots, sliced

1 medium onion, sliced

1 rib celery, sliced

3-lb. boneless chuck roast, trimmed of fat

¼ tsp. pepper

1 envelope dry onion soup mix

2 cups water

1 Tbsp. vinegar

1 bay leaf

half a small head of cabbage, cut in wedges

2 Tbsp. melted margarine, or butter

2 Tbsp. flour

1 Tbsp. dried minced onion

2 Tbsp. prepared horseradish

½ tsp. salt

1. Place carrots, onion, and celery in slow cooker. Place roast on top. Sprinkle with pepper. Add soup mix, water, vinegar, and bay leaf.

2. Cover. Cook on Low 7–9 hours. Remove beef and keep warm. Just before serving, cut into pieces or thin slices.

3. Discard bay leaf. Add cabbage to juice in slow cooker.

4. Cover. Cook on High 1 hour, or until cabbage is tender.

5. Melt margarine in saucepan. Stir in flour and onion. Add 1½ cups liquid from slow cooker. Stir in horseradish and ½ tsp. salt. Bring to boil. Cook over Low heat until thick and smooth, about 2 minutes.

6. Return to cooker and blend with remaining sauce in cooker. When blended, serve over or alongside meat and vegetables.

Exchange List Values: Vegetable 2.0, Meat, lean 3.0, Fat 0.5

Basic Nutritional Values: Calories 234 (Calories from Fat 85), Total Fat 9 gm (Saturated Fat 2.7 gm, Polyunsat Fat 1.3 gm, Monounsat Fat 4.0 gm, Cholesterol 74 mg), Sodium 607 mg, Total Carbohydrate 11 gm, Dietary Fiber 3 gm, Sugars 6 gm, Protein 26 gm

If you're taking a long car trip alone, take special care to avoid high or low blood sugars. Check your levels every 2–4 hours, and always keep some form of sugar with you, whether it's glucose tablets, regular soda, or a candy.

Easy Beef Stew

Connie Johnson • Loudon, NH

Makes 6 servings (Ideal slow cooker size: 4–5-quart)

1 lb. stewing beef

1 cup cubed turnip

2 medium potatoes, cubed, unpeeled

1 large onion, sliced

1 clove garlic, minced

2 large carrots, sliced

½ cup green beans, cut up

½ cup peas

1 bay leaf

½ tsp. dried thyme

1 tsp. chopped parsley

2 Tbsp. tomato paste

2 Tbsp. celery leaves

¼ tsp. salt

¼ tsp. pepper

1 qt., or 2 14½-oz. cans, lower-sodium beef broth

1. Place meat, vegetables, and seasonings in slow cooker. Pour broth over all.

2. Cover. Cook on Low 6–8 hours.

Exchange List Values: Starch 1.0, Vegetable 2.0, Meat, lean 1.0

Basic Nutritional Values: Calories 175 (Calories from Fat 29), Total Fat 3 gm (Saturated Fat 0.9 gm, Polyunsat Fat 0.3 gm, Monounsat Fat 1.4 gm, Cholesterol 38 mg), Sodium 466 mg, Total Carbohydrate 21 gm, Dietary Fiber 5 gm, Sugars 6 gm, Protein 16 gm

Pot Roast with Gravy and Vegetables

Irene Klaeger • Inverness, FL /
Jan Pembleton • Arlington, TX

Makes 4–6 servings (Ideal slow cooker size: 4-quart)

3–4-lb. bottom round, rump, or arm roast, trimmed of fat

¼ tsp. salt

2–3 tsp. pepper

2 Tbsp. flour

¼ cup cold water

1 tsp. kitchen bouquet, or gravy browning seasoning sauce

1 clove garlic, minced

2 medium onions, cut in wedges

4 medium potatoes, cubed, unpeeled

2 carrots, quartered

1 green pepper, sliced

1. Place roast in slow cooker. Sprinkle with salt and pepper.

2. Make paste of flour and cold water. Stir in kitchen bouquet and spread over roast.

3. Add garlic, onions, potatoes, carrots, and green pepper.

4. Cover. Cook on Low 8–10 hours, or High 4–5 hours.

5. Taste and adjust seasonings before serving.

Exchange List Values: Starch 1.5, Vegetable 2.0, Meat, lean 3.0

Basic Nutritional Values: Calories 336 (Calories from Fat 75), Total Fat 8 gm (Saturated Fat 2.9 gm, Polyunsat Fat 0.5 gm, Monounsat Fat 3.4 gm, Cholesterol 98 mg), Sodium 577 mg, Total Carbohydrate 28 gm, Dietary Fiber 4 gm, Sugars 7 gm, Protein 36 gm

"Smothered" Steak

Susan Yoder Graber • Eureka, IL

Makes 6 servings (Ideal slow cooker size: 4-quart)

1½ lbs. chuck, or round, steak, trimmed of fat, cut into strips

⅓ cup flour

¼ tsp. pepper

1 large onion, sliced

1 green pepper, sliced

14½-oz. can stewed tomatoes

4-oz. can mushrooms, drained

2 Tbsp. soy sauce

10-oz. pkg. frozen French-style green beans

1. Layer steak in bottom of slow cooker. Sprinkle with flour and pepper. Stir well to coat steak.

2. Add remaining ingredients. Mix together gently.

3. Cover. Cook on Low 8 hours.

4. Serve over rice.

Exchange List Values: Vegetable 4.0, Meat, lean 2.0

Basic Nutritional Values: Calories 222 (Calories from Fat 50), Total Fat 6 gm (Saturated Fat 1.7 gm, Polyunsat Fat 0.4 gm, Monounsat Fat 2.3 gm, Cholesterol 64 mg), Sodium 613 mg, Total Carbohydrate 19 gm, Dietary Fiber 4 gm, Sugars 7 gm, Protein 25 gm

VARIATIONS:

1. Use 8-oz. can tomato sauce instead of stewed tomatoes.
2. Substitute 1 Tbsp. Worcestershire sauce in place of soy sauce.

Mary E. Martin • Goshen, IN

Veal and Peppers

Irma H. Schoen • Windsor, CT

Makes 4 servings (Ideal slow cooker size: 4-quart)

1½ lbs. boneless veal, cubed

3 green peppers, quartered

2 onions, thinly sliced

½ lb. fresh mushrooms, sliced

1 tsp. salt

½ tsp. dried basil

2 cloves garlic, minced

28-oz. can tomatoes

1. Combine all ingredients in slow cooker.

2. Cover. Cook on Low 7 hours, or on High 4 hours.

3. Serve over rice or noodles.

Exchange List Values: Vegetable 3.0, Meat, very lean 3.0, Fat 0.5

Basic Nutritional Values: Calories 194 (Calories from Fat 31), Total Fat 3 gm (Saturated Fat 0.9 gm, Polyunsat Fat 0.5 gm, Monounsat Fat 1.0 gm, Cholesterol 95 mg), Sodium 555 mg, Total Carbohydrate 16 gm, Dietary Fiber 4 gm, Sugars 9 gm, Protein 26 gm

VARIATION: Use boneless, skinless chicken breast, cut into chunks, instead of veal.

Beef and Beans

Robin Schrock • Millersburg, OH

Makes 8 servings (Ideal slow cooker size: 4-quart)

1 Tbsp. prepared mustard

1 Tbsp. chili powder

½ tsp. salt

¼ tsp. pepper

1½-lb. boneless round steak, trimmed of fat, cut into thin slices

2 14½-oz. cans diced tomatoes, undrained

1 medium onion, chopped

1 beef bouillon cube, crushed

16-oz. can kidney beans, rinsed and drained

1. Combine mustard, chili powder, salt, and pepper. Add beef slices and toss to coat. Place meat in slow cooker.

2. Add tomatoes, onion, and bouillon.

3. Cover. Cook on Low 6–8 hours.

4. Stir in beans. Cook 30 minutes longer.

5. Serve over rice.

Exchange List Values: Starch 0.5, Vegetable 1.0, Meat, lean 2.0

Basic Nutritional Values: Calories 182 (Calories from Fat 40), Total Fat 4 gm (Saturated Fat 1.3 gm, Polyunsat Fat 0.4 gm, Monounsat Fat 1.8 gm, Cholesterol 48 mg), Sodium 582 mg, Total Carbohydrate 16 gm, Dietary Fiber 4 gm, Sugars 6 gm, Protein 21 gm

Have your lipids (blood fats or cholesterol) checked once a year. HDL cholesterol is Healthy, so you want the number to be high; LDL cholesterol is Lousy, so the number should be low.

Three-Bean Burrito Bake

Darla Sathre • Baxter, MN

Recipe photo appears in color section.

Makes 8 servings (Ideal slow cooker size: 4-quart)

1 onion, chopped

1 green bell pepper, chopped

2 cloves garlic, minced

1 Tbsp. canola oil

16-oz. can pinto beans, drained

16-oz. can kidney beans, drained

15-oz. can black beans, drained

4-oz. can sliced black olives, drained

4-oz. can green chilies

2 15-oz. cans no-salt-added diced tomatoes

1 tsp. chili powder

1 tsp. ground cumin

6 6" flour tortillas

1 cup shredded Co-Jack cheese

sour cream

1. Saute onions, green peppers, and garlic in large skillet in oil.

2. Add beans, olives, chilies, tomatoes, chili powder, and cumin.

3. In greased slow cooker, layer ¾ cup vegetables, a tortilla, ⅓ cup cheese. Repeat layers until all those ingredients are used, ending with sauce.

4. Cover. Cook on Low 8–10 hours.

5. Serve with dollops of sour cream on individual servings.

Exchange List Values: Starch 2.5, Vegetable 2.0, Meat, lean 1.0, Fat 1.0

Basic Nutritional Values: Calories 346 (Calories from Fat 99), Total Fat 11 gm (Saturated Fat 3.3 gm, Polyunsat Fat 1.5 gm, Monounsat Fat 4.8 gm, Cholesterol 15 mg), Sodium 573 mg, Total Carbohydrate 48 gm, Dietary Fiber 12 gm, Sugars 8 gm, Protein 16 gm

Beef Stew Bourguignonne

Jo Haberkamp • Fairbank, IA

Makes 6 servings (Ideal slow cooker size: 4-quart)

2 lbs. stewing beef, trimmed of fat, cut in 1" cubes

2 Tbsp. cooking oil

10¾-oz. can condensed golden cream of mushroom soup

1 tsp. Worcestershire sauce

⅓ cup dry red wine

½ tsp. dried oregano

¼ tsp. salt

½ tsp. pepper

½ cup chopped onions

½ cup chopped carrots

4-oz. can mushroom pieces, drained

½ cup cold water

¼ cup flour

1. Brown meat in oil in saucepan. Transfer to slow cooker.

2. Mix together soup, Worcestershire sauce, wine, oregano, salt, pepper, onions, carrots, and mushrooms. Pour over meat.

3. Cover. Cook on Low 10–12 hours.

4. Combine water and flour. Stir into beef mixture. Turn cooker to High.

5. Cook and stir until thickened and bubbly.

6. Serve over noodles.

Exchange List Values: Carbohydrate 1.0, Meat, lean 3.0, Fat 0.5

Basic Nutritional Values: Calories 266 (Calories from Fat 106), Total Fat 12 gm (Saturated Fat 2.5 gm, Polyunsat Fat 2.5 gm, Monounsat Fat 5.7 gm, Cholesterol 77 mg), Sodium 585 mg, Total Carbohydrate 12 gm, Dietary Fiber 2 gm, Sugars 2 gm, Protein 26 gm

Succulent Steak

Betty B. Dennison • Grove City, PA

Makes 4 servings (Ideal slow cooker size: 4-quart)

1/4 cup flour

1/2 tsp. salt

1/4 tsp. pepper

1/4 tsp. paprika

1 1/2-lb. round steak, trimmed of fat,
    cut 1/2"-3/4" thick

2 medium onions, sliced

4-oz. can sliced mushrooms, drained

1/2 cup beef broth

2 tsp. Worcestershire sauce

2 Tbsp. flour

3 Tbsp. water

1. Mix together 1/4 cup flour, salt, pepper, and paprika.

2. Cut steak into 5–6 pieces. Dredge steak pieces in seasoned flour until lightly coated.

3. Layer half of onions, half of steak, and half of mushrooms into cooker. Repeat.

4. Combine beef broth and Worcestershire sauce. Pour over mixture in slow cooker.

5. Cover. Cook on Low 8–10 hours.

6. Remove steak to serving platter and keep warm. Mix together 2 Tbsp. flour and water. Stir into drippings and cook on High until thickened, about 10 minutes. Pour over steak and serve.

Exchange List Values: Starch 0.5, Vegetable 2.0, Meat, lean 4.0

Basic Nutritional Values: Calories 295 (Calories from Fat 73), Total Fat 8 gm (Saturated Fat 2.6 gm, Polyunsat Fat 0.5 gm, Monounsat Fat 3.4 gm, Cholesterol 96 mg), Sodium 601 mg, Total Carbohydrate 18 gm, Dietary Fiber 3 gm, Sugars 6 gm, Protein 36 gm

Steak Hi-Hat

Bonita Ensenberger • Albuquerque, NM

Makes 8–10 servings (Ideal slow cooker size: 4-quart)

10 3/4-oz. can 98%-fat-free, reduced-sodium cream of chicken soup

10 3/4-oz. can 98%-fat-free, reduced-sodium cream of mushroom soup

1 1/2 Tbsp. Worcestershire sauce

1/2 tsp. black pepper

1 tsp. paprika

2 cups chopped onion

1 clove garlic, minced

1 cup fresh, small button mushrooms, quartered

2 lbs. round steak, trimmed of fat, cubed

1 cup fat-free sour cream

crisp bacon bits, optional

1. Combine chicken soup, mushroom soup, Worcestershire sauce, pepper, paprika, onion, garlic, and mushrooms in slow cooker.

2. Stir in steak.

3. Cover. Cook on Low 8–9 hours.

4. Stir in sour cream during the last 20–30 minutes.

5. Serve on hot buttered noodles sprinkled with poppy seeds. Garnish with bacon bits.

Exchange List Values: Carbohydrate 1.0, Meat, lean 2.0

Basic Nutritional Values: Calories 178 (Calories from Fat 49), Total Fat 5 gm (Saturated Fat 1.8 gm, Polyunsat Fat 0.6 gm, Monounsat Fat 2.0 gm, Cholesterol 56 mg), Sodium 321 mg, Total Carbohydrate 12 gm, Dietary Fiber 1 gm, Sugars 4 gm, Protein 19 gm

VARIATION: Add 1 tsp. salt with seasonings in Step 1.

Steak Stroganoff

Marie Morucci • Glen Lyon, PA

Makes 6 servings (Ideal slow cooker size: 4-quart)

2 Tbsp. flour

$\frac{1}{2}$ tsp. garlic powder

$\frac{1}{2}$ tsp. pepper

$\frac{1}{4}$ tsp. paprika

1$\frac{3}{4}$-lb. boneless beef round steak, trimmed of fat

10$\frac{3}{4}$-oz. can 98%-fat-free, reduced-sodium cream of mushroom soup

$\frac{1}{2}$ cup water

1 envelope sodium-free dried onion soup mix

9-oz. jar sliced mushrooms, drained

$\frac{1}{2}$ cup fat-free sour cream

1 Tbsp. minced fresh parsley

1. Combine flour, garlic powder, pepper, and paprika in slow cooker.

2. Cut meat into 1$\frac{1}{2}$" x $\frac{1}{2}$" strips. Place in flour mixture and toss until meat is well coated.

3. Add mushroom soup, water, and soup mix. Stir until well blended.

4. Cover. Cook on High 3–3$\frac{1}{2}$ hours, or Low 6–7 hours.

5. Stir in mushrooms, sour cream, and parsley. Cover and cook on High 10–15 minutes, or until heated through.

6. Serve with rice.

Exchange List Values: Carbohydrate 1.0, Meat, lean 3.0

Basic Nutritional Values: Calories 256 (Calories from Fat 66), Total Fat 7 gm (Saturated Fat 2.4 gm, Polyunsat Fat 0.5 gm, Monounsat Fat 2.8 gm, Cholesterol 77 mg), Sodium 390 mg, Total Carbohydrate 17 gm, Dietary Fiber 2 gm, Sugars 5 gm, Protein 29 gm

Garlic Beef Stroganoff

Sharon Miller • Holmesville, OH

Makes 6 servings (Ideal slow cooker size: 4–5-quart)

2 tsp. sodium-free beef bouillon powder

2 4$\frac{1}{2}$-oz. jars sliced mushrooms, drained, with juice reserved

1 cup mushroom juice, with boiling water added to make a full cup

10$\frac{3}{4}$-oz. can 98%-fat-free, reduced-sodium cream of mushroom soup

1 large onion, chopped

3 cloves garlic, minced

1 Tbsp. Worcestershire sauce

1$\frac{1}{2}$- lb. boneless round steak, trimmed of fat, cut into thin strips

2 Tbsp. canola oil

6 ozs. fat-free cream cheese, cubed and softened

1. Dissolve bouillon in mushroom juice and water in slow cooker.

2. Add soup, mushrooms, onion, garlic, and Worcestershire sauce.

3. Saute beef in oil in skillet. Transfer to slow cooker and stir into sauce.

4. Cover. Cook on Low 7–8 hours. Turn off heat.

5. Stir in cream cheese until smooth.

6. Serve over noodles.

Exchange List Values: Carbohydrate 0.5, Vegetable 1.0, Meat, lean 2.0, Fat 0.5

Basic Nutritional Values: Calories 202 (Calories from Fat 73), Total Fat 8 gm (Saturated Fat 1.8 gm, Polyunsat Fat 1.4 gm, Monounsat Fat 3.9 gm, Cholesterol 51 mg), Sodium 474 mg, Total Carbohydrate 10 gm, Dietary Fiber 2 gm, Sugars 4 gm, Protein 21 gm

Machaca Beef

Jeanne Allen • Rye, CO

Makes 12 servings (Ideal slow cooker size: 4-quart)

1½-lb. beef roast

1 large onion, sliced

4-oz. can chopped green chilies

2 beef bouillon cubes

1½ tsp. dry mustard

½ tsp. garlic powder

1 tsp. seasoning salt

½ tsp. pepper

1 cup salsa

1. Combine all ingredients except salsa in slow cooker. Add just enough water to cover.

2. Cover cooker and cook on Low 10–12 hours, or until beef is tender. Drain and reserve liquid.

3. Shred beef using two forks to pull it apart.

4. Combine beef, salsa, and enough of the reserved liquid to make desired consistency.

5. Use this filling for burritos, chalupas, quesadillas, or tacos.

Exchange List Values: Meat, lean 1.0

Basic Nutritional Values: Calories 69 (Calories from Fat 20), Total Fat 2 gm (Saturated Fat 0.7 gm, Polyunsat Fat 0.1 gm, Monounsat Fat 0.9 gm, Cholesterol 24 mg), Sodium 392 mg, Total Carbohydrate 3 gm, Dietary Fiber 1 gm, Sugars 2 gm, Protein 9 gm

Roast

Tracey Yohn •Harrisburg, PA

Makes 6 servings (Ideal slow cooker size: 4-quart)

2-lb. shoulder roast, trimmed of fat

1 tsp. pepper

1 tsp. garlic salt

1 small onion, sliced in rings

1 beef bouillon cube

1 cup boiling water

1. Place roast in slow cooker. Sprinkle with pepper and garlic salt. Place onion rings on top.

2. Dissolve bouillon cube in water. Pour over roast.

3. Cover. Cook on Low 10–12 hours, or on High 5–6 hours.

Exchange List Values: Meat, lean 3.0

Basic Nutritional Values: Calories 148 (Calories from Fat 49), Total Fat 5 gm (Saturated Fat 1.9 gm, Polyunsat Fat 0.2 gm, Monounsat Fat 2.3 gm, Cholesterol 65 mg), Sodium 407 mg, Total Carbohydrate 2 gm, Dietary Fiber 0 gm, Sugars 1 gm, Protein 22 gm

Apple and Onion Beef Pot Roast

Betty K. Drescher • Quakertown, PA

Makes 8 servings (Ideal slow cooker size: 4-quart)

3-lb. boneless beef roast, cut in half, trimmed of fat

2 Tbsp. canola oil

1 cup water

1 tsp. seasoning salt

½ tsp. soy sauce

½ tsp. Worcestershire sauce

¼ tsp. garlic powder

1 large tart apple, quartered

1 large onion, sliced

2 Tbsp. cornstarch

2 Tbsp. water

1. Brown roast on all sides in oil in skillet. Transfer to slow cooker.

2. Add water to skillet to loosen browned bits. Pour over roast.

3. Sprinkle with seasoning salt, soy sauce, Worcestershire sauce, and garlic powder.

4. Top with apple and onion.

5. Cover. Cook on Low 5–6 hours.

6. Remove roast and onion. Discard apple. Let stand 15 minutes.

7. To make gravy, pour juices from roast into saucepan and simmer until reduced to 2 cups. Combine cornstarch and water until smooth in small bowl. Stir into beef broth. Bring to boil. Cook and stir for 2 minutes until thickened.

8. Slice pot roast and serve with gravy.

Exchange List Values: Carbohydrate 0.5, Meat, lean 3.0

Basic Nutritional Values: Calories 208 (Calories from Fat 85), Total Fat 9 gm (Saturated Fat 2.4 gm, Polyunsat Fat 1.3 gm, Monounsat Fat 4.6 gm, Cholesterol 73 mg), Sodium 265 mg, Total Carbohydrate 5 gm, Dietary Fiber 1 gm, Sugars 2 gm, Protein 24 gm

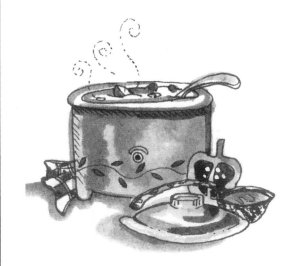

Savory Sweet Roast

Martha Ann Auker • Landisburg, PA

Makes 6-8 servings (Ideal slow cooker size: 4-quart)

3-lb. blade, or chuck, roast, trimmed of fat

2 Tbsp. canola oil

1 onion, chopped

10¾-oz. can 99%-fat-free, reduced-sodium cream of mushroom soup

½ cup water

¼ cup sugar

¼ cup vinegar

¾ tsp. salt

1 tsp. prepared mustard

1 tsp. Worcestershire sauce

1. Brown meat in oil on both sides in saucepan. Put in slow cooker.

2. Blend together remaining ingredients. Pour over meat.

3. Cover. Cook on Low 12–16 hours.

Exchange List Values: Carbohydrate 1.0, Meat, lean 3.0

Basic Nutritional Values: Calories 241 (Calories from Fat 92), Total Fat 10 gm (Saturated Fat 2.7 gm, Polyunsat Fat 1.4 gm, Monounsat Fat 4.7 gm, Cholesterol 74 mg), Sodium 424 mg, Total Carbohydrate 11 gm, Dietary Fiber 0 gm, Sugars 8 gm, Protein 25 gm

Dilled Pot Roast

C. J. Slagle • Roann, IN

Makes 6 servings (Ideal slow cooker size: 4-quart)

3-lb. beef pot roast, trimmed of fat

¾ tsp. salt

¼ tsp. pepper

2 tsp. dried dillweed, divided

¼ cup water

1 Tbsp. vinegar

3 Tbsp. flour

½ cup water

1 cup fat-free sour cream

1. Sprinkle both sides of meat with salt, pepper, and 1 tsp. dill. Place in slow cooker. Add water and vinegar.

2. Cover. Cook on Low 7–9 hours, or until tender. Remove meat from pot. Turn to High.

3. Dissolve flour in water. Stir into meat drippings. Stir in additional 1 tsp. dill. Cook on High 5 minutes. Stir in sour cream. Cook on High another 5 minutes.

4. Slice meat and serve with sour cream sauce over top.

Exchange List Values: Carbohydrate 0.5, Meat, lean 4.0

Basic Nutritional Values: Calories 260 (Calories from Fat 73), Total Fat 8 gm (Saturated Fat 2.9 gm, Polyunsat Fat 0.3 gm, Monounsat Fat 3.4 gm, Cholesterol 101 mg), Sodium 403 mg, Total Carbohydrate 10 gm, Dietary Fiber 0 gm, Sugars 3 gm, Protein 34 gm

Beef Burgundy

Jacqueline Stefl • East Bethany, NY

Makes 6 servings (Ideal slow cooker size: 4-quart)

5 medium onions, thinly sliced

2 lbs. stewing meat, trimmed of fat, cubed

1½ Tbsp. flour

½ lb. fresh mushrooms, sliced

1 tsp. salt

¼ tsp. dried marjoram

¼ tsp. dried thyme

⅛ tsp. pepper

¾ cup beef broth

1½ cups burgundy wine

1. Place onions in slow cooker.

2. Dredge meat in flour. Put in slow cooker.

3. Add mushrooms, salt, marjoram, thyme, and pepper.

4. Pour in broth and wine.

5. Cover. Cook on Low 8–10 hours.

6. Serve over cooked noodles.

Exchange List Values: Vegetable 3.0, Meat, lean 3.0

Basic Nutritional Values: Calories 219 (Calories from Fat 54), Total Fat 6 gm (Saturated Fat 1.9 gm, Polyunsat Fat 0.4 gm, Monounsat Fat 2.8 gm, Cholesterol 75 mg), Sodium 576 mg, Total Carbohydrate 14 gm, Dietary Fiber 2 gm, Sugars 5 gm, Protein 26 gm

Goodtime Beef Brisket

AmyMarlene Jensen • Fountain, CO

Makes 10 servings (Ideal slow cooker size: 4–5-quart)

3½-lb. beef brisket, trimmed of fat

1 can beer

2 cups tomato sauce

2 tsp. prepared mustard

2 Tbsp. balsamic vinegar

2 Tbsp. Worcestershire sauce

1 tsp. garlic powder

½ tsp. ground allspice

2 Tbsp. brown sugar

1 small green, or red, bell pepper, chopped

1 medium onion, chopped

¼ tsp. salt

½ tsp. pepper

1. Place brisket in slow cooker.

2. Combine remaining ingredients. Pour over meat.

3. Cover. Cook on Low 8–10 hours.

4. Remove meat from sauce. Slice very thin.

5. Serve on rolls or over couscous.

Exchange List Values: Carbohydrate 0.5, Vegetable 1.0, Meat, lean 3.0

Basic Nutritional Values: Calories 247 (Calories from Fat 85), Total Fat 9 gm (Saturated Fat 3.4 gm, Polyunsat Fat 0.3 gm, Monounsat Fat 4.3 gm, Cholesterol 86 mg), Sodium 472 mg, Total Carbohydrate 11 gm, Dietary Fiber 1 gm, Sugars 9 gm, Protein 29 gm

Zippy Beef Tips

Maryann Westerberg • Rosamond, CA

Recipe photo appears in color section.

Makes 6–8 servings (Ideal slow cooker size: 4-quart)

2 lbs. stewing meat, trimmed of fat, cubed

2 cups sliced fresh mushrooms

10¾-oz. can cream of mushroom soup

1 envelope fat-free dry onion soup mix

1 cup sugar-free 7Up, or other sugar-free
   lemon-lime carbonated drink

1. Place meat and mushrooms in slow cooker.

2. Combine mushroom soup, soup mix, and soda. Pour over meat.

3. Cover. Cook on Low 8 hours.

4. Serve over rice.

Exchange List Values: Carbohydrate 0.5, Meat, lean 2.0

Basic Nutritional Values: Calories 166 (Calories from Fat 59), Total Fat 7 gm (Saturated Fat 2.1 gm, Polyunsat Fat 1.2 gm, Monounsat Fat 2.5 gm, Cholesterol 58 mg), Sodium 349 mg, Total Carbohydrate 7 gm, Dietary Fiber 1 gm, Sugars 2 gm, Protein 19 gm

Don't let diabetes stop you from
living life to the fullest.

Horseradish Beef

Barbara Nolan • Pleasant Valley, NY

Makes 6–8 servings (Ideal slow cooker size: 4-quart)

3-lb. pot roast, trimmed of fat

1 Tbsp. canola oil

½ tsp. salt

½ tsp. pepper

1 medium onion, chopped

6-oz. can tomato paste

¼ cup horseradish sauce

1. Brown roast on all sides in oil in skillet. Place in slow cooker. Add remaining ingredients.

2. Cover. Cook on Low 8–10 hours.

Exchange List Values: Vegetable 1.0, Meat, lean 3.0, Fat 0.5

Basic Nutritional Values: Calories 220 (Calories from Fat 92), Total Fat 10 gm (Saturated Fat 3.3 gm, Polyunsat Fat 0.9 gm, Monounsat Fat 4.0 gm, Cholesterol 77 mg), Sodium 268 mg, Total Carbohydrate 6 gm, Dietary Fiber 1 gm, Sugars 2 gm, Protein 25 gm

Hungarian Goulash

Audrey Romonosky • Austin, TX

Makes 5–6 servings (Ideal slow cooker size: 4-quart)

2 lbs. beef chuck, trimmed of fat, cubed

1 medium onion, sliced

1/2 tsp. garlic powder

1/2 cup ketchup

2 Tbsp. Worcestershire sauce

1 Tbsp. brown sugar

1/4 tsp. salt

2 tsp. paprika

1/2 tsp. dry mustard

1 cup cold water

1/4 cup flour

1/2 cup water

1. Place meat in slow cooker. Add onion.

2. Combine garlic powder, ketchup, Worcestershire sauce, brown sugar, salt, paprika, mustard, and 1 cup water. Pour over meat.

3. Cover. Cook on Low 8 hours.

4. Dissolve flour in 1/2 cup water. Stir into meat mixture. Cook on High until thickened, about 10 minutes.

5. Serve over noodles.

Exchange List Values: Carbohydrate 1.0, Meat, lean 2.0

Basic Nutritional Values: Calories 207 (Calories from Fat 52), Total Fat 6 gm (Saturated Fat 2.0 gm, Polyunsat Fat 0.3 gm, Monounsat Fat 2.3 gm, Cholesterol 65 mg), Sodium 444 mg, Total Carbohydrate 15 gm, Dietary Fiber 1 gm, Sugars 7 gm, Protein 23 gm

Chinese Pot Roast

Marsha Sabus • Fallbrook, CA

Makes 6 servings (Ideal slow cooker size: 4-quart)

3-lb. boneless beef pot roast, trimmed of fat

2 Tbsp. flour

1 Tbsp. canola oil

2 large onions, chopped

1/4 cup light soy sauce

1/4 cup water

1/2 tsp. ground ginger

1. Dip roast in flour and brown on both sides in oil in saucepan. Place in slow cooker.

2. Top with onions.

3. Combine soy sauce, water, and ginger. Pour over meat.

4. Cover. Cook on High 10 minutes. Reduce heat to Low and cook 8–10 hours.

5. Slice and serve with rice.

Exchange List Values: Carbohydrate 0.5, Meat, lean 4.0

Basic Nutritional Values: Calories 272 (Calories from Fat 94), Total Fat 10 gm (Saturated Fat 3.1 gm, Polyunsat Fat 1.1 gm, Monounsat Fat 4.7 gm, Cholesterol 98 mg), Sodium 446 mg, Total Carbohydrate 9 gm, Dietary Fiber 1 gm, Sugars 4 gm, Protein 34 gm

Peppery Roast

Lovina Baer • Conrath, WI

Makes 8–10 servings (Ideal slow cooker size: 4–5-quart)

4-lb. beef, or venison, roast, trimmed of fat

½ tsp. garlic salt

½ tsp. onion salt

½ tsp. celery salt

2 tsp. Worcestershire sauce

2 tsp. pepper

½ cup ketchup

1 Tbsp. liquid smoke

3 Tbsp. brown sugar

1 Tbsp. dry mustard

dash nutmeg

1 Tbsp. light soy sauce

1 Tbsp. lemon juice

3 drops hot pepper sauce

1. Place roast in slow cooker.

2. Combine remaining ingredients and pour over roast.

3. Cover. Cook on High 6–8 hours.

Exchange List Values: Carbohydrate 0.5, Meat, lean 3.0

Basic Nutritional Values: Calories 202 (Calories from Fat 61), Total Fat 7 gm (Saturated Fat 2.3 gm, Polyunsat Fat 0.3 gm, Monounsat Fat 2.7 gm, Cholesterol 78 mg), Sodium 422 mg, Total Carbohydrate 8 gm, Dietary Fiber 0 gm, Sugars 6 gm, Protein 26 gm

Mexican Pot Roast

Bernice A. Esau • North Newton, KS

Makes 10 servings (Ideal slow cooker size: 4-quart)

3 lbs. boneless beef brisket, trimmed of fat, cubed

2 Tbsp. canola oil

½ cup slivered almonds

1½ cups mild picante sauce, or hot, if you prefer

2 Tbsp. vinegar

1 tsp. garlic powder

¼ tsp. cinnamon

¼ tsp. dried thyme

¼ tsp. dried oregano

⅛ tsp. ground cloves

⅛ tsp. pepper

1–1¼ cups water, as needed

1. Brown beef in oil in skillet. Place in slow cooker.

2. Combine remaining ingredients. Pour over meat.

3. Cover. Cook on Low 10–12 hours. Add water as needed.

4. Serve with potatoes, noodles, or rice.

Exchange List Values: Vegetable 1.0, Meat, lean 3.0, Fat 1.0

Basic Nutritional Values: Calories 244 (Calories from Fat 124), Total Fat 14 gm (Saturated Fat 3.3 gm, Polyunsat Fat 1.8 gm, Monounsat Fat 7.2 gm, Cholesterol 74 mg), Sodium 339 mg, Total Carbohydrate 4 gm, Dietary Fiber 1 gm, Sugars 1 gm, Protein 25 gm

Chuck Wagon Beef

Charlotte Bull • Cassville, MO

Makes 10 servings (Ideal slow cooker size: 4-quart)

4-lb. boneless chuck roast, trimmed of fat

1 tsp. garlic salt

1/4 tsp. black pepper

2 Tbsp. canola oil

6 cloves garlic, minced

1 large onion, sliced

1 cup water

1 bouillon cube

2 tsp. instant coffee

1 bay leaf, or 1 Tbsp. mixed Italian herbs

3 Tbsp. cold water

2 Tbsp. cornstarch

1. Sprinkle roast with garlic salt and pepper. Brown on all sides in oil in saucepan. Place in slow cooker. Reserve drippings.

2. Sauté garlic and onion in meat drippings in saucepan. Add 1 cup water, bouillon cube, and coffee. Cook over Low heat for several minutes, stirring until drippings loosen. Pour over meat in cooker.

3. Add bay leaf or herbs.

4. Cover. Cook on Low 8–10 hours, or until very tender. Remove bay leaf and discard. Remove meat to serving platter and keep warm.

5. Mix 3 Tbsp. water and cornstarch together until paste forms. Stir into hot liquid and onions in cooker. Cover. Cook 10 minutes on High or until thickened.

6. Slice meat and serve with gravy over top or on the side.

Exchange List Values: Vegetable 1.0, Meat, lean 3.0

Basic Nutritional Values: Calories 211 (Calories from Fat 83), Total Fat 9 gm (Saturated Fat 2.5 gm, Polyunsat Fat 1.1 gm, Monounsat Fat 4.3 gm, Cholesterol 78 mg), Sodium 271 mg, Total Carbohydrate 4 gm, Dietary Fiber 1 gm, Sugars 2 gm, Protein 26 gm

French Dip Roast

Patti Boston • Newark, OH

Makes 8 servings (Ideal slow cooker size: 4-quart)

1 large onion, sliced

3-lb. beef bottom roast, trimmed of fat

1/2 cup dry white wine, or water

half 1-oz. pkg. dry au jus gravy mix

2 cups 100%-fat-free, lower-sodium beef broth

1. Place onion in slow cooker. Add roast.

2. Combine wine and gravy mix. Pour over roast.

3. Add enough broth to cover roast.

4. Cover. Cook on High 5–6 hours, or Low 10–12 hours.

5. Remove meat from liquid. Let stand 5 minutes before slicing thinly across grain.

Exchange List Values: Meat, lean 3.0

Basic Nutritional Values: Calories 177 (Calories from Fat 55), Total Fat 6 gm (Saturated Fat 2.2 gm, Polyunsat Fat 0.3 gm, Monounsat Fat 2.5 gm, Cholesterol 74 mg), Sodium 376 mg, Total Carbohydrate 3 gm, Dietary Fiber 1 gm, Sugars 2 gm, Protein 25 gm

Dripped Beef

Mitzi McGlynchey • Downingtown, PA

Makes 8 servings (Ideal slow cooker size: 4-quart)

3-lb. chuck roast, trimmed of fat

½ tsp. salt

1 tsp. seasoned salt

1 tsp. white pepper

1 Tbsp. rosemary

1 Tbsp. dried oregano

1 Tbsp. garlic powder

1 cup water

1. Combine all ingredients in slow cooker.

2. Cover. Cook on Low 6–7 hours.

3. Shred meat using two forks. Strain liquid and return liquid and meat to slow cooker. Serve meat and au jus over mashed potatoes, noodles, or rice.

Exchange List Values: Meat, lean 3.0

Basic Nutritional Values: Calories 165 (Calories from Fat 56), Total Fat 6 gm (Saturated Fat 2.2 gm, Polyunsat Fat 0.3 gm, Mounsat Fat 2.5 gm, Cholesterol 73 mg), Sodium 384 mg, Total Carbohydrate 2 gm, Dietary Fiber 1 gm, Sugars 0 gm, Protein 24 gm

Exercise helps your body use insulin more efficiently, so it lowers your blood sugars more than normal—that's why insulin doses can usually be decreased before and after exercise.

Barbecued Roast Beef

Kim Stoltzfus • New Holland, PA

Makes 10 servings (Ideal slow cooker size: 4-5-quart)

4-lb. chuck roast, trimmed of fat

1 cup no-salt-added ketchup

1 cup barbecue sauce

2 cups chopped celery

2 cups water

1 cup chopped onions

4 Tbsp. vinegar

2 Tbsp. brown sugar

2 Tbsp. Worcestershire sauce

1 tsp. chili powder

1 tsp. garlic powder

¼ tsp. salt

5 cups cooked brown rice

1. Combine all ingredients except rice in large bowl. Spoon into 5-quart cooker, or 2 3½-quart cookers.

2. Cover. Cook on Low 6–8 hours, or High 3–4 hours.

3. Slice meat into thin slices and serve in barbecue sauce over rice.

Exchange List Values: Starch 1.5, Carbohydrate 1.0, Meat, lean 3.0

Basic Nutritional Values: Calories 352 (Calories from Fat 72), Total Fat 8 gm (Saturated Fat 2.6 gm, Polyunsat Fat 0.8 gm, Mounsat Fat 3.2 gm, Cholesterol 78 mg), Sodium 388 mg, Total Carbohydrate 40 gm, Dietary Fiber 3 gm, Sugars 15 gm, Protein 29 gm

Sour Beef

Rosanne Hankins • Stevensville, MD

Makes 6–8 servings (Ideal slow cooker size: 4-quart)

3-lb. pot roast, trimmed of fat

1/3 cup cider vinegar

1 large onion, sliced

3 bay leaves

1/2 tsp. salt

1/4 tsp. ground cloves

1/4 tsp. garlic powder

1. Place roast in slow cooker. Add remaining ingredients.

2. Cover. Cook on Low 8–10 hours.

Exchange List Values: Meat, lean 3.0

Basic Nutritional Values: Calories 169 (Calories from Fat 55), Total Fat 6 gm (Saturated Fat 2.2 gm, Polyunsat Fat 0.3 gm, Monounsat Fat 2.5 gm, Cholesterol 73 mg), Sodium 194 mg, Total Carbohydrate 3 gm, Dietary Fiber 1 gm, Sugars 2 gm, Protein 24 gm

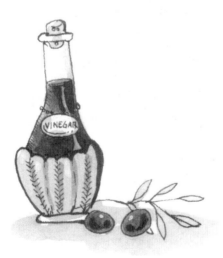

Old World Sauerbraten

C. J. Slagle • Roann, IN / Angeline Lang • Greeley, CO

Makes 8 servings (Ideal slow cooker size: 4-quart)

3 1/2-lb. beef rump roast, trimmed of fat

1 cup water

1 cup vinegar

1 lemon, sliced but unpeeled

10 whole cloves

1 large onion, sliced

4 bay leaves

6 whole peppercorns

1 Tbsp. salt

2 Tbsp. sugar

12 gingersnaps, crumbled

1. Place meat in deep ceramic or glass bowl.

2. Combine water, vinegar, lemon, cloves, onion, bay leaves, peppercorns, salt, and sugar. Pour over meat. Cover and refrigerate 24–36 hours. Turn meat several times during marinating.

3. Place beef in slow cooker. Pour 1 cup marinade over meat.

4. Cover. Cook on Low 6–8 hours. Remove meat.

5. Strain meat juices and return to pot. Turn to High. Stir in gingersnaps. Cover and cook on High 10–14 minutes. Slice meat. Pour finished sauce over meat.

Exchange List Values: Carbohydrate 0.5, Meat, lean 4.0

Basic Nutritional Values: Calories 235 (Calories from Fat 73), Total Fat 8 gm (Saturated Fat 2.6 gm, Polyunsat Fat 0.4 gm, Monounsat Fat 3.5 gm, Cholesterol 86 mg), Sodium 416 mg, Total Carbohydrate 10 gm, Dietary Fiber 0 gm, Sugars 4 gm, Protein 29 gm

Chili and Cheese on Rice

Dale and Shari Mast • Harrisonburg, VA

Recipe photo appears in color section.

Makes 6 servings (Ideal slow cooker size: 4-quart)

1 lb. extra-lean ground beef

1 medium onion, diced

1 tsp. dried basil

1 tsp. dried oregano

16-oz. can light red kidney beans

15½-oz. can chili beans

1½ cups stewed tomatoes, drained

2 cups cooked rice

6 Tbsp. fat-free grated cheddar cheese

1. Brown ground beef and onion in skillet. Drain. Season with basil and oregano.

2. Combine all ingredients except rice and cheese in slow cooker.

3. Cover. Cook on Low 4 hours.

4. Serve over cooked rice. Top with cheese.

Exchange List Values: Starch 2.5, Vegetable 2.0, Meat, lean 2.0, Fat 0.5

Basic Nutritional Values: Calories 371 (Calories from Fat 78), Total Fat 9 gm (Saturated Fat 3.2 gm, Polyunsat Fat 0.6 gm, Monounsat Fat 3.6 gm, Cholesterol 49 mg), Sodium 745 mg, Total Carbohydrate 46 gm, Dietary Fiber 9 gm, Sugars 7 gm, Protein 26 gm

Loretta's Spanish Rice

Loretta Krahn • Mt. Lake, MN

Makes 8 servings (Ideal slow cooker size: 4-5-quart)

1¾ lbs. 90%-lean ground beef, browned

2 medium onions, chopped

2 medium green peppers, chopped

28-oz. can tomatoes

8-oz. can tomato sauce

1½ cups water

2½ tsp. chili powder

½ tsp. salt

2 tsp. Worcestershire sauce

1½ cups rice, uncooked

1. Combine all ingredients in slow cooker.

2. Cover. Cook on Low 8–10 hours, or High 6 hours.

Exchange List Values: Starch 2.0, Vegetable 2.0, Meat, lean 2.0, Fat 0.5

Basic Nutritional Values: Calories 335 (Calories from Fat 79), Total Fat 9 gm (Saturated Fat 3.3 gm, Polyunsat Fat 0.6 gm, Monounsat Fat 3.7 gm, Cholesterol 60 mg), Sodium 550 mg, Total Carbohydrate 40 gm, Dietary Fiber 3 gm, Sugars 8 gm, Protein 24 gm

Just for today, add up the calories from all your beverages, including alcohol. Pay special attention to serving sizes, since many sodas and juice bottles contain 2 servings, but the calories listed are for 1 serving.

A Hearty Western Casserole

Karen Ashworth • Duenweg, MO

Makes 7 servings (Ideal slow cooker size: 4-quart)

1 lb. 90%-lean ground beef, browned, drained of fat, patted dry

16-oz. can whole corn, drained

15-oz. can no-salt-added red kidney beans, drained

10³⁄₄-oz. can reduced-sodium condensed tomato soup

¹⁄₂ cup (2 ozs.) reduced-fat Colby cheese

¹⁄₄ cup fat-free milk

1 tsp. minced dry onion flakes

¹⁄₂ tsp. chili powder

1. Combine beef, corn, beans, soup, cheese, milk, onion, and chili powder in slow cooker.

2. Cover. Cook on Low 1 hour.

Exchange List Values: Starch 1.0, Carbohydrate 0.5, Meat, lean 2.0, Fat 0.5

Basic Nutritional Values: Calories 241 (Calories from Fat 72), Total Fat 8 gm (Saturated Fat 3.5 gm, Polyunsat Fat 0.7 gm, Monounsat Fat 3.0 gm, Cholesterol 45 mg), Sodium 348 mg, Total Carbohydrate 23 gm, Dietary Fiber 4 gm, Sugars 6 gm, Protein 20 gm

VARIATION:

1 pkg. (of 10) refrigerator biscuits

2 Tbsp. margarine

¹⁄₄ cup yellow cornmeal

Dip biscuits in margarine and then in cornmeal. Bake 20 minutes or until brown. Top beef mixture with biscuits before serving.

Green Chili Stew

Jeanne Allen • Rye, CO

Makes 8 servings (Ideal slow cooker size: 4-quart)

2 cloves garlic, minced

1 large onion, diced

1 lb. extra-lean ground sirloin

¹⁄₃ lb. ground pork

2 Tbsp. oil

3 cups reduced-sodium chicken broth

2 cups water

2 4-oz. cans diced green chilies

4 large potatoes, diced

10-oz. pkg. frozen corn

1 tsp. black pepper

1 tsp. crushed dried oregano

¹⁄₂ tsp. ground cumin

¹⁄₂ tsp. salt

1. Brown garlic, onion, sirloin, and pork in oil in skillet. Cook until meat is no longer pink. Drain.

2. Combine all ingredients in slow cooker.

3. Cover. Cook on Low 4–6 hours, or until potatoes are soft.

Exchange List Values: Starch 2.0, Vegetable 1.0, Meat, lean 2.0, Fat 0.5

Basic Nutritional Values: Calories 309 (Calories from Fat 99), Total Fat 11 gm (Saturated Fat 3.1 gm, Polyunsat Fat 1.6 gm, Monounsat Fat 5.3 gm, Cholesterol 47 mg), Sodium 529 mg, Total Carbohydrate 33 gm, Dietary Fiber 5 gm, Sugars 5 gm, Protein 20 gm

Note: Excellent served with warm tortillas or corn bread.

Cowboy Casserole

Lori Berezovsky • Salina, KS

Makes 4–6 servings (Ideal slow cooker size: 4-quart)

1 medium onion, chopped

1¼ lbs. 90%-lean ground beef, browned, drained, and patted dry

6 medium potatoes, sliced, unpeeled

1 clove garlic, minced

16-oz. can kidney beans

15-oz. can diced tomatoes mixed with 2 Tbsp. flour, or 10¾-oz. can tomato soup

¼ tsp. salt

¼ tsp. pepper

1. Layer onions, ground beef, potatoes, garlic, and beans in slow cooker.

2. Spread tomatoes or soup over all. Sprinkle with salt and pepper.

3. Cover. Cook on Low 5–6 hours, or until potatoes are tender.

Exchange List Values: Starch 2.5, Vegetable 2.0, Meat, lean 2.0

Basic Nutritional Values: Calories 373 (Calories from Fat 73), Total Fat 8 gm (Saturated Fat 3.2 gm, Polyunsat Fat 0.6 gm, Monounsat Fat 3.4 gm, Cholesterol 57 mg), Sodium 567 mg, Total Carbohydrate 48 gm, Dietary Fiber 7 gm, Sugars 8 gm, Protein 27 gm

Eat more beans (kidney, pinto, chickpeas, etc.)—they're an excellent alternative to meat, providing protein and fiber with no saturated fat or cholesterol.

10-Layer Slow Cooker Dish

Norma Saltzman • Shickley, NE

Makes 8 servings (Ideal slow cooker size: 4-quart)

6 medium potatoes, thinly sliced, unpeeled

1 medium onion, thinly sliced

15-oz. can corn, drained

15-oz. can peas, drained

¼ cup water

1½ lbs. ground beef, browned and drained

10¾-oz. can cream of mushroom soup

1. Layer 1: ¼ of potatoes, ½ of onion.

2. Layer 2: ½ can of corn.

3. Layer 3: ¼ of potatoes.

4. Layer 4: ½ can peas.

5. Layer 5: ¼ of potatoes, ½ of onion.

6. Layer 6: remaining corn.

7. Layer 7: remaining potatoes.

8. Layer 8: remaining peas and water.

9. Layer 9: ground beef.

10. Layer 10: soup.

11. Cover. Cook on High 4 hours.

Exchange List Values: Starch 2.5, Meat, lean 2.0, Fat 0.5

Basic Nutritional Values: Calories 333 (Calories from Fat 101), Total Fat 11 gm (Saturated Fat 4.2 gm, Polyunsat Fat 1.6 gm, Monounsat Fat 4.2 gm, Cholesterol 52 mg), Sodium 525 mg, Total Carbohydrate 37 gm, Dietary Fiber 5 gm, Sugars 6 gm, Protein 22 gm

Beef and Lentils

Esther Porter • Minneapolis, MN

Makes 12 servings (Ideal slow cooker size: 4–5-quart)

3 whole cloves

1 medium onion

5 cups water

1 lb. lentils

1 tsp. salt

1 bay leaf

1 lb. (or less) ground beef, browned and drained

$1/2$ cup ketchup

$1/4$ cup molasses

2 Tbsp. brown sugar

1 tsp. dry mustard

$1/4$ tsp. Worcestershire sauce

1 medium onion, finely chopped

1. Stick cloves into whole onion. Set aside.

2. In large saucepan, combine water, lentils, salt, bay leaf, and whole onion with cloves. Simmer 30 minutes.

3. Meanwhile, combine all remaining ingredients in slow cooker. Stir in simmered ingredients from saucepan. Add additional water if mixture seems dry.

4. Cover. Cook on Low 6–8 hours (check to see if lentils are tender).

Exchange List Values: Starch 1.5, Carbohydrate 0.5, Vegetable 1.0, Meat, lean 1.0

Basic Nutritional Values: Calories 230 (Calories from Fat 39), Total Fat 4 gm (Saturated Fat 1.5 gm, Polyunsat Fat 0.3 gm, Monounsat Fat 1.7 gm, Cholesterol 22 mg), Sodium 342 mg, Total Carbohydrate 32 gm, Dietary Fiber 9 gm, Sugars 11 gm, Protein 17 gm

VARIATION: Top with sour cream and/or salsa when serving.

Note: This dish freezes well.

Hamburger Potatoes

Juanita Marner • Shipshewana, IN

Makes 3–4 servings (Ideal slow cooker size: 4-quart)

3 medium potatoes, sliced, unpeeled

3 medium carrots, sliced

1 small onion, sliced

2 Tbsp. dry rice

$1/4$ tsp. salt

$1/2$ tsp. pepper

$3/4$ lb. 85%-lean ground beef, browned and drained

$1^1/2$–2 cups tomato juice, as needed to keep dish from getting too dry

1. Combine all ingredients in slow cooker.

2. Cover. Cook on Low 6–8 hours.

Exchange List Values: Starch 2.0, Vegetable 1.0, Meat, lean 2.0, Fat 0.5

Basic Nutritional Values: Calories 311 (Calories from Fat 80), Total Fat 9 gm (Saturated Fat 3.4 gm, Polyunsat Fat 0.4 gm, Monounsat Fat 3.8 gm, Cholesterol 50 mg), Sodium 576 mg, Total Carbohydrate 38 gm, Dietary Fiber 5 gm, Sugars 9 gm, Protein 20 gm

Find out if your local shopping mall opens early so people can walk the mall before the stores open. If it has a walking club, join it!

Supper-in-a-Dish

Martha Hershey • Ronks, PA

Recipe photo appears in color section.

Makes 8 servings (Ideal slow cooker size: 4-quart)

1 lb. ground beef, browned and drained

1½ cups sliced raw potatoes

1 cup sliced carrots

1 cup fresh or frozen peas

½ cup chopped onions

½ cup chopped celery

¼ cup chopped green peppers

¼ tsp. salt

¼ tsp. pepper

10¾-oz. can 98%-fat-free reduced-sodium cream of chicken, or mushroom, soup

¼ cup fat-free milk

2 ozs. grated fat-free sharp cheddar cheese

1. Layer ground beef, potatoes, carrots, peas, onions, celery, green peppers, salt, and pepper in slow cooker.

2. Combine soup and milk. Pour over layered ingredients. Sprinkle with cheese.

3. Cover. Cook on High 4 hours.

Exchange List Values: Starch 1.0, Vegetable 1.0, Meat, lean 2.0, Fat 0.5

Basic Nutritional Values: Calories 246 (Calories from Fat 79), Total Fat 9 gm (Saturated Fat 3.4 gm, Polyunsat Fat 0.7 gm, Monounsat Fat 3.5 gm, Cholesterol 50 mg), Sodium 462 mg, Total Carbohydrate 20 gm, Dietary Fiber 3 gm, Sugars 6 gm, Protein 21 gm

Meal-in-One-Casserole

Elizabeth Yoder • Millersburg, OH / Marcella Stalter • Flanagan, IL

Makes 8 servings (Ideal slow cooker size: 4-quart)

1 lb. ground beef

1 medium onion, chopped

1 medium green pepper, chopped

15¼-oz. can whole kernel corn, drained

4-oz. can mushrooms, drained

¼ tsp. pepper

11-oz. jar salsa

5 cups uncooked medium egg noodles

28-oz. can no-salt-added diced tomatoes, undrained

1 cup shredded fat-free cheddar cheese

1. Cook beef and onion in saucepan over medium heat until meat is no longer pink. Drain. Transfer to slow cooker.

2. Top with green pepper, corn, and mushrooms. Sprinkle with pepper. Pour salsa over mushrooms. Cover and cook on Low 3 hours.

3. Cook noodles according to package in separate pan. Drain and add to slow cooker after mixture in cooker has cooked for 3 hours. Top with tomatoes. Sprinkle with cheese.

Exchange List Values: Starch 1.5, Vegetable 2.0, Meat, lean 2.0

Basic Nutritional Values: Calories 282 (Calories from Fat 67), Total Fat 7 gm (Saturated Fat 2.7 gm, Polyunsat Fat 0.8 gm, Monounsat Fat 2.9 gm, Cholesterol 58 mg), Sodium 393 mg, Total Carbohydrate 34 gm, Dietary Fiber 4 gm, Sugars 8 gm, Protein 21 gm

Yum-e-setti

Elsie Schlabach • Millersburg, OH

Makes 9 servings (Ideal slow cooker size: 4–5-quart)

1¼ lbs. 90%-lean ground beef, browned, drained, and patted dry

10¾-oz. can 98%-fat-free, reduced-sodium tomato soup

8-oz. pkg. wide noodles, cooked

10¾-oz. can 98%-fat-free, reduced-sodium cream of chicken soup

1 cup chopped celery, cooked tender

1-lb. pkg. frozen mixed vegetables (including corn)

3 ozs. Velveeta Light cheese, cubed

1. Combine ground beef and tomato soup.

2. Combine noodles, chicken soup, and celery.

3. Layer beef mixture, chicken mixture, and vegetables into slow cooker. Lay cheese over top.

4. Cover. Cook on Low 2–3 hours.

Exchange List Values: Starch 2.0, Vegetable 1.0, Meat, lean 2.0

Basic Nutritional Values: Calories 293 (Calories from Fat 76), Total Fat 8 gm (Saturated Fat 3.5 gm, Polyunsat Fat 1.0 gm, Monounsat Fat 3.0 gm, Cholesterol 68 mg), Sodium 478 mg, Total Carbohydrate 34 gm, Dietary Fiber 3 gm, Sugars 7 gm, Protein 20 gm

VARIATION: For more "bite," use shredded cheddar cheese instead of cubed Velveeta.

Meatball Stew

Nanci Keatley • Salem, OR / Ada Miller • Sugarcreek, OH

Makes 8 servings (Ideal slow cooker size: 4-quart)

1¾ lbs. 98%-lean ground beef

½ tsp. pepper

6 medium potatoes, cubed, unpeeled

1 large onion, sliced

6 medium carrots, sliced

1 cup ketchup

1 cup water

1½ tsp. balsamic vinegar

1 tsp. dried basil

1 tsp. dried oregano

½ tsp. pepper

1. Combine beef and ½ tsp. pepper. Mix well. Shape into 1" balls. Brown meatballs in saucepan over medium heat. Drain. Pat dry.

2. Place potatoes, onion, and carrots in slow cooker. Top with meatballs.

3. Combine ketchup, water, vinegar, basil, oregano, and ½ tsp. pepper. Pour over meatballs.

4. Cover. Cook on High 4–5 hours, or until vegetables are tender.

Exchange List Values: Starch 1.5, Carbohydrate 0.5, Vegetable 2.0, Meat, lean 2.0

Basic Nutritional Values: Calories 318 (Calories from Fat 77), Total Fat 9 gm (Saturated Fat 3.3 gm, Polyunsat Fat 0.4 gm, Monounsat Fat 3.5 gm, Cholesterol 60 mg), Sodium 610 mg, Total Carbohydrate 38 gm, Dietary Fiber 5 gm, Sugars 9 gm, Protein 23 gm

Mary Ellen's Barbecued Meatballs

Mary Ellen Wilcox • Scatia, NY

**Makes about 60 small meatballs (10 servings)
(Ideal slow cooker size: 4-quart)**

MEATBALLS:

¾ lb. ground beef

¾ cup bread crumbs

1½ Tbsp. minced onion

½ tsp. horseradish

3 drops Tabasco sauce

2 eggs, beaten

¼ tsp. salt

½ tsp. pepper

1 Tbsp. canola oil

SAUCE:

¾ cup ketchup

½ cup water

¼ cup cider vinegar

2 Tbsp. brown sugar

1 Tbsp. minced onion

2 tsp. horseradish

1 tsp. dry mustard

3 drops Tabasco

dash pepper

1. Combine all meatball ingredients. Shape into ¾" balls. Brown in nonstick skillet. Place in slow cooker.

2. Combine all sauce ingredients. Pour over meatballs.

3. Cover. Cook on Low 5 hours.

Exchange List Values: Starch 0.5, Carbohydrate 0.5, Meat, lean 1.0, Fat 0.5

Basic Nutritional Values: Calories 148 (Calories from Fat 57), Total Fat 6 gm (Saturated Fat 1.8 gm, Polyunsat Fat 0.8 gm, Monounsat Fat 2.8 gm, Cholesterol 63 mg), Sodium 378 mg, Total Carbohydrate 14 gm, Dietary Fiber 1 gm, Sugars 6 gm, Protein 9 gm

*Keep healthy snacks handy!
A delayed meal or change in your
schedule can happen anytime, so keep
snacks in your desk, briefcase,
pocketbook, or glove compartment.*

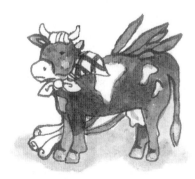

Cocktail Meatballs

Irene Klaeger • Inverness, FL

Makes 20 appetizer servings (Ideal slow cooker size: 4-quart)

2 lbs. ground beef

$\frac{1}{3}$ cup ketchup

3 tsp. dry bread crumbs

1 egg, beaten

2 tsp. onion flakes

$\frac{3}{4}$ tsp. garlic salt

$\frac{1}{2}$ tsp. pepper

1 cup ketchup

$\frac{1}{2}$ cup packed brown sugar

6-oz. can tomato paste

$\frac{1}{4}$ cup light soy sauce

$\frac{1}{4}$ cup cider vinegar

1–1$\frac{1}{2}$ tsp. hot pepper sauce

1. Combine ground beef, $\frac{1}{3}$ cup ketchup, bread crumbs, egg, onion flakes, garlic salt, and pepper. Mix well. Shape into 1" meatballs. Place on jelly roll pan. Bake at 350° for 18 minutes, or until brown. Place in slow cooker.

2. Combine 1 cup ketchup, brown sugar, tomato paste, soy sauce, vinegar, and hot pepper sauce. Pour over meatballs.

3. Cover. Cook on Low 4 hours.

Exchange List Values: Carbohydrate 1.0, Meat, lean 1.0

Basic Nutritional Values: Calories 128 (Calories from Fat 45), Total Fat 5 gm (Saturated Fat 1.9 gm, Polyunsat Fat 0.2 gm, Monounsat Fat 2.1 gm, Cholesterol 37 mg), Sodium 318 mg, Total Carbohydrate 12 gm, Dietary Fiber 1 gm, Sugars 8 gm, Protein 9 gm

Swedish Meatballs

Zona Mae Bontrager • Kokomo, IN

Makes 12 servings (Ideal slow cooker size: 4-quart)

MEATBALLS:

$\frac{3}{4}$ lb. ground beef

$\frac{1}{2}$ lb. ground pork

$\frac{1}{2}$ cup minced onions

$\frac{3}{4}$ cup fine dry bread crumbs

1 Tbsp. minced parsley

1 tsp. salt

$\frac{1}{8}$ tsp. pepper

$\frac{1}{2}$ tsp. garlic powder

1 Tbsp. Worcestershire sauce

1 egg

$\frac{1}{2}$ cup fat-free milk

2 Tbsp. canola oil

GRAVY:

$\frac{1}{4}$ cup flour

$\frac{1}{4}$ tsp. salt

$\frac{1}{4}$ tsp. garlic powder

$\frac{1}{8}$ tsp. pepper

1 tsp. paprika

2 cups boiling water

$\frac{3}{4}$ cup fat-free sour cream

1. Combine meats, onions, bread crumbs, parsley, salt, pepper, garlic powder, Worcestershire sauce, egg, and milk.

2. Shape into balls the size of a walnut. Brown in oil in skillet. Reserve drippings, and place meatballs in slow cooker.

3. Cover. Cook on High 10–15 minutes.

4. Stir flour, salt, garlic powder, pepper, and paprika into hot drippings in skillet. Stir in water and sour cream. Pour over meatballs.

5. Cover. Reduce heat to Low. Cook 4–5 hours.

6. Serve over rice or noodles.

Exchange List Values: Starch 1.0, Meat, lean 1.0, Fat 1.0

Basic Nutritional Values: Calories 168 (Calories from Fat 78), Total Fat 9 gm (Saturated Fat 2.5 gm, Polyunsat Fat 1.2 gm, Monounsat Fat 4.1 gm, Cholesterol 48 mg), Sodium 368 mg, Total Carbohydrate 11 gm, Dietary Fiber 0 gm, Sugars 2 gm, Protein 11 gm

Italian Meatball Subs

Bonnie Miller • Louisville, OH

Makes 9 servings (Ideal slow cooker size: 4-5-quart)

MEATBALLS:

1 egg, beaten

$\frac{1}{4}$ cup fat-free milk

$\frac{1}{2}$ cup dry bread crumbs

2 Tbsp. freshly grated Parmesan cheese

$\frac{1}{2}$ tsp. salt

$\frac{1}{4}$ tsp. pepper

$\frac{1}{8}$ tsp. garlic powder

$\frac{3}{4}$ lb. 85%-lean ground beef

$\frac{1}{2}$ lb. bulk pork sausage

SAUCE:

15-oz. can no-salt-added tomato sauce

6-oz. can tomato paste

1 small onion, chopped

$\frac{1}{2}$ cup chopped green bell pepper

$\frac{1}{2}$ cup red wine, or beef broth

$\frac{1}{3}$ cup water

2 cloves garlic, minced

1 tsp. dried oregano

$\frac{1}{2}$ tsp. salt

$\frac{1}{2}$ tsp. pepper

$\frac{1}{2}$ tsp. sugar

1. Make meatballs by combining egg and milk. Add bread crumbs, cheese, and seasonings. Add meats. Mix well. Shape into 1" balls. Broil or saute until brown. Put in slow cooker.

2. Combine sauce ingredients. Pour over meatballs.

3. Cover. Cook on Low 4–6 hours.

4. Serve on rolls with creamy red potatoes, salad, and dessert.

Exchange List Values: Starch 0.5, Vegetable 1.0, Meat, medium fat 1.0, Fat 1.0

Basic Nutritional Values: Calories 186 (Calories from Fat 81), Total Fat 9 gm (Saturated Fat 3.3 gm, Polyunsat Fat 0.9 gm, Monounsat Fat 3.8 gm, Cholesterol 57 mg), Sodium 403 mg, Total Carbohydrate 14 gm, Dietary Fiber 2 gm, Sugars 5 gm, Protein 13 gm

Sweet and Sour Meatballs

Elaine Unruh • Minneapolis, MN

Makes 6–8 main-dish servings, or 20 appetizer servings (Ideal slow cooker size: 4-quart)

MEATBALLS:

2 lbs. ground beef

1¼ cups bread crumbs

¼ tsp. salt

1 tsp. pepper

2–3 Tbsp. Worcestershire sauce

1 egg

½ tsp. garlic salt

¼ cup finely chopped onions

SAUCE:

20-oz. can pineapple chunks, juice reserved

3 Tbsp. cornstarch

¼ cup cold water

1 cup ketchup

2 Tbsp. Worcestershire sauce

¼ tsp. salt

¼ tsp. pepper

¼ tsp. garlic salt

½ cup chopped green peppers

1. Combine all meatball ingredients. Shape into 60 meatballs. Brown in nonstick skillet, rolling so all sides are browned. Place meatballs in slow cooker.

2. Pour juice from pineapples into skillet. Stir into drippings.

3. Combine cornstarch and cold water. Add to skillet and stir until thickened.

4. Stir in ketchup and Worcestershire sauce. Season with salt, pepper, and garlic salt. Add green peppers and pineapples. Pour over meatballs.

5. Cover. Cook on Low 6 hours.

Exchange List Values: Carbohydrate 1.0, Meat, lean 1.0, Fat 0.5

Basic Nutritional Values: Calories 150 (Calories from Fat 48), Total Fat 5 gm (Saturated Fat 1.9 gm, Polyunsat Fat 0.3 gm, Monounsat Fat 2.2 gm, Cholesterol 37 mg), Sodium 430 mg, Total Carbohydrate 16 gm, Dietary Fiber 1 gm, Sugars 7 gm, Protein 10 gm

In addition to your regular doctor, have someone— a certified diabetes educator, nurse practitioner, or nurse case manager— whom you can contact on short notice to discuss problems or questions that come up, such as unexplained high blood sugars or sudden illness.

Swedish Cabbage Rolls

Fean Butzer • Batavia, NY /
Pam Hochstedler • Kalona, IA

**Makes 6 servings (1 serving = 2 cabbage rolls)
(Ideal slow cooker size: 4–5-quart)**

12 large cabbage leaves

1 egg, beaten

¼ cup fat-free milk

¼ cup finely chopped onions

¾ tsp. salt

¼ tsp. pepper

1 lb. ground beef, browned and drained

1 cup cooked rice

8-oz. can tomato sauce

1 Tbsp. brown sugar

1 Tbsp. lemon juice

1 tsp. Worcestershire sauce

1. Immerse cabbage leaves in boiling water for about 3 minutes, or until limp. Drain.

2. Combine egg, milk, onions, salt, pepper, beef, and rice. Place about ¼ cup meat mixture in center of each leaf. Fold in sides and roll ends over meat. Place in slow cooker.

3. Combine tomato sauce, brown sugar, lemon juice, and Worcestershire sauce. Pour over cabbage rolls.

4. Cover. Cook on Low 7–9 hours.

Exchange List Values: Starch 0.5, Vegetable 2.0, Meat, lean 2.0, Fat 0.5

Basic Nutritional Values: Calories 219 (Calories from Fat 79), Total Fat 9 gm (Saturated Fat 3.4 gm, Polyunsat Fat 0.5 gm, Monounsat Fat 3.7 gm, Cholesterol 80 mg), Sodium 603 mg, Total Carbohydrate 18 gm, Dietary Fiber 2 gm, Sugars 7 gm, Protein 17 gm

Stuffed Cabbage

Barbara Nolan • Pleasant Valley, NY

Makes 6 servings (Ideal slow cooker size: 4–5-quart)

4 cups water

12 large cabbage leaves

1 lb. ground beef, lamb, or turkey

½ cup cooked rice

½ tsp. salt

⅛ tsp. pepper

¼ tsp. dried thyme

¼ tsp. nutmeg

¼ tsp. cinnamon

6-oz. can tomato paste

¾ cup water

1. Boil 4 cups water in deep kettle. Remove kettle from heat. Soak cabbage leaves in hot water for 5 minutes, or just until softened. Remove. Drain. Cool.

2. Combine meat, rice, salt, pepper, thyme, nutmeg, and cinnamon. Place 2 Tbsp. of mixture on each leaf. Roll up firmly. Stack stuffed leaves in slow cooker.

3. Combine tomato paste and ¾ cup water until smooth. Pour over cabbage rolls.

4. Cover. Cook on Low 6–8 hours.

Exchange List Values: Vegetable 2.0, Meat, lean 2.0, Fat 0.5

Basic Nutritional Values: Calories 186 (Calories from Fat 73), Total Fat 8 gm (Saturated Fat 3.0 gm, Polyunsat Fat 0.4 gm, Monounsat Fat 3.4 gm, Cholesterol 45 mg), Sodium 269 mg, Total Carbohydrate 13 gm, Dietary Fiber 3 gm, Sugars 3 gm, Protein 16 gm

*Make exercise fun—
do something silly today.*

Stuffed Green Peppers

Lois Stoltzfus • Honey Brook, PA

Makes 6 servings (Ideal slow cooker size: 6-quart oval, so the peppers can each sit on the bottom of the cooker)

6 large green peppers

¾ lb. 85%-lean ground beef, browned and drained

2 Tbsp. minced onion

⅛ tsp. salt

⅛ tsp. garlic powder

2 cups cooked rice

15-oz. can tomato sauce

½ cup reduced-fat shredded mozzarella cheese

1. Cut peppers in half and remove seeds.

2. Combine all ingredients except peppers and cheese.

3. Stuff peppers with ground beef mixture. Place in slow cooker.

4. Cover. Cook on Low 6–8 hours, or on High 3–4 hours. Sprinkle with cheese during last 30 minutes.

Exchange List Values: Starch 1.0, Vegetable 3.0, Meat, lean 1.0, Fat 1.0

Basic Nutritional Values: Calories 253 (Calories from Fat 69), Total Fat 8 gm (Saturated Fat 3.2 gm, Polyunsat Fat 0.5 gm, Monounsat Fat 2.8 gm, Cholesterol 39 mg), Sodium 585 mg, Total Carbohydrate 30 gm, Dietary Fiber 5 gm, Sugars 9 gm, Protein 17 gm

Beef Enchiladas

Jane Talso • Albuquerque, NM

Makes 12–16 servings (Ideal slow cooker size: 5–6-quart)

4-lb. boneless chuck roast, trimmed of fat

2 Tbsp. canola oil

4 cups sliced onions

2 tsp. black pepper

2 tsp. cumin seeds

2 4½-oz. cans peeled, diced green chilies

14½-oz. can no-salt-added, peeled, diced tomatoes

8 large tortillas (10" size)

4 cups green, or red, enchilada sauce

1 cup (4 ozs.) reduced-fat cheddar cheese, shredded

1. Brown roast on all sides in oil in saucepan. Place roast in slow cooker.

2. Add remaining ingredients except tortillas, cheese, and sauce.

3. Cover. Cook on High 4–5 hours.

4. Shred meat with fork and return to slow cooker.

5. Warm tortillas in oven. Heat enchilada sauce. Fill each tortilla with ¾ cup beef mixture and ⅛ cup cheese. Roll up and serve with sauce.

Exchange List Values: Starch 1.0, Vegetable 2.0, Meat, lean 3.0, Fat 1.0

Basic Nutritional Values: Calories 336 (Calories from Fat 114), Total Fat 13 gm (Saturated Fat 3.5 gm, Polyunsat Fat 1.5 gm, Monounsat Fat 5.1 gm, Cholesterol 69 mg), Sodium 542 mg, Total Carbohydrate 29 gm, Dietary Fiber 4 gm, Sugars 5 gm, Protein 27 gm

VARIATION: Use 2 lbs. ground beef instead of chuck roast. Brown without oil in saucepan, along with onions.

Slow Cooker Enchiladas

Lori Berezovsky • Salina, KS /
Tracy Clark • Mt. Crawford, VA /
Mary E. Herr and Michelle Reineck •
Three Rivers, MI / Marcia S. Myer •
Manheim, PA / Renee Shirk • Mt. Joy, PA /
Janice Showalter • Flint, MI

Makes 8 servings (Ideal slow cooker size: 4-quart)

1 lb. 90%-lean ground beef

1 cup chopped onions

$\frac{1}{2}$ cup chopped green peppers

16-oz. can no-salt-added red kidney beans, rinsed and drained

15-oz. can no-salt-added black beans, rinsed and drained

10-oz. can diced tomatoes with green chilies, undrained

$\frac{1}{3}$ cup water

$1\frac{1}{2}$ tsp. chili powder

$\frac{1}{2}$ tsp. ground cumin

$\frac{1}{4}$ tsp. pepper

4 ozs. (1 cup) shredded fat-free sharp cheddar cheese

2 ozs. ($\frac{1}{2}$ cup) shredded reduced-fat Monterey Jack cheese

8 flour tortillas (6"–7" in diameter)

1. Cook beef, onions, and green peppers in skillet until beef is browned and vegetables are tender. Drain. Pat dry.

2. Add next 7 ingredients and bring to a boil. Reduce heat. Cover and simmer 10 minutes.

3. Combine cheeses.

4. In slow cooker, layer about $\frac{3}{4}$ cup beef mixture, one tortilla, and about $\frac{1}{3}$ cup cheeses. Repeat layers.

5. Cover. Cook on Low 5–7 hours or until heated through.

6. To serve, reach to bottom with each spoonful to get all the layers, or carefully invert onto large platter and cut into wedges. Serve with sour cream and/or guacamole.

Exchange List Values: Starch 2.0, Vegetable 1.0, Meat, lean 3.0

Basic Nutritional Values: Calories 335 (Calories from Fat 76), Total Fat 8 gm (Saturated Fat 3.5 gm, Polyunsat Fat 0.7 gm, Monounsat Fat 3.6 gm, Cholesterol 41 mg), Sodium 484 mg, Total Carbohydrate 38 gm, Dietary Fiber 6 gm, Sugars 5 gm, Protein 27 gm

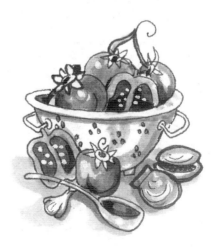

Shredded Beef for Tacos

Dawn Day • Westminster, CA

Makes 6–8 servings (Ideal slow cooker size: 4-quart)

2-lb. round roast, trimmed of fat, cut into large chunks

1 large onion, chopped

2 Tbsp. canola oil

2 serrano chilies, chopped

3 cloves garlic, minced

1 tsp. salt

1 cup water

1. Brown meat and onion in oil. Transfer to slow cooker.

2. Add chilies, garlic, salt, and water.

3. Cover. Cook on High 6–8 hours.

4. Pull meat apart with two forks until shredded.

5. Serve with fresh tortillas, lettuce, tomatoes, cheese, and guacamole.

Exchange List Values: Meat, lean 3.0

Basic Nutritional Values: Calories 184 (Calories from Fat 79), Total Fat 9 gm (Saturated Fat 2.1 gm, Polyunsat Fat 1.2 gm, Monounsat Fat 4.2 gm, Cholesterol 64 mg), Sodium 335 mg, Total Carbohydrate 4 gm, Dietary Fiber 1 gm, Sugars 3 gm, Protein 22 gm

Tamale Pie

Jeannine Janzen • Elbing, KS

Makes 8 servings (Ideal slow cooker size: 4-quart)

¾ cup cornmeal

1½ cups fat-free milk

1 egg, beaten

1 lb. ground beef, browned and drained

1.25-oz. envelope dry chili seasoning mix

16-oz. can diced tomatoes

16-oz. can corn, drained

1 cup grated fat-free cheddar cheese

1. Combine cornmeal, milk, and egg.

2. Stir in meat, chili seasoning mix, tomatoes, and corn until well blended. Pour into slow cooker.

3. Cover. Cook on High 1 hour, then on Low 3 hours.

4. Sprinkle with cheese. Cook another 5 minutes until cheese is melted.

Exchange List Values: Starch 1.0, Carbohydrate 0.5, Vegetable 1.0, Meat, lean 2.0

Basic Nutritional Values: Calories 244 (Calories from Fat 65), Total Fat 7 gm (Saturated Fat 2.6 gm, Polyunsat Fat 0.6 gm, Monounsat Fat 2.9 gm, Cholesterol 63 mg), Sodium 500 mg, Total Carbohydrate 25 gm, Dietary Fiber 3 gm, Sugars 6 gm, Protein 20 gm

Mexican Corn Bread

Jeanne Heyerly • Chenoa, IL

Makes 8 servings (Ideal slow cooker size: 4-quart)

16-oz. can no-salt-added cream-style corn

1 cup cornmeal

½ tsp. baking soda

½ tsp. salt

¼ cup canola oil

1 cup fat-free milk

2 eggs, beaten

½ cup taco sauce

4 ozs. (1 cup) shredded fat-free cheddar cheese

1 medium onion, chopped

1 clove garlic, minced

4-oz. can diced green chilies

1 lb. 85%-lean ground beef, lightly cooked, drained, and patted dry

1. Combine corn, cornmeal, baking soda, salt, oil, milk, eggs, and taco sauce. Pour half of mixture into slow cooker.

2. Layer cheese, onion, garlic, green chilies, and ground beef on top of cornmeal mixture. Cover with remaining cornmeal mixture.

3. Cover. Cook on High 1 hour and on Low 3½–4 hours, or only on Low 6 hours.

Exchange List Values: Starch 2.0, Meat, lean 2.0, Fat 1.5

Basic Nutritional Values: Calories 320 (Calories from Fat 134), Total Fat 15 gm (Saturated Fat 3.3 gm, Polyunsat Fat 2.7 gm, Monounsat Fat 7.3 gm, Cholesterol 89 mg), Sodium 575 mg, Total Carbohydrate 27 gm, Dietary Fiber 3 gm, Sugars 7 gm, Protein 20 gm

Jean & Tammy's Sloppy Joes

Jean Shaner • York, PA /
Tammy Smoker • Cochranville, PA

Makes 14 servings (Ideal slow cooker size: 4-quart)

2¾ lbs. 85%-lean ground beef, browned, drained, and patted dry

1 onion, finely chopped

1 green pepper, chopped

8-oz. can tomato sauce

8-oz. can no-salt-added tomato sauce

¾ cup ketchup

1 Tbsp. Worcestershire sauce

1 tsp. chili powder

¼ tsp. pepper

¼ tsp. garlic powder

1. Combine all ingredients in slow cooker.

2. Cover. Cook on Low 8–10 hours, or on High 3–4 hours.

3. Serve in sandwich rolls.

Exchange List Values: Carbohydrate 0.5, Meat, lean 3.0, Fat 0.5

Basic Nutritional Values: Calories 227 (Calories from Fat 104), Total Fat 12 gm (Saturated Fat 4.5 gm, Polyunsat Fat 0.4 gm, Monounsat Fat 5.0 gm, Cholesterol 67 mg), Sodium 383 mg, Total Carbohydrate 9 gm, Dietary Fiber 1 gm, Sugars 5 gm, Protein 21 gm

Mile-High Shredded Beef Sandwiches

Miriam Christophel • Battle Creek, MI /
Mary Seielstad • Sparks, NV

Makes 8 servings (Ideal slow cooker size: 4-quart)

3 lbs. chuck roast, or round steak, trimmed of fat

2 Tbsp. oil

1 cup chopped onions

½ cup sliced celery

2 cups lower-sodium, 98%-fat-free beef broth

1 clove garlic

¾ cup ketchup

2 Tbsp. brown sugar

2 Tbsp. vinegar

1 tsp. dry mustard

½ tsp. chili powder

3 drops Tabasco sauce

1 bay leaf

¼ tsp. paprika

¼ tsp. garlic powder

1 tsp. Worcestershire sauce

1. In skillet brown both sides of meat in oil. Add onions and celery and saute briefly. Transfer to slow cooker. Add broth.

2. Cover. Cook on Low 6–8 hours, or until tender. Remove meat from cooker and cool. Shred beef.

3. Remove vegetables from cooker and drain, reserving 1½ cups broth. Combine vegetables and meat.

4. Return shredded meat and vegetables to cooker. Add broth and remaining ingredients and combine well.

5. Cover. Cook on High 1 hour. Remove bay leaf.

6. Pile into 8 sandwich rolls and serve.

Exchange List Values: Carbohydrate 1.0, Meat, lean 3.0

Basic Nutritional Values: Calories 239 (Calories from Fat 88), Total Fat 10 gm (Saturated Fat 2.4 gm, Polyunsat Fat 1.3 gm, Monounsat Fat 4.6 gm, Cholesterol 73 mg), Sodium 444 mg, Total Carbohydrate 12 gm, Dietary Fiber 1 gm, Sugars 8 gm, Protein 25 gm

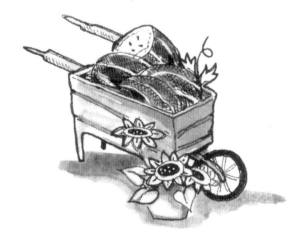

Corned Beef

Elaine Vigoda • Rochester, NY

Makes 12 servings (Ideal slow cooker size: 4–5-quart)

3 large carrots, cut into chunks

1 cup chopped celery

½ tsp. pepper

1 cup water

2-lb. piece of corned beef, trimmed of fat

1 large onion, cut into pieces

half a small head of cabbage, cut in wedges

4 medium potatoes, peeled and chunked

1. Place carrots, celery, pepper, and water in slow cooker.

2. Add beef. Cover with onions.

3. Cover. Cook on Low 8–10 hours, or on High 5–6 hours.

4. Lift corned beef out of cooker and add cabbage and potatoes, pushing them to bottom of slow cooker. Return beef to cooker.

5. Cover. Cook on High 2 hours.

6. Remove corned beef. Cool and slice on the diagonal. Serve surrounded by vegetables.

Exchange List Values: Starch 0.5, Vegetable 1.0, Meat, medium fat 1.0, Fat 1.0

Basic Nutritional Values: Calories 194 (Calories from Fat 93), Total Fat 10 gm (Saturated Fat 3.4 gm, Polyunsat Fat 0.5 gm, Monounsat Fat 4.9 gm, Cholesterol 52 mg), Sodium 639 mg, Total Carbohydrate 14 gm, Dietary Fiber 3 gm, Sugars 4 gm, Protein 11 gm

Corned Beef and Cabbage

Rhoda Burgoon • Collingswood, NJ /
Jo Ellen Moore • Pendleton, IN

Makes 12 servings (Ideal slow cooker size: 4–5-quart)

3 carrots, cut in 3" pieces

2-lb. corned beef brisket, trimmed of all fat

2-3 medium onions, quartered

¾-1¼ cups water

half a small head of cabbage, cut in wedges

1. Layer all ingredients except cabbage in slow cooker.

2. Cover. Cook on Low 8–10 hours, or on High 5–6 hours.

3. Add cabbage wedges to liquid, pushing down to moisten. Turn to High and cook an additional 2–3 hours.

Exchange List Values: Vegetable 1.0, Meat, medium fat 2.0

Basic Nutritional Values: Calories 159 (Calories from Fat 93), Total Fat 10 gm (Saturated Fat 3.4 gm, Polyunsat Fat 0.4 gm, Monounsat Fat 4.9 gm, Cholesterol 52 mg), Sodium 624 mg, Total Carbohydrate 6 gm, Dietary Fiber 2 gm, Sugars 3 gm, Protein 11 gm

VARIATIONS:

1. Add 4 medium potatoes, halved, with the onions.

2. Top individual servings with mixture of sour cream and horseradish.

Kathi Rogge • Alexandria, IN

Note: To cook more cabbage than slow cooker will hold, cook separately in skillet. Remove 1 cup broth from slow cooker during last hour of cooking. Pour over cabbage wedges in skillet. Cover and cook slowly for 20–30 minutes.

Corned Beef

Margaret Jarrett • Anderson, IN

Makes 12 servings (Ideal slow cooker size: 4-quart)

2-lb. cut of marinated corned beef

2–3 cloves garlic, minced

10–12 peppercorns

1. Place meat in bottom of cooker. Top with garlic and peppercorns. Cover with water.

2. Cover. Cook on High 4–5 hours, or until tender.

3. Cool meat, slice thin, and use to make Reuben sandwiches.

Exchange List Values: Meat, medium fat 2.0

Basic Nutritional Values: Calories 135 (Calories from Fat 91), Total Fat 10 gm (Saturated Fat 3.4 gm, Polyunsat Fat 0.4 gm, Monounsat Fat 4.9 gm, Cholesterol 52 mg), Sodium 605 mg, Total Carbohydrate 0 gm, Dietary Fiber 0 gm, Sugars 0 gm, Protein 10 gm

We suggest your sandwiches include a slice of Swiss cheese, sauerkraut, and Thousand Island dressing on toasted pumpernickel bread.

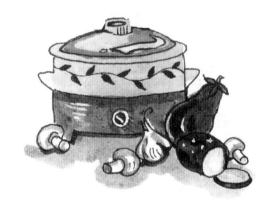

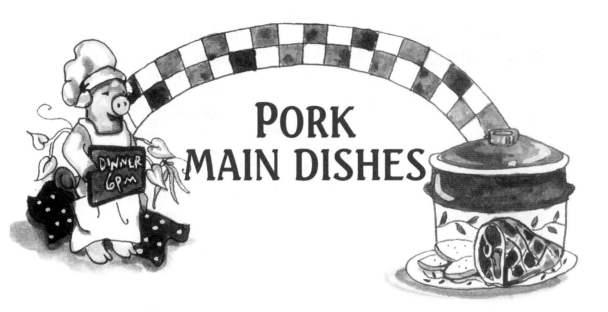

PORK MAIN DISHES

Cranberry Pork Roast

Barbara Aston • Ashdown, AR

Recipe photo appears in color section.

Makes 9 servings (Ideal slow cooker size: 4-quart)

2¾-lb. boneless pork roast, trimmed of fat

pepper to taste

1 cup ground, or finely chopped, cranberries

3 Tbsp. honey

1 tsp. grated orange peel

⅛ tsp. ground cloves

⅛ tsp. ground nutmeg

1. Sprinkle roast with pepper. Place in slow cooker.

2. Combine remaining ingredients. Pour over roast.

3. Cover. Cook on Low 8–10 hours.

Exchange List Values: Carbohydrate 0.5, Meat, lean 3.0

Basic Nutritional Values: Calories 214 (Calories from Fat 81), Total Fat 9 gm (Saturated Fat 3.5 gm, Polyunsat Fat 0.6 gm, Monounsat Fat 4.3 gm, Cholesterol 63 mg), Sodium 37 mg, Total Carbohydrate 7 gm, Dietary Fiber 1 gm, Sugars 7 gm, Protein 25 gm

Note: You may want to add a little salt to this recipe if you generally use it in your diet.

Drinking less alcohol, quitting smoking, and getting more exercise are not only better for your health, they will also save you money on health care, since you may be able to use less insulin.

Barbara Jean's Whole Pork Tenderloin

Barbara Jean Fabel • Wausau, WI

Makes 6–8 servings (Ideal slow cooker size: 4-5-quart)

½ cup sliced celery

¼ lb. fresh mushrooms, quartered

1 medium onion, sliced

2 Tbsp. margarine

2 1¼-lb. pork tenderloins, trimmed of fat

1 Tbsp. canola oil

½ cup beef broth

¾ tsp. salt

¼ tsp. pepper

½ tsp. sodium-free beef-flavored instant bouillon

1 Tbsp. flour

1. Place celery, mushrooms, onion, and margarine in slow cooker.

2. Brown tenderloins in skillet in 1 Tbsp. canola oil. Layer over vegetables in slow cooker.

3. Pour beef broth over tenderloins. Sprinkle with salt and pepper.

4. Combine bouillon and flour. Pour over tenderloins.

5. Cover. Cook on High 3 hours, or on Low 4–5 hours.

Exchange List Values: Meat, lean 4.0

Basic Nutritional Values: Calories 228 (Calories from Fat 87), Total Fat 10 gm (Saturated Fat 2.4 gm, Polyunsat Fat 1.9 gm, Monounsat Fat 4.3 gm, Cholesterol 82 mg), Sodium 385 mg, Total Carbohydrate 3 gm, Dietary Fiber 1 gm, Sugars 2 gm, Protein 30 gm

Autumn Harvest Pork Loin

Stacy Schmucker Stoltzfus • Enola, PA

Makes 4–6 servings (Ideal slow cooker size: 4-quart)

1 cup cider or apple juice

1½-lb. boneless pork loin, trimmed of fat

½ tsp. salt

¼ tsp. pepper

2 large Granny Smith apples, peeled and sliced

1½ whole medium butternut squashes, peeled and cubed

2 Tbsp. brown sugar

¼ tsp. cinnamon

¼ tsp. dried thyme

¼ tsp. dried sage

1. Heat cider in hot skillet. Sear pork loin on all sides in cider.

2. Sprinkle meat with salt and pepper on all sides. Place in slow cooker, along with juices.

3. Combine apples and squash. Sprinkle with sugar, cinnamon, and herbs. Stir. Place around pork loin.

4. Cover. Cook on Low 5–6 hours.

5. Remove pork from cooker. Let stand 10–15 minutes. Slice into ½"-thick slices.

6. Serve topped with apples and squash.

Exchange List Values: Starch 1.0, Fruit 1.0, Meat, lean 2.0, Fat 0.5

Basic Nutritional Values: Calories 280 (Calories from Fat 68), Total Fat 8 gm (Saturated Fat 2.7 gm, Polyunsat Fat 0.7 gm, Monounsat Fat 3.3 gm, Cholesterol 63 mg), Sodium 241 mg, Total Carbohydrate 31 gm, Dietary Fiber 3 gm, Sugars 19 gm, Protein 24 gm

Teriyaki Pork Roast

Janice Yoskovich • Carmichaels, PA

Makes 10 servings (Ideal slow cooker size: 4-quart)

¾ cup unsweetened apple juice

2 Tbsp. sugar

2 Tbsp. soy sauce

1 Tbsp. vinegar

1 tsp. ground ginger

¼ tsp. garlic powder

⅛ tsp. pepper

3-lb. boneless pork loin roast, halved, trimmed of fat

2½ Tbsp. cornstarch

3 Tbsp. cold water

1. Combine apple juice, sugar, soy sauce, vinegar, ginger, garlic powder, and pepper in greased slow cooker.

2. Add roast. Turn to coat.

3. Cover. Cook on Low 7–8 hours. Remove roast and keep warm.

4. In saucepan, combine cornstarch and cold water until smooth. Stir in juices from roast. Bring to boil. Cook and stir for 2 minutes or until thickened. Serve with roast.

Exchange List Values: Carbohydrate 0.5, Meat, lean 3.0

Basic Nutritional Values: Calories 211 (Calories from Fat 79), Total Fat 9 gm (Saturated Fat 3.4 gm, Polyunsat Fat 0.6 gm, Monounsat Fat 4.2 gm, Cholesterol 62 mg), Sodium 241 mg, Total Carbohydrate 7 gm, Dietary Fiber 0 gm, Sugars 5 gm, Protein 24 gm

Pork Roast with Potatoes and Onions

Trudy Kutter • Corfu, NY

Makes 6–8 servings (Ideal slow cooker size: 4-quart)

2½–3-lb. boneless pork loin roast, trimmed of fat

1 large clove garlic, slivered

5 potatoes, cubed, unpeeled

1 large onion, sliced

¾ cup broth, tomato juice, or water

1½ Tbsp. soy sauce

1 Tbsp. cornstarch

1 Tbsp. cold water

1. Make slits in roast and insert slivers of garlic. Put under broiler to brown.

2. Put potatoes in slow cooker. Add half of onions. Place roast on onions and potatoes. Cover with remaining onions.

3. Combine broth and soy sauce. Pour over roast.

4. Cover. Cook on Low 8 hours. Remove roast and vegetables from liquid.

5. Combine cornstarch and water. Add to liquid in slow cooker. Turn to High and cook until thickened. Serve over sliced meat and vegetables.

Exchange List Values: Starch 1.5, Meat, lean 3.0

Basic Nutritional Values: Calories 289 (Calories from Fat 83), Total Fat 9 gm (Saturated Fat 3.6 gm, Polyunsat Fat 0.7 gm, Monounsat Fat 4.4 gm, Cholesterol 64 mg), Sodium 339 mg, Total Carbohydrate 22 gm, Dietary Fiber 3 gm, Sugars 4 gm, Protein 28 gm

VARIATION: Use sweet potatoes instead of white potatoes.

Savory Pork Roast

Betty A. Holt • St. Charles, MO

Makes 8–10 servings (Ideal slow cooker size: 4-quart)

3-lb. boneless pork loin roast, trimmed of fat

1 large onion, sliced

1 bay leaf

2 Tbsp. soy sauce

1 Tbsp. garlic powder

1. Place roast and onion in slow cooker. Add bay leaf, soy sauce, and garlic powder.

2. Cover. Cook on High 1 hour and then on Low 6 hours.

3. Slice and serve.

Exchange List Values: Meat, lean 3.0

Basic Nutritional Values: Calories 187 (Calories from Fat 79), Total Fat 9 gm (Saturated Fat 3.4 gm, Polyunsat Fat 0.6 gm, Monounsat Fat 4.2 gm, Cholesterol 62 mg), Sodium 241 mg, Total Carbohydrate 1 gm, Dietary Fiber 0 gm, Sugars 0 gm, Protein 24 gm

Are you taking a drug that could be interfering with another drug you take? Make an appointment with your pharmacist for a pill check; most will do it for free or for a small fee.

Flautas with Pork Filling

Donna Lantgen • Rapid City, SD

Makes 6–8 servings (Ideal slow cooker size: 4-quart)

1-lb. pork roast or chops, cubed

¼ cup chopped onions

4-oz. can diced green chilies

7-oz. can green or red chili salsa

1 tsp. cocoa powder

16-oz. can chili with beans

1. Brown cubed pork in nonstick skillet. Drain. Place in slow cooker.

2. Add remaining ingredients except chili.

3. Cover. Cook on Low 2–3 hours.

4. Add chili. Cook 2–3 hours longer on Low.

5. Serve on flour tortillas with guacamole dip.

Exchange List Values: Starch 0.5, Meat, lean 2.0

Basic Nutritional Values: Calories 153 (Calories from Fat 62), Total Fat 7 gm (Saturated Fat 2.8 gm, Polyunsat Fat 0.5 gm, Monounsat Fat 3.1 gm, Cholesterol 35 mg), Sodium 566 mg, Total Carbohydrate 9 gm, Dietary Fiber 3 gm, Sugars 2 gm, Protein 14 gm

Note: This is especially good on spinach-herb tortillas.

Shepherd's Pie

Melanie Thrower • McPherson, KS

Makes 6 servings (Ideal slow cooker size: 3–4-quart)

¾ lb. ground pork

1 Tbsp. vinegar

¾ tsp. salt

¼ tsp. hot pepper

1 tsp. paprika

¼ tsp. dried oregano

¼ tsp. black pepper

1 tsp. chili powder

1 small onion, chopped

15-oz. can corn, drained

3 large potatoes, unpeeled

¼ cup fat-free milk

1 tsp. margarine

¼ tsp. salt

dash pepper

shredded cheese

1. Combine pork, vinegar, and spices. Cook in skillet until brown. Add onion and cook until onions begin to glaze. Spread in bottom of slow cooker.

2. Spread corn over meat.

3. Boil potatoes until soft. Mash with milk, margarine, ¼ tsp. salt, and dash of pepper. Spread over meat and corn.

4. Cover. Cook on Low 3 hours. Sprinkle top with cheese a few minutes before serving.

Exchange List Values: Starch 2.0, Meat, lean 1.0, Fat 1.0

Basic Nutritional Values: Calories 269 (Calories from Fat 85), Total Fat 9 gm (Saturated Fat 3.2 gm, Polyunsat Fat 1.3 gm, Monounsat Fat 4.0 gm, Cholesterol 38 mg), Sodium 538 mg, Total Carbohydrate 33 gm, Dietary Fiber 4 gm, Sugars 5 gm, Protein 15 gm

VARIATION: You can substitute ground beef for the pork. This is my 9-year-old son's favorite dish.

Verenike Casserole

Jennifer Yoder Sommers • Harrisonburg, VA

Makes 8-10 servings (Ideal slow cooker size: 4–5-quart)

24 ozs. 1% (low-fat) cottage cheese

3 eggs

1 tsp. salt

½ tsp. pepper

1 cup fat-free sour cream

2 cups fat-free evaporated milk

2 cups cubed, cooked, extra-lean, lower-sodium ham

7 dry lasagna noodles

1. Combine all ingredients except noodles.

2. Place half of creamy ham mixture in bottom of cooker. Add uncooked noodles. Cover with remaining half of creamy ham sauce. Be sure noodles are fully submerged in sauce.

3. Cover. Cook on Low 5–6 hours.

4. Serve with green salad, peas, and zwiebach or bread.

Exchange List Values: Starch 1.0, Milk, fat-free 1.0, Meat, lean 1.0

Basic Nutritional Values: Calories 222 (Calories from Fat 28), Total Fat 3 gm (Saturated Fat 0.8 gm, Polyunsat Fat 0.4 gm, Monounsat Fat 1.0 gm, Cholesterol 81 mg), Sodium 604 mg, Total Carbohydrate 26 gm, Dietary Fiber 1 gm, Sugars 11 gm, Protein 22 gm

Chalupa

Jeannine Janzen • Elbing, KS

Makes 12-16 servings (Ideal slow cooker size: 5-quart)

1 lb. dry pinto beans

3-lb. pork roast, trimmed of fat

2 cloves garlic, minced

1 Tbsp. ground cumin

1 Tbsp. dried oregano

2 Tbsp. chili powder

1 Tbsp. salt

4-oz. can chopped green chilies

water

1. Cover beans with water and soak overnight in slow cooker.

2. In the morning, remove beans (reserve soaking water) and put roast in bottom of cooker. Add remaining ingredients (including the beans and their soaking water) and more water if needed to cover all the ingredients.

3. Cook on High 1 hour, and then on Low 6 hours. Remove meat and shred with two forks. Return meat to slow cooker.

4. Cook on High 1 more hour.

5. Serve over a bed of lettuce. Top with grated cheese and chopped onions and tomatoes.

Exchange List Values: Starch 1.0, Meat, lean 2.0

Basic Nutritional Values: Calories 200 (Calories from Fat 55), Total Fat 6 gm (Saturated Fat 2.2 gm, Polyunsat Fat 0.6 gm, Monounsat Fat 2.8 gm, Cholesterol 38 mg), Sodium 501 mg, Total Carbohydrate 16 gm, Dietary Fiber 6 gm, Sugars 2 gm, Protein 20 gm

Tangy Pork Chops

Tracy Clark • Mt. Crawford, VA / Lois M. Martin • Lititz, PA / Becky Oswald • Broadway, PA

Makes 4 servings (Ideal slow cooker size: 4-quart)

4 pork chops ($\frac{1}{2}$"-thick each), bone in, trimmed of fat

$\frac{1}{8}$ tsp. pepper

2 medium onions, chopped

2 ribs celery, chopped

1 large green pepper, sliced

$14\frac{1}{2}$-oz. can no-salt-added stewed tomatoes

$\frac{1}{3}$ cup ketchup

2 Tbsp. cider vinegar

2 Tbsp. brown sugar

2 Tbsp. Worcestershire sauce

1 Tbsp. lemon juice

1 reduced-sodium beef bouillon cube

2 Tbsp. cornstarch

2 Tbsp. water

1. Place chops in slow cooker. Sprinkle with pepper.

2. Add onions, celery, pepper, and tomatoes.

3. Combine ketchup, vinegar, brown sugar, Worcestershire sauce, lemon juice, and bouillon. Pour over vegetables.

4. Cover. Cook on Low 5–6 hours.

5. Combine cornstarch and water until smooth. Stir into slow cooker.

6. Cover. Cook on High 30 minutes, or until thickened.

7. Serve over rice.

Exchange List Values: Carbohydrate 1.5, Vegetable 3.0, Meat, lean 1.0

Basic Nutritional Values: Calories 254 (Calories from Fat 47), Total Fat 5 gm (Saturated Fat 1.7 gm, Polyunsat Fat 0.5 gm, Monounsat Fat 2.1 gm, Cholesterol 47 mg), Sodium 546 mg, Total Carbohydrate 35 gm, Dietary Fiber 4 gm, Sugars 20 gm, Protein 19 gm

VARIATION: Use chunks of beef or chicken legs and thighs instead of pork.

Exercise is like a miracle drug—it boosts your metabolism, increases muscle mass so you burn more calories, improves your body's response to insulin, and naturally lowers glucose.

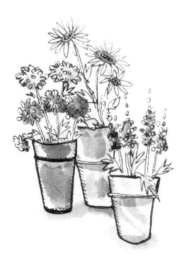

Chops and Beans

Mary L. Casey • Scranton, PA

Makes 4–6 servings (Ideal slow cooker size: 4-quart)

2 1-lb. cans pork and beans

¼ cup no-salt-added ketchup

2 slices bacon, browned and crumbled

½ cup chopped onions, sauteed

1 Tbsp. Worcestershire sauce

1 Tbsp. brown sugar

brown sugar substitute to equal 1 Tbsp

6 (1½ lbs.) pork chops, bone in, trimmed of fat

2 tsp. prepared mustard

1 Tbsp. brown sugar

2 Tbsp. no-salt-added ketchup

1 lemon

1. Combine beans, ¼ cup ketchup, bacon, onions, Worcestershire sauce, 1 Tbsp. brown sugar, and 1 Tbsp. brown sugar substitute in slow cooker.

2. Brown chops in nonstick skillet. In separate bowl, mix together 2 tsp. mustard, 1 Tbsp. brown sugar, and 2 Tbsp. ketchup. Brush each chop with sauce, then carefully stack into cooker, placing a slice of lemon on each chop. Submerge in bean/bacon mixture.

3. Cover. Cook on Low 4–6 hours.

Exchange List Values: Starch 2.0, Carbohydrate 0.5, Meat, lean 2.0, Fat 0.5

Basic Nutritional Values: Calories 323 (Calories from Fat 73), Total Fat 8 gm (Saturated Fat 2.0 gm, Polyunsat Fat 1.0 gm, Monounsat Fat 3.5 gm, Cholesterol 55 mg), Sodium 790 mg, Total Carbohydrate 40 gm, Dietary Fiber 8 gm, Sugars 20 gm, Protein 23 gm

Perfect Pork Chops

Brenda Pope • Dundee, OH

Makes 2 servings (Ideal slow cooker size: 4-quart)

2 small onions

1/2 lb. boneless, center loin pork chops, frozen, trimmed of fat

fresh ground pepper to taste

3/4 tsp. reduced-sodium bouillon granules

1/4 cup hot water

2 Tbsp. prepared mustard with white wine

fresh parsley sprigs, or lemon slices, optional

1. Cut off ends of onions and peel. Cut onions in half crosswise to make 4 thick wheels. Place in bottom of slow cooker.

2. Sear both sides of frozen chops in heavy skillet. Place in cooker on top of onions. Sprinkle with pepper.

3. Dissolve bouillon granules in hot water. Stir in mustard. Pour into slow cooker.

4. Cover. Cook on High 3–4 hours.

5. Serve topped with fresh parsley sprigs or lemon slices, if desired.

Exchange List Values: Carbohydrate 0.5, Meat, lean 3.0

Basic Nutritional Values: Calories 204 (Calories from Fat 72), Total Fat 8 gm (Saturated Fat 2.9 gm, Polyunsat Fat 0.7 gm, Monounsat Fat 3.9 gm, Cholesterol 51 mg), Sodium 392 mg, Total Carbohydrate 11 gm, Dietary Fiber 2 gm, Sugars 7 gm, Protein 22 gm

Pork Chops with Mushroom Sauce

Jennifer J. Gehman • Harrisburg, PA

Makes 6 servings (Ideal slow cooker size: 4-quart)

6 boneless pork chops, 1/2"-thick (1/4 lb. each)

10 3/4-oz. can 98%-fat-free, reduced-sodium cream of mushroom soup

3/4 cup white wine

4-oz. can sliced mushrooms

2 Tbsp. quick-cooking tapioca

2 tsp. Worcestershire sauce

1 tsp. beef bouillon granules, or 1 beef bouillon cube

1/4 tsp. minced garlic

3/4 tsp. dried thyme, optional

1. Place pork chops in slow cooker.

2. Combine remaining ingredients and pour over pork chops.

3. Cook on Low 8–10 hours, or on High 4 1/2–5 hours.

Exchange List Values: Carbohydrate 0.5, Meat, lean 3.0

Basic Nutritional Values: Calories 207 (Calories from Fat 76), Total Fat 8 gm (Saturated Fat 3.3 gm, Polyunsat Fat 0.8 gm, Monounsat Fat 3.7 gm, Cholesterol 52 mg), Sodium 452 mg, Total Carbohydrate 9 gm, Dietary Fiber 1 gm, Sugars 2 gm, Protein 22 gm

Make a backup plan of things you will do when you are tempted to overeat or smoke— take a walk, play some music and dance, suck on a mint, or knit.

Pork Chops on Rice

Hannah D. Burkholder • Bridgewater, VA

Makes 4 servings (Ideal slow cooker size: 4-quart)

½ cup brown rice, uncooked

⅔ cup converted white rice, uncooked

1 Tbsp. olive oil

½ cup chopped onions

4-oz. can sliced mushrooms, drained

½ tsp. dried thyme

½ tsp. sage

¼ tsp. black pepper

4 small (about 4 ozs. each) boneless pork chops

¾ cup beef consommé

½ cup water

2 Tbsp. Worcestershire sauce

½ tsp. dried thyme

½ tsp. paprika

¼ tsp. ground nutmeg

1. Saute brown and white rice in olive oil in skillet until rice is golden brown.

2. Remove from heat and stir in onions, mushrooms, ½ tsp. thyme, sage, and pepper. Pour into greased slow cooker.

3. Arrange chops over rice.

4. Combine consommé, water, and Worcestershire sauce. Pour over chops.

5. Combine ½ tsp. thyme, paprika, and nutmeg. Sprinkle over chops.

6. Cover. Cook on Low 7–9 hours, or on High 4–5 hours.

Exchange List Values: Starch 3.0, Vegetable 1.0, Meat, lean 2.0, Fat 1.0

Basic Nutritional Values: Calories 425 (Calories from Fat 107), Total Fat 12 gm (Saturated Fat 3.5 gm, Polyunsat Fat 1.2 gm, Monounsat Fat 6.3 gm, Cholesterol 52 mg), Sodium 528 mg, Total Carbohydrate 50 gm, Dietary Fiber 3 gm, Sugars 4 gm, Protein 28 gm

Pork and Cabbage Dinner

Mrs. Paul Gray • Beatrice, NE

Makes 8 servings (Ideal slow cooker size: 4-5-quart)

2 lbs. pork steaks, or chops, or shoulder, bone-in, trimmed of fat

¾ cup chopped onions

¼ cup chopped fresh parsley, or 2 Tbsp. dried parsley

4 cups shredded cabbage

1 tsp. salt

⅛ tsp. pepper

½ tsp. caraway seeds

⅛ tsp. allspice

½ cup beef broth

2 medium cooking apples, cored and sliced ¼" thick

1. Place pork in slow cooker. Layer onions, parsley, and cabbage over pork.

2. Combine salt, pepper, caraway seeds, and allspice. Sprinkle over cabbage. Pour broth over cabbage.

3. Cover. Cook on Low 5–6 hours.

4. Add apple slices 30 minutes before serving.

Exchange List Values: Fruit 0.5, Vegetable 1.0, Meat, lean 2.0

Basic Nutritional Values: Calories 149 (Calories from Fat 44), Total Fat 5 gm (Saturated Fat 1.7 gm, Polyunsat Fat 0.4 gm, Monounsat Fat 2.1 gm, Cholesterol 47 mg), Sodium 382 mg, Total Carbohydrate 9 gm, Dietary Fiber 2 gm, Sugars 6 gm, Protein 18 gm

Creamy Ham Topping (for baked potatoes)

Judy Buller • Bluffton, OH

Makes 12 servings (Ideal slow cooker size: 4-quart)

2 Tbsp. margarine

¼ cup flour

2 cups fat-free milk

¼ cup fat-free half-and-half

1 Tbsp. chopped parsley

1 Tbsp. sodium-free chicken bouillon granules

½ tsp. Italian seasoning

2 cups diced cooked ham

¼ cup grated Romano cheese

1 cup sliced mushrooms

1. Melt butter in saucepan. Stir in flour. Add milk and half-and-half.

2. Stir in remaining ingredients. Pour into slow cooker.

3. Cover. Cook on Low 1–2 hours.

4. Serve over baked potatoes. Top with shredded cheese and sour cream, if you wish.

Exchange List Values: Carbohydrate 0.5, Meat, lean 1.0

Basic Nutritional Values: Calories 93 (Calories from Fat 36), Total Fat 4 gm (Saturated Fat 1.3 gm, Polyunsat Fat 0.8 gm, Monounsat Fat 1.6 gm, Cholesterol 17 mg), Sodium 386 mg, Total Carbohydrate 5 gm, Dietary Fiber 0 gm, Sugars 3 gm

Black Beans with Ham

Colleen Heatwole • Burton, MI

Makes 8–10 servings (Ideal slow cooker size: 5-quart)

4 cups dry black beans

1 cup diced ham

1 tsp. cumin

½–1 cup minced onion

2 cloves garlic, minced

3 bay leaves

1 qt. fresh diced tomatoes

1 Tbsp. brown sugar

1. Cover black beans with water and soak for 8 hours, or overnight. Drain and pour beans into slow cooker.

2. Add all remaining ingredients and stir well. Cover with water.

3. Cover cooker. Cook on Low 10–12 hours.

4. Serve over rice.

Exchange List Values: Starch 3.0, Vegetable 1.0, Meat, very lean 1.0

Basic Nutritional Values: Calories 302 (Calories from Fat 19), Total Fat 2 gm (Saturated Fat 0.5 gm, Polyunsat Fat 0.6 gm, Monounsat Fat 0.5 gm, Cholesterol 8 mg), Sodium 196 mg, Total Carbohydrate 51 gm, Dietary Fiber 18 gm, Sugars 8 gm, Protein 21 gm

This is our favorite black bean recipe. We make it frequently in the winter.

Ham and Lima Beans

Charlotte Shaffer • East Earl, PA

Makes 6 servings (Ideal slow cooker size: 4-quart)

1 lb. dry lima beans

1 medium onion, chopped

1 medium bell pepper, chopped

1 tsp. dry mustard

1 tsp. pepper

6 ozs. ham, finely cubed

1 cup water

10¾-oz. can 98%-fat-free, reduced-sodium tomato soup

1. Cover beans with water. Soak 8 hours. Drain.

2. Combine ingredients in slow cooker.

3. Cover. Cook on Low 7 hours, or High 4 hours.

4. If mixture begins to dry out, add ½ cup water or more and stir well.

5. This is delicious served with hot corn bread.

Exchange List Values: Starch 2.5, Carbohydrate 0.5, Vegetable 1.0, Meat, lean 1.0

Basic Nutritional Values: Calories 313 (Calories from Fat 27), Total Fat 3 gm (Saturated Fat 0.9 gm, Polyunsat Fat 0.8 gm, Monounsat Fat 0.8 gm, Cholesterol 16 mg), Sodium 561 mg, Total Carbohydrate 50 gm, Dietary Fiber 15 gm, Sugars 12 gm, Protein 23 gm

Ham and Corn Slow Cooker Casserole

Vicki Dinkel • Sharon Springs, KS

Makes 8 servings (Ideal slow cooker size: 4-5-quart)

1 small green pepper, chopped

1 medium onion, chopped

¼ cup canola oil

½ cup flour

½ tsp. paprika

½ tsp. pepper

¼ tsp. dried thyme

1 tsp. dry mustard

4 cups fat-free milk

8-oz. can cream-style corn

2 cups diced, slightly cooked potatoes

3 cups diced, cooked, extra-lean, reduced-sodium ham

3 ozs. shredded reduced-fat cheddar cheese

1. Saute green pepper and onion in canola oil in skillet.

2. Stir in flour and seasonings.

3. Gradually stir in milk and cook until thickened. Pour into slow cooker.

4. Stir in remaining ingredients.

5. Cover. Cook on Low 8 hours, or High 4 hours.

Exchange List Values: Starch 1.0, Milk, fat-free 0.5, Meat, lean 2.0, Fat 0.5

Basic Nutritional Values: Calories 255 (Calories from Fat 95), Total Fat 11 gm (Saturated Fat 2.3 gm, Polyunsat Fat 2.4 gm, Monounsat Fat 5.3 gm, Cholesterol 34 mg), Sodium 596 mg, Total Carbohydrate 24 gm, Dietary Fiber 2 gm, Sugars 11 gm, Protein 18 gm

Ham and Scalloped Potatoes

Penny Blosser • Beavercreek, OH / Jo Haberkamp • Fairbank, IA / Ruth Hofstetter • Versailles, MO / Rachel Kauffman • Alto, MI / Mary E. Martin • Goshen, IN / Brenda Pope • Dundee, OH / Joyce Slaymaker, Strasburg, PA

Makes 6-8 servings (Ideal slow cooker size: 4-5-quart)

6-8 (1 lb. total) slices ham

8 medium potatoes, thinly sliced

2 medium onions, thinly sliced

1 cup grated reduced-fat cheddar, or American, cheese

10¾-oz. can 98%-fat-free, reduced-sodium cream of celery, or mushroom, soup

paprika

1. Put half of ham, potatoes, and onions in slow cooker. Sprinkle with cheese. Repeat layers.

2. Spoon soup over top. Sprinkle with paprika.

3. Cover. Cook on Low 8-10 hours, or High 4 hours.

Exchange List Values: Starch 2.0, Meat, lean 2.0

Basic Nutritional Values: Calories 229 (Calories from Fat 45), Total Fat 5 gm (Saturated Fat 2.5 gm, Polyunsat Fat 0.6 gm, Monounsat Fat 1.4 gm, Cholesterol 36 mg), Sodium 733 mg, Total Carbohydrate 32 gm, Dietary Fiber 3 gm, Sugars 7 gm, Protein 17 gm

VARIATION: If you like a lot of creamy sauce with your ham and potatoes, stir three-quarters of soup can of milk into the soup before pouring it over the layers.

Alma Z. Weaver • Ephrata, PA

Note: You may want to add salt and pepper to taste if you generally use them in your diet.

Ham in Cider

Dorothy M. Van Deest • Memphis, TN

Makes 6-8 servings (Ideal slow cooker size: 4-5-quart)

3-lb. boneless, precooked, extra-lean, lower-sodium ham, trimmed of fat

4 cups sweet cider, or apple juice

¼ cup brown sugar

brown sugar substitute to equal ¼ cup

2 tsp. dry mustard

1 tsp. ground cloves

1 cup white seedless raisins

1. Place ham and cider in slow cooker.

2. Cover. Cook on Low 8-10 hours.

3. Remove ham from cider and place in baking pan.

4. Make a paste of brown sugar, sugar substitute, mustard, cloves, and a little hot cider. Brush over ham. Pour ½ cup of juice from slow cooker into baking pan. Stir in raisins.

5. Bake at 375° for 30 minutes, until the paste has turned into a glaze.

Exchange List Values: Carbohydrate 2.0, Meat, very lean 3.0

Basic Nutritional Values: Calories 255 (Calories from Fat 26), Total Fat 3 gm (Saturated Fat 1.0 gm, Polyunsat Fat 0.6 gm, Monounsat Fat 1.0 gm, Cholesterol 67 mg), Sodium 1194 mg, Total Carbohydrate 31 gm, Dietary Fiber 1 gm, Sugars 28 gm, Protein 27 gm

Two tablespoons (one ladle) of salad dressing alone can add 150–200 calories to your salad. Instead, choose low-calorie salad dressing or add a little oil and vinegar.

Sweet-Sour Pork

Mary W. Stauffer • Ephrata, PA

Makes 4–6 servings (Ideal slow cooker size: 4-quart)

2 lbs. boneless pork shoulder, cut in strips, trimmed of fat

1 green pepper, cut in strips

half a medium onion, thinly sliced

¾ cup shredded carrots

2 Tbsp. coarsely chopped sweet pickles

2 Tbsp. brown sugar

brown sugar substitute to equal 1 Tbsp.

2 Tbsp. cornstarch

¼ cup water

1 cup pineapple juice (reserved from pineapple chunks)

¼ cup cider vinegar

1 Tbsp. soy sauce

2 cups (20-oz. can) pineapple chunks, canned in juice

1. Place pork strips in slow cooker.

2. Add green pepper, onion, carrots, and pickles.

3. In bowl, mix together brown sugar, sugar substitute, and cornstarch. Add water, pineapple juice, vinegar, and soy sauce. Stir until smooth.

4. Pour over ingredients in slow cooker.

5. Cover. Cook on Low 5–7 hours. One hour before serving, add pineapple chunks. Stir.

6. Serve over buttered noodles with an additional dash of vinegar or garlic to taste.

Exchange List Values: Fruit 1.0, Carbohydrate 0.5, Vegetable 1.0, Meat, lean 3.0

Basic Nutritional Values: Calories 270 (Calories from Fat 74), Total Fat 8 gm (Saturated Fat 2.8 gm, Polyunsat Fat 0.8 gm, Monounsat Fat 3.8 gm, Cholesterol 75 mg), Sodium 285 mg, Total Carbohydrate 27 gm, Dietary Fiber 2 gm, Sugars 21 gm, Protein 22 gm

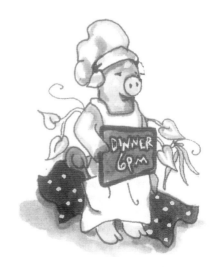

Schnitz und Knepp

Jean Robinson • Cinnaminson, NJ

Makes 12 servings (Ideal slow cooker size: 5-quart)

SCHNITZ:

1 qt. dried sweet apples

3 lbs. extra-lean, lower-sodium, boneless ham slices, cut into 2" cubes

2 Tbsp. brown sugar

1 cinnamon stick

KNEPP (DUMPLINGS):

2 cups flour

4 tsp. baking powder

1 egg, well beaten

3 Tbsp. melted margarine

scant ½ cup fat-free milk

¼ tsp. pepper

1. Cover apples with water in large bowl and let soak for a few hours.

2. Place ham in slow cooker. Cover with water.

3. Cover cooker. Cook on High 2 hours.

4. Add apples and water in which they have been soaking.

5. Add brown sugar and cinnamon stick. Mix until dissolved.

6. Cover. Cook on Low 3 hours.

7. Combine dumpling ingredients in bowl. Drop into hot liquid in cooker by tablespoonfuls. Turn to High. Cover. Do not lift lid for 15 minutes.

8. Serve piping hot on a large platter. A celery-carrot jello salad rounds out the meal well.

Exchange List Values: Starch 1.5, Fruit 1.0, Meat, lean 2.0

Basic Nutritional Values: Calories 293 (Calories from Fat 48), Total Fat 5 gm (Saturated Fat 1.4 gm, Polyunsat Fat 1.4 gm, Monounsat Fat 2.1 gm, Cholesterol 63 mg), Sodium 980 mg, Total Carbohydrate 41 gm, Dietary Fiber 3 gm, Sugars 19 gm, Protein 20 gm

Note: This was my grandmother's recipe, and she had no slow cooker. Schnitz und Knepp cooked on the back of the woodstove till the quilting was done. I was allowed to drop in the dumplings.

Keep a bottle of uncoated aspirin handy. If someone shows signs of having a heart attack, give the person an aspirin with water while you call 911.

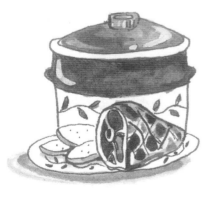

Barbecued Pork

Grace Ketcham • Marietta, GA /
Mary Seielstad • Sparks, NV

Recipe photo appears in color section.

Makes 10 servings (Ideal slow cooker size: 4-quart)

3 lbs. pork, trimmed of fat, cubed

2 cups chopped onions

3 medium green peppers, chopped

¼ cup brown sugar

brown sugar substitute to equal 2 Tbsp.

¼ cup vinegar

6-oz. can tomato paste

1½ Tbsp. chili powder

1 tsp. dry mustard

2 tsp. Worcestershire sauce

1¼ tsp. salt

1. Combine all ingredients in slow cooker.

2. Cover. Cook on High 8 hours.

3. Shred meat with fork. Mix into sauce and heat through.

4. Serve on hamburger buns with grated cheese and cole slaw on top.

Exchange List Values: Carbohydrate 0.5, Vegetable 2.0, Meat, lean 3.0

Basic Nutritional Values: Calories 246 (Calories from Fat 84), Total Fat 9 gm (Saturated Fat 3.5 gm, Polyunsat Fat 0.8 gm, Monounsat Fat 4.3 gm, Cholesterol 62 mg), Sodium 367 mg, Total Carbohydrate 15 gm, Dietary Fiber 3 gm, Sugars 9 gm, Protein 26 gm

VARIATION: Substitute cubed chuck roast or stewing beef for the pork, or use half beef, half pork.

Rice and Beans— and Sausage

Marcia S. Myer • Manheim, PA

Makes 8 servings (Ideal slow cooker size: 4-quart)

3 ribs celery, chopped

1 onion, chopped

2 cloves garlic, minced

1¾ cups tomato juice

2 16-oz. cans kidney beans, drained

¾ tsp. dried oregano

¾ tsp. dried thyme

¼ tsp. red pepper flakes

¼ tsp. pepper

½ lb. (or more) fully cooked smoked turkey sausage, or kielbasa, cut into ¼" slices

3 cups cooked rice

shredded cheese, optional

1. Combine all ingredients except rice and shredded cheese in slow cooker.

2. Cover. Cook on Low 4–6 hours.

3. Serve over rice. Garnish with shredded cheese, if you wish.

Exchange List Values: Starch 2.5, Vegetable 1.0, Meat, lean 1.0

Basic Nutritional Values: Calories 241 (Calories from Fat 33), Total Fat 4 gm (Saturated Fat 1.0 gm, Polyunsat Fat 0.8 gm, Monounsat Fat 0.8 gm, Cholesterol 18 mg), Sodium 611 mg, Total Carbohydrate 42 gm, Dietary Fiber 6 gm, Sugars 6 gm, Protein 13 gm

Sausage-Potato Slow Cooker Dinner

Deborah Swartz • Grottoes, VA

Makes 6–8 servings (Ideal slow cooker size: 4–5-quart)

1 cup water

1/2 tsp. cream of tartar

6 medium potatoes, unpeeled, thinly sliced

3/4 lb. sausage, casings removed and browned

1 onion, chopped

1/4 cup flour

salt to taste

pepper to taste

1 1/2 cups grated fat-free cheddar cheese, divided

1 Tbsp. margarine

10 3/4-oz. can 98%-fat-free, reduced-sodium cream of mushroom soup

1. Combine water and cream of tartar. Toss sliced potatoes in water. Drain.

2. Layer half of potatoes, sausage, onion, and flour, a sprinkling of salt and pepper, and one-third of cheddar cheese in slow cooker. Repeat layers until ingredients are used, reserving one-third of cheese for top.

3. Dot margarine over top. Pour soup over all.

4. Cover. Cook on Low 7–9 hours, or on High 3–4 hours.

5. Sprinkle reserved cheese over top just before serving.

Exchange List Values: Starch 2.0, Meat, medium fat 1.0, Fat 0.5

Basic Nutritional Values: Calories 262 (Calories from Fat 77), Total Fat 9 gm (Saturated Fat 2.8 gm, Polyunsat Fat 1.5 gm, Monounsat Fat 3.6 gm, Cholesterol 19 mg), Sodium 579 mg, Total Carbohydrate 32 gm, Dietary Fiber 3 gm, Sugars 5 gm, Protein 15 gm

Election Lunch

Alix Nancy Botsford • Seminole, OK

Makes 12 servings (Ideal slow cooker size: 6-quart)

1 large onion, chopped

1 lb. sausage, cut into thin slices, or casings removed and crumbled

2 Tbsp. olive oil

1 rib celery, sliced

1 Tbsp. Worcestershire sauce

1 1/2 tsp. dry mustard

2 Tbsp. honey

1 Tbsp. sugar substitute

10-oz. can tomatoes with green chili peppers

1-lb. can lima or butter beans, drained, with liquid reserved

1-lb. can red kidney beans, drained, with liquid reserved

1-lb. can garbanzo beans, drained, rinsed

1. Brown onion and sausage in oil.

2. Combine ingredients in 6-qt. slow cooker, or divide between 2 4-qt. cookers and stir to combine. Add reserved juice from lima and kidney beans if there's enough room in the cooker(s).

3. Cover. Cook on Low 2–4 hours.

Exchange List Values: Starch 1.5, Meat, medium fat 1.0, Fat 0.5

Basic Nutritional Values: Calories 204 (Calories from Fat 79), Total Fat 9 gm (Saturated Fat 2.4 gm, Polyunsat Fat 1.3 gm, Monounsat Fat 4.3 gm, Cholesterol 14 mg), Sodium 613 mg, Total Carbohydrate 23 gm, Dietary Fiber 5 gm, Sugars 8 gm, Protein 9 gm

Note: I mixed up this hearty stew the night before Election Day and took it to the voting site the next morning. I plugged it in, and all day long we could smell the stew cooking. I work at a very sparsely populated, country poling place and ended up giving out the recipe and little water-cup samples to many voters!

I have four different sizes of slow cookers. One is very tiny, with only an on and off switch, for keeping cheese sauce hot. One I use for heating gravy. Another I often use to keep mashed potatoes warm.

Golden Autumn Stew

Naomi E. Fast • Hesston, KS

Recipe photo appears in color section.

Makes 8–10 servings (Ideal slow cooker size: 4–5-quart)

2 cups cubed Yukon gold potatoes

2 cups cubed, peeled sweet potatoes

2 cups cubed, peeled butternut squash

1 cup cubed, peeled rutabaga

1 cup diced carrots

1 cup sliced celery

1 lb. low-fat smoked sausage

2 cups apple juice or cider

1 tart apple, thinly sliced

salt to taste

pepper to taste

1 Tbsp. sugar or honey

1. Combine vegetables in slow cooker.

2. Place ring of sausage on top.

3. Add apple juice and apple slices.

4. Cover. Cook on High 2 hours and on Low 4 hours, or until vegetables are tender. Do not stir.

5. To serve, remove sausage ring. Season with salt, pepper, and sugar as desired. Place vegetables in bowl. Slice meat into rings and place on top.

6. Serve with hot baking-powder biscuits and honey, and a green salad or cole slaw.

Exchange List Values: Starch 1.0, Fruit 0.5, Vegetable 1.0, Meat, lean 1.0

Basic Nutritional Values: Calories 172 (Calories from Fat 21), Total Fat 2 gm (Saturated Fat 0.8 gm, Polyunsat Fat 0.9 gm, Monounsat Fat 0.5 gm, Cholesterol 19 mg), Sodium 413 mg, Total Carbohydrate 31 gm, Dietary Fiber 3 gm, Sugars 15 gm, Protein 7 gm

Don't omit the rutabaga! Get acquainted with its rich uniqueness. It will surprise and please your taste buds.

Melt-in-Your-Mouth Sausages

Ruth Ann Gingrich • New Holland, PA / Ruth Hershey • Paradise, PA / Carol Sherwood • Batavia, NY / Nancy Zimmerman • Loysville, PA

Recipe photo appears in color section.

Makes 8 servings (Ideal slow cooker size: 4-quart)

1¾ lbs. sweet turkey Italian sausage, cut into 5" lengths

48-oz. jar fat-free, low-sodium pasta sauce

6-oz. can no-salt-added tomato paste

1 large green bell pepper, thinly sliced

1 large onion, thinly sliced

1 Tbsp. grated Parmesan cheese

1 tsp. dried parsley, or 1 Tbsp. chopped fresh parsley

1 cup water

1. Place sausage in skillet. Cover with water. Simmer 10 minutes. Drain.

2. Combine remaining ingredients in slow cooker. Add sausage.

3. Cover. Cook on Low 6 hours.

4. Serve in buns, or cut sausage into bite-sized pieces and serve over cooked spaghetti. Sprinkle with more Parmesan cheese, if you wish.

Exchange List Values: Carbohydrate 1.5, Meat, lean 3.0, Fat 0.5

Basic Nutritional Values: Calories 288 (Calories from Fat 111), Total Fat 12 gm (Saturated Fat 3.5 gm, Polyunsat Fat 1.5 gm, Monounsat Fat 2.2 gm, Cholesterol 79 mg), Sodium 692 mg, Total Carbohydrate 21 gm, Dietary Fiber 3 gm, Sugars 12 gm, Protein 25 gm

Polish Kraut 'n Apples

Lori Berezovsky • Salina, KS / Marie Morucci • Glen Lyon, PA

Makes 6 servings (Ideal slow cooker size: 4-quart)

1 lb. fresh, or canned, sauerkraut

1 lb. low-fat, smoked Polish sausage

3 tart cooking apples, unpeeled, thinly sliced

2 Tbsp. brown sugar

brown sugar substitute to equal 3 Tbsp.

⅛ tsp. pepper

½ tsp. caraway seeds, optional

¾ cup apple juice, or cider

1. Rinse sauerkraut and squeeze dry. Place half in slow cooker.

2. Cut sausage into 2" lengths and add to cooker.

3. Continue to layer remaining ingredients in slow cooker in order given. Top with remaining sauerkraut. Do not stir.

4. Cover. Cook on High 3–3½ hours, or Low 6–7 hours.

Exchange List Values: Fruit 1.0, Carbohydrate 1.0, Meat, lean 1.0

Basic Nutritional Values: Calories 195 (Calories from Fat 33), Total Fat 4 gm (Saturated Fat 1.4 gm, Polyunsat Fat 0.3 gm, Monounsat Fat 1.9 gm, Cholesterol 35 mg), Sodium 945 mg, Total Carbohydrate 31 gm, Dietary Fiber 4 gm, Sugars 20 gm, Protein 10 gm

Many people resist going on insulin injections, even though their doctor wants them to, but it may be just what they need to feel their best, ensure tight control, and avoid future complications.

Dawn's Sausage and Peppers

Dawn Day • Westminster, CA

Makes 8-10 servings (Ideal slow cooker size: 4-5-quart)

3 medium onions, sliced

1 medium sweet red pepper, sliced

1 medium sweet green pepper, sliced

1 medium sweet yellow pepper, sliced

4 cloves garlic, minced

1 Tbsp. canola oil

28-oz. can no-salt-added chopped tomatoes

½ tsp. crushed red pepper

2 lbs. fresh turkey sweet Italian sausage, cut into 3" pieces

1. Saute onions, peppers, and garlic in oil in skillet. When just softened, place in slow cooker.

2. Add tomatoes and crushed pepper. Mix well.

3. Add sausage links.

4. Cover. Cook on Low 6 hours.

5. Serve on rolls, or over pasta or baked potatoes.

Exchange List Values: Vegetable 2.0, Meat, medium fat 2.0, Fat 0.5

Basic Nutritional Values: Calories 237 (Calories from Fat 112), Total Fat 12 gm (Saturated Fat 3.1 gm, Polyunsat Fat 1.8 gm, Monounsat Fat 2.7 gm, Cholesterol 72 mg), Sodium 619 mg, Total Carbohydrate 12 gm, Dietary Fiber 3 gm, Sugars 7 gm, Protein 21 gm

VARIATION: For a thicker sauce, stir in 3 Tbsp. ClearJel during the last 15 minutes of the cooking time.

Sausage Sauerkraut Supper

Ruth Ann Hoover • New Holland, PA / Robin Schrock • Millersburg, OH

Makes 10-12 servings (Ideal slow cooker size: 4-5-quart)

4 cups cubed carrots

4 cups cubed red potatoes

2 14-oz. cans sauerkraut, rinsed and drained

1 lb. fresh Polish sausage, cut into 3" pieces

1 medium onion, thinly sliced

3 cloves garlic, minced

1½ cups dry white wine, or chicken broth

½ tsp. pepper

1 tsp. caraway seeds

1. Layer carrots, potatoes, and sauerkraut in slow cooker.

2. Brown sausage in skillet. Transfer to slow cooker. Reserve 1 Tbsp. drippings in skillet.

3. Saute onion and garlic in drippings until tender. Stir in wine. Bring to boil. Stir to loosen brown bits. Stir in pepper and caraway seeds. Pour over sausage.

4. Cover. Cook on Low 8-9 hours.

Exchange List Values: Starch 1.0, Vegetable 1.0, Meat, high fat 1.0

Basic Nutritional Values: Calories 195 (Calories from Fat 86), Total Fat 10 gm (Saturated Fat 3.4 gm, Polyunsat Fat 1.0 gm, Monounsat Fat 5.2 gm, Cholesterol 24 mg), Sodium 689 mg, Total Carbohydrate 18 gm, Dietary Fiber 5 gm, Sugars 5 gm, Protein 8 gm

Kielbasa and Cabbage

Barbara McGinnis • Jupiter, FL

Makes 6 servings (Ideal slow cooker size: 4–5-quart)

1½ lb.-head green cabbage, shredded

2 medium onions, chopped

3 medium red potatoes, peeled and cubed

1 red bell pepper, chopped

2 cloves garlic, minced

⅔ cup dry white wine

1 lb. low-fat Polish kielbasa, cut into 3"-long links

28-oz. can cut-up no-salt-added tomatoes with juice

1 Tbsp. Dijon mustard

¾ tsp. caraway seeds

½ tsp. pepper

1. Combine all ingredients in slow cooker.

2. Cover. Cook on Low 7–8 hours, or until cabbage is tender.

Exchange List Values: Starch 0.5, Carbohydrate 0.5, Vegetable 3.0, Meat, lean 1.0

Basic Nutritional Values: Calories 226 (Calories from Fat 39), Total Fat 4 gm (Saturated Fat 1.4 gm, Polyunsat Fat 0.6 gm, Monounsat Fat 2.0 gm, Cholesterol 35 mg), Sodium 781 mg, Total Carbohydrate 34 gm, Dietary Fiber 7 gm, Sugars 15 gm, Protein 14 gm

Aunt Lavina's Sauerkraut

Pat Unternahrer • Wayland, IA

Makes 8–12 servings (Ideal slow cooker size: 4-quart)

2 lbs. smoked low-fat sausage, cut into 1" pieces

2 bell peppers, chopped

2 onions, sliced

½ lb. fresh mushrooms, sliced

2 Tbsp. water, or oil

1 qt. sauerkraut, drained

2 14½-oz. cans no-salt-added diced tomatoes with green peppers

½ tsp. pepper

2 Tbsp. brown sugar

1. Place sausage in slow cooker. Heat on Low while you prepare other ingredients.

2. Saute peppers, onions, and mushrooms in small amount of water or oil in saucepan.

3. Combine all ingredients in slow cooker.

4. Cover. Cook on Low 5–6 hours, or High 3–4 hours.

5. Serve with mashed potatoes.

Exchange List Values: Carbohydrate 0.5, Vegetable 2.0, Meat, lean 1.0

Basic Nutritional Values: Calories 163 (Calories from Fat 34), Total Fat 4 gm (Saturated Fat 1.4 gm, Polyunsat Fat 1.5 gm, Monounsat Fat 0.8 gm, Cholesterol 32 mg), Sodium 984 mg, Total Carbohydrate 21 gm, Dietary Fiber 4 gm, Sugars 11 gm, Protein 12 gm

Pork Spareribs with Sauerkraut

Char Hagner • Montague, MI

Makes 4–6 servings (Ideal slow cooker size: 4-quart)

2 small cooking apples, sliced in rings

1½–2 lbs. country-style spareribs, trimmed of fat, cut into serving-size pieces and browned

2 cups canned sauerkraut, drained and rinsed

½ cup apple cider, or juice

½ tsp. caraway seeds, optional

1. Layer apples, ribs, and sauerkraut in slow cooker. Pour on juice. Sprinkle with caraway seeds.

2. Cover. Cook on Low 8 hours, or High 4 hours.

Exchange List Values: Fruit 0.5, Vegetable 1.0, Meat, medium fat 2.0

Basic Nutritional Values: Calories 198 (Calories from Fat 82), Total Fat 9 gm (Saturated Fat 3.3 gm, Polyunsat Fat 0.8 gm, Monounsat Fat 3.9 gm, Cholesterol 57 mg), Sodium 356 mg, Total Carbohydrate 11 gm, Dietary Fiber 3 gm, Sugars 7 gm, Protein 18 gm

Check your blood sugar as soon as you get up, before you do anything else, and then treat as needed. Starting the day with a normal blood sugar level will make it easier to keep your level under control throughout the day.

Sauerkraut and Ribs

Margaret H. Moffitt • Bartlett, TN

Makes 6 servings (Ideal slow cooker size: 4-quart)

27-oz. can sauerkraut, drained (juice reserved) and rinsed

1 small onion, chopped

2 lbs. country-style pork ribs, trimmed of fat, cut into serving-size pieces

¼ tsp. pepper

half a sauerkraut can of water

1. Pour sauerkraut and juice into slow cooker. Add onion.

2. Season ribs with pepper. Place on top of kraut. Add water.

3. Cover. Cook on High until mixture boils. Reduce heat to Low and cook 4 hours.

4. Serve with mashed potatoes.

Exchange List Values: Vegetable 1.0, Meat, medium fat 2.0

Basic Nutritional Values: Calories 185 (Calories from Fat 82), Total Fat 9 gm (Saturated Fat 3.3 gm, Polyunsat Fat 0.8 gm, Monounsat Fat 3.9 gm, Cholesterol 57 mg), Sodium 548 mg, Total Carbohydrate 7 gm, Dietary Fiber 4 gm, Sugars 3 gm, Protein 19 gm

Chops and Kraut

Willard E. Roth • Elkhart, IN

Makes 6 servings (Ideal slow cooker size: 4-quart)

1-lb. bag fresh sauerkraut, drained and rinsed

2 large Vidalia onions, sliced

6 (¼ lb. each) pork chops, bone-in, trimmed of fat

⅓ cup water

1. Make 3 layers in well-greased cooker: kraut, onions, and chops. Pour water over top.

2. Cover. Cook on Low 6 hours.

3. Serve with mashed potatoes and applesauce or cranberry sauce.

Exchange List Values: Vegetable 2.0, Meat, lean 2.0

Basic Nutritional Values: Calories 156 (Calories from Fat 43), Total Fat 5 gm (Saturated Fat 1.7 gm, Polyunsat Fat 0.4 gm, Monounsat Fat 2.1 gm, Cholesterol 47 mg), Sodium 336 mg, Total Carbohydrate 10 gm, Dietary Fiber 3 gm, Sugars 6 gm, Protein 18 gm

Smothered Lentils

Tracey B. Stenger • Gretna, LA

Makes 6 servings (Ideal slow cooker size: 4-quart)

2 cups dry lentils, rinsed and sorted

1 medium onion, chopped

½ cup chopped celery

2 cloves garlic, minced

1 cup ham, cooked and chopped

½ cup chopped carrots

1 cup diced fresh tomatoes

1 tsp. dried marjoram

1 tsp. ground coriander

3 cups water

1. Combine all ingredients in slow cooker.

2. Cover. Cook on Low 8 hours. (Check lentils after 5 hours of cooking. If they've absorbed all the water, stir in 1 more cup water.)

Exchange List Values: Starch 2.0, Vegetable 1.0, Meat, very lean 2.0

Basic Nutritional Values: Calories 239 (Calories from Fat 19), Total Fat 2 gm (Saturated Fat 0.5 gm, Polyunsat Fat 0.5 gm, Monounsat Fat 0.7 gm, Cholesterol 13 mg), Sodium 333 mg, Total Carbohydrate 36 gm, Dietary Fiber 14 gm, Sugars 6 gm, Protein 21 gm

You may want to add salt and pepper if you regularly use them in your diet.

Green Beans and Sausage

Alma Weaver • Ephrata, PA

Makes 4–6 servings (Ideal slow cooker size: 4-quart)

1 qt. green beans, cut into 2" pieces

1 carrot, chopped

1 small green pepper, chopped

8-oz. can no-salt-added tomato sauce

¼ tsp. dried thyme

¼ tsp. salt

½ lb. bulk pork sausage, browned and drained

1. Combine all ingredients except sausage in slow cooker.

2. Cover. Cook on High 3–4 hours. Add sausage and cook another 2 hours on Low.

Exchange List Values: Vegetable 2.0, Meat, medium fat 1.0

Basic Nutritional Values: Calories 114 (Calories from Fat 53), Total Fat 6 gm (Saturated Fat 2.0 gm, Polyunsat Fat 0.8 gm, Monounsat Fat 2.5 gm, Cholesterol 14 mg), Sodium 350 mg, Total Carbohydrate 11 gm, Dietary Fiber 4 gm, Sugars 5 gm, Protein 6 gm

Brats and Spuds

Kathi Rogge • Alexandria, IN

Makes 6 servings (Ideal slow cooker size: 4-quart)

5–6 bratwurst links, cut into 1" pieces

5 medium-sized potatoes, peeled and cubed

27-oz. can sauerkraut, rinsed and drained

1 medium tart apple, unpeeled, chopped

1 small onion, chopped

2 Tbsp. brown sugar

brown sugar substitute to equal 1 Tbsp.

1. Brown bratwurst on all sides in skillet.

2. Combine remaining ingredients in slow cooker. Stir in bratwurst.

3. Cover. Cook on High 4–6 hours, or until potatoes and apples are tender.

Exchange List Values: Starch 1.5, Carbohydrate 0.5, Vegetable 1.0, Meat, high fat 1.0

Basic Nutritional Values: Calories 273 (Calories from Fat 88), Total Fat 10 gm (Saturated Fat 3.5 gm, Polyunsat Fat 1.1 gm, Monounsat Fat 5.4 gm, Cholesterol 25 mg), Sodium 920 mg, Total Carbohydrate 36 gm, Dietary Fiber 6 gm, Sugars 13 gm, Protein 10 gm

VARIATION: Add a small amount of caraway seeds or crisp bacon pieces, just before serving.

Ham Balls

Jo Haberkamp • Fairbank, IA

Makes 24 servings (Ideal slow cooker size: 6-quart)

HAM BALLS:

3 eggs

3 cups crushed graham crackers

2 cups milk

2 tsp. dried minced onion

1/4 tsp. pepper

2 lbs. extra-lean, reduced-sodium ground ham

1 1/2 lbs. 90%-lean ground beef

1 1/2 lbs. ground pork, trimmed of fat

TOPPING:

1/2 cup no-salt-added ketchup

1/4 cup water

1/2 cup brown sugar

1/4 cup plus 2 Tbsp. vinegar

1/2 tsp. dry mustard

1. Beat eggs slightly in large bowl. Add graham crackers, milk, minced onion, pepper, and ground meats. Mix well.

2. Form into 24 balls, using a 1/2-cup measuring cup for each ball.

3. Combine topping ingredients.

4. Layer meatballs and topping in greased slow cooker.

5. Cover. Cook on High 1 hour. Reduce heat to Low and cook 3–4 hours more.

Exchange List Values: Carbohydrate 1.0, Meat, medium fat 2.0

Basic Nutritional Values: Calories 220 (Calories from Fat 63), Total Fat 7 gm (Saturated Fat 2.5 gm, Polyunsat Fat 0.9 gm, Monounsat Fat 2.9 gm, Cholesterol 82 mg), Sodium 429 mg, Total Carbohydrate 17 gm, Dietary Fiber 0 gm, Sugars 10 gm, Protein 21 gm

Hot Dogs and Noodles

Dolores Kratz • Souderton, PA

Makes 6 servings (Ideal slow cooker size: 4-quart)

8-oz. pkg. medium egg noodles, cooked and drained

1 cup freshly grated Parmesan cheese

1 cup fat-free milk

1 Tbsp. flour

1-lb. pkg. fat-free hot dogs, sliced

2 Tbsp. brown sugar

brown sugar substitute to equal 1 Tbsp.

1/4 cup fat-free mayonnaise

2 Tbsp. prepared mustard

1. Place noodles, cheese, milk, and flour in slow cooker. Mix well.

2. Combine hot dogs with remaining ingredients. Spoon evenly over noodles.

3. Cover. Cook on Low 5–6 hours.

Exchange List Values: Starch 2.0, Carbohydrate 1.0, Meat, lean 2.0

Basic Nutritional Values: Calories 326 (Calories from Fat 59), Total Fat 7 gm (Saturated Fat 3.4 gm, Polyunsat Fat 0.8 gm, Monounsat Fat 2.2 gm, Cholesterol 65 mg), Sodium 1036 mg, Total Carbohydrate 44 gm, Dietary Fiber 1 gm, Sugars 12 gm, Protein 22 gm

Foods with trans fats are bad for your heart. If the label says partially hydrogenated vegetable oil, shortening, or margarine, beware!

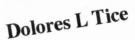

Dolores L Tice

Chicken and Sa... Cacciatore

Joyce Ka...

Recipe photo appears in color secti...

Makes 4–6 servings (Ideal slow ... 4-quart)

1 large green pepper, sliced in 1"...

1 cup sliced mushrooms

1 medium onion, sliced in rings

1 lb. boneless, skinless chicken brea...

1 lb. lean fresh, sweet Italian turkey ...
   links, browned

½ tsp. dried oregano

½ tsp. dried basil

2 Tbsp. Italian Seasoning Mix (see rec...
   on page 333)

1½ cups no-salt-added tomato sauce

... getables in slow cooker.

... meat.

... with oregano, basil, and Italian
... mix.

... omato sauce.

... on Low 8 hours.

... during last 30 minutes of
... to allow sauce to cook off

... ked spiral pasta.

... lues: Vegetable 2.0,

... ues: Calories 278 (Calories
... t 11 gm (Saturated Fat 3.1 gm,
... Monounsat Fat 2.3 gm,
... odium 547 mg, Total
... ietary Fiber 2 gm, Sugars

Wild Rice Hot Dish

Barbara Tenney • Delta, PA

Makes 8-10 side-dish servings (Ideal slow cooker size: 4-quart)

2 cups wild rice, uncooked

½ cup slivered almonds

½ cup chopped onions

½ cup chopped celery

8-12-oz. can mushrooms, drained

2 cups cut-up cooked chicken

6 cups 98%-fat-free, lower-sodium chicken broth

¼ tsp. pepper

¼ tsp. garlic powder

1 Tbsp. parsley

1. Wash and drain rice.

2. Combine all ingredients in slow cooker. Mix well.

3. Cover. Cook on Low 4–6 hours, or until rice is finished. Do not remove lid before rice has cooked 4 hours.

Exchange List Values: Starch 2.0, Meat, lean 1.0, Fat 0.5

Basic Nutritional Values: Calories 227 (Calories from Fat 51), Total Fat 6 gm (Saturated Fat 0.8 gm, Polyunsat Fat 1.4 gm, Monounsat Fat 2.7 gm, Cholesterol 25 mg), Sodium 403 mg, Total Carbohydrate 28 gm, Dietary Fiber 4 gm, Sugars 2 gm, Protein 17 gm

Frances's Roast Chicken

Frances Schrag • Newton, KS

Makes 6 servings (Ideal slow cooker size: 4-5-quart)

3-lb. whole frying chicken

salt to taste

pepper to taste

½ tsp. poultry seasoning

half an onion, chopped

1 rib celery, chopped

¼ tsp. dried basil

1. Sprinkle chicken cavity with salt, pepper, and poultry seasoning. Put onion and celery inside cavity. Put chicken in slow cooker. Sprinkle with basil.

2. Cover. Cook on Low 8–10 hours, or High 4–6 hours.

3. Remove skin from chicken and discard liquid.

Exchange List Values: Meat, lean 3.0

Basic Nutritional Values: Calories 140 (Calories from Fat 48), Total Fat 5 gm (Saturated Fat 1.4 gm, Polyunsat Fat 1.2 gm, Monounsat Fat 1.9 gm, Cholesterol 65 mg), Sodium 56 mg, Total Carbohydrate 0 gm, Dietary Fiber 0 gm, Sugars 0 gm, Protein 21 gm

Donna's Cooked Chicken

Donna Treloar • Gaston, IN

(Ideal slow cooker size: 5-quart)

1 medium onion, sliced

2½ lbs. boneless, skinless chicken breasts

½ tsp. seasoned salt

¼ tsp. pepper

½ tsp. garlic powder

1. Layer onion in bottom of slow cooker. Add chicken and sprinkle with seasoned salt, pepper, and garlic powder.

2. Cook on Low 4 hours, or until done but not dry.

3. Use in stir-fries, chicken salads, or casseroles; slice for sandwiches; shred for enchiladas; or cut up and freeze for later use.

Exchange List Values: Meat, very lean 4.0

Basic Nutritional Values: Calories 138 (Calories from Fat 24), Total Fat 3 gm (Saturated Fat 0.7 gm, Polyunsat Fat 0.6 gm, Monounsat Fat 0.9 gm, Cholesterol 67 mg), Sodium 131 mg, Total Carbohydrate 1 gm, Dietary Fiber 0 gm, Sugars 1 gm, Protein 25 gm

VARIATION: Splash chicken with 2 Tbsp. light soy sauce before cooking.

If you lose just 10 pounds and keep it off, your blood pressure, blood sugars, and cholesterol levels are likely to improve.

Chicken in a Pot

Carolyn Baer • Conrath, WI / Evie Hershey • Atglen, PA / Judy Koczo • Plano, IL / Mary Puskar • Forest Hill, MD / Mary Wheatley • Mashpee, MA

Makes 6 servings (Ideal slow cooker size: 5-quart)

2 medium carrots, sliced

2 medium onions, sliced

2 ribs celery, cut in 1" pieces

3-lb. chicken, whole or cut up, skin removed

¾ tsp. salt

½ tsp. coarse black pepper

1 tsp. dried basil

½ cup water, chicken broth, or white cooking wine

1. Place vegetables in bottom of slow cooker. Place chicken on top of vegetables. Add seasonings and water.

2. Cover. Cook on Low 8–10 hours, or High 3½ hours (use 1 cup liquid if cooking on High).

3. This is a great foundation for soups— chicken vegetable, chicken noodle, chicken rice, chicken corn, and other favorites.

Exchange List Values: Vegetable 1.0, Meat, lean 3.0

Basic Nutritional Values: Calories 172 (Calories from Fat 49), Total Fat 5 gm (Saturated Fat 1.5 gm, Polyunsat Fat 1.3 gm, Monounsat Fat 1.9 gm, Cholesterol 65 mg), Sodium 381 mg, Total Carbohydrate 8 gm, Dietary Fiber 2 gm, Sugars 4 gm, Protein 22 gm

Note: To make this a full meal, add 2 medium-sized potatoes, quartered, to vegetables before cooking.

Another Chicken in a Pot

Jennifer J. Gehman • Harrisburg, PA

Makes 4–6 servings (Ideal slow cooker size: 4–5-quart)

1-lb. pkg. baby carrots

1 small onion, diced

10-oz. pkg. frozen green beans, thawed

3-lb. whole chicken, cut into serving-size pieces, skin and fat removed

$\frac{1}{2}$ tsp. salt

$\frac{1}{2}$ tsp. black pepper

$\frac{1}{2}$ cup chicken broth

$\frac{1}{4}$ cup white wine

$\frac{1}{2}$–1 tsp. dried basil

1. Put carrots, onion, and beans on bottom of slow cooker. Add chicken. Top with salt, pepper, broth, and wine. Sprinkle with basil.

2. Cover. Cook on Low 8–10 hours, or High 3$\frac{1}{2}$–5 hours.

Exchange List Values: Vegetable 2.0, Meat, lean 3.0

Basic Nutritional Values: Calories 194 (Calories from Fat 51), Total Fat 6 gm (Saturated Fat 1.5 gm, Polyunsat Fat 1.4 gm, Monounsat Fat 2.0 gm, Cholesterol 66 mg), Sodium 434 mg, Total Carbohydrate 12 gm, Dietary Fiber 4 gm, Sugars 6 gm, Protein 23 gm

Savory Slow Cooker Chicken

Sara Harter Fredette • Williamsburg, MA

Makes 4 servings (Ideal slow cooker size: 4–5-quart)

2$\frac{1}{2}$ lbs. chicken pieces, skinned

1 lb. fresh tomatoes, chopped, or 15-oz. can stewed tomatoes

2 Tbsp. white wine

1 bay leaf

$\frac{1}{4}$ tsp. pepper

2 cloves garlic, minced

1 onion, chopped

$\frac{1}{2}$ cup chicken broth

1 tsp. dried thyme

$\frac{1}{4}$ tsp. salt

2 cups broccoli, cut into bite-sized pieces

1. Combine all ingredients except broccoli in slow cooker.

2. Cover. Cook on Low 8–10 hours.

3. Add broccoli 30 minutes before serving.

Exchange List Values: Vegetable 2.0, Meat, lean 3.0

Basic Nutritional Values: Calories 230 (Calories from Fat 67), Total Fat 7 gm (Saturated Fat 1.9 gm, Polyunsat Fat 1.8 gm, Monounsat Fat 2.5 gm, Cholesterol 82 mg), Sodium 427 mg, Total Carbohydrate 11 gm, Dietary Fiber 3 gm, Sugars 7 gm, Protein 30 gm

Chicken and Vegetables

Rosanne Hankins • Stevensville, MD

Makes 6 servings (Ideal slow cooker size: 4–5-quart)

salt to taste

pepper to taste

3 lbs. chicken, cut up, skin and fat trimmed

1 bay leaf

2 tsp. lemon juice

1/4 cup diced onions

1/4 cup diced celery

1-lb. pkg. frozen mixed vegetables, including corn

1. Sprinkle salt and pepper over chicken and place chicken in slow cooker. Add bay leaf and lemon juice.

2. Cover. Cook on Low 6–8 hours, or High 3–5 hours. Remove chicken from bones. Reserve liquid, skimming fat if desired.

3. Cook 1/2 cup liquid, onions, and celery in microwave on High for 2 minutes. Add frozen vegetables and microwave until cooked through.

4. Return all ingredients to slow cooker and cook on High 30 minutes.

5. Serve over cooked rice.

Exchange List Values: Vegetable 2.0, Meat, lean 3.0

Basic Nutritional Values: Calories 187 (Calories from Fat 49), Total Fat 5 gm (Saturated Fat 1.4 gm, Polyunsat Fat 1.3 gm, Monounsat Fat 1.9 gm, Cholesterol 65 mg), Sodium 105 mg, Total Carbohydrate 11 gm, Dietary Fiber 2 gm, Sugars 3 gm, Protein 24 gm

Baked Chicken Breasts

Janice Crist • Quinter, KS /
Tracy Supcoe • Barclay, MD

Makes 4–6 servings (Ideal slow cooker size: 4-quart)

3 whole chicken breasts, halved

10 3/4-oz. can 98%-fat-free, reduced-sodium cream of chicken soup

1/2 cup dry sherry

1 tsp. dried tarragon, or rosemary, or both

1 tsp. Worcestershire sauce

1/4 tsp. garlic powder

4-oz. can sliced mushrooms, drained

1. Place chicken breasts in slow cooker.

2. In saucepan, combine remaining ingredients. Heat until smooth and hot. Pour over chicken.

3. Cover. Cook on Low 8–10 hours.

Exchange List Values: Carbohydrate 0.5, Meat, very lean 4.0, Fat 0.5

Basic Nutritional Values: Calories 214 (Calories from Fat 40), Total Fat 4 gm (Saturated Fat 1.3 gm, Polyunsat Fat 1.2 gm, Monounsat Fat 1.3 gm, Cholesterol 88 mg), Sodium 339 mg, Total Carbohydrate 7 gm, Dietary Fiber 1 gm, Sugars 2 gm, Protein 34 gm

When you eat out, ask for a to-go box. Before you take a single bite of your meal, put half of it in the box. Out of sight, out of mind!

Chicken Delicious

Janice Crist • Quinter, KS

Makes 8–12 servings (Ideal slow cooker size: 4–5-quart)

6 whole boneless, skinless chicken breasts, halved, visible fat removed

10¾-oz. can 98%-fat-free, reduced-sodium cream of mushroom soup

10¾-oz. can cream of celery soup

⅓ cup dry sherry, or white wine

1. Place chicken in slow cooker.

2. Combine soups with sherry. Pour over chicken.

3. Cover. Cook on Low 8–10 hours.

4. Serve with rice.

Exchange List Values: Carbohydrate 0.5, Meat, very lean 4.0, Fat 0.5

Basic Nutritional Values: Calories 203 (Calories from Fat 48), Total Fat 5 gm (Saturated Fat 1.6 gm, Polyunsat Fat 1.4 gm, Monounsat Fat 1.5 gm, Cholesterol 85 mg), Sodium 352 mg, Total Carbohydrate 4 gm, Dietary Fiber 0 gm, Sugars 1 gm, Protein 32 gm

This recipe is best if seasoned with lemon juice, salt, pepper, celery salt, and paprika before cooking. You can also sprinkle with grated Parmesan cheese.

Chicken in Wine

Mary Seielstad • Sparks, NV

Makes 4–6 servings (Ideal slow cooker size: 4-quart)

2 lbs. chicken breasts, or pieces, trimmed of skin and fat

10¾-oz. can 98%-fat-free, reduced-sodium cream of mushroom soup

10¾-oz. can French onion soup

1 cup dry white wine, or chicken broth

1. Put chicken in slow cooker.

2. Combine soups and wine. Pour over chicken.

3. Cover. Cook on Low 6–8 hours.

4. Serve over rice, pasta, or potatoes.

Exchange List Values: Carbohydrate 0.5, Meat, very lean 5.0

Basic Nutritional Values: Calories 225 (Calories from Fat 47), Total Fat 5 gm (Saturated Fat 1.4 gm, Polyunsat Fat 1.2 gm, Monounsat Fat 1.6 gm, Cholesterol 91 mg), Sodium 645 mg, Total Carbohydrate 7 gm, Dietary Fiber 1 gm, Sugars 3 gm, Protein 35 gm

Creamy Chicken and Noodles

Rhonda Burgoon • Collingswood, NJ

Recipe photo appears in color section.

Makes 4–6 servings (Ideal slow cooker size: 4-quart)

2 cups sliced carrots

1 1/2 cups chopped onions

1 cup sliced celery

2 Tbsp. snipped fresh parsley

1 bay leaf

3 medium-sized chicken legs and thighs (about 2 lbs.), skin removed

2 10 3/4-oz. cans 98%-fat-free, reduced-sodium cream of chicken soup

1/2 cup water

1 tsp. dried thyme

1/4 tsp. salt

1/4 tsp. pepper

1 cup peas

8 ozs. dry wide noodles, cooked

1. Place carrots, onions, celery, parsley, and bay leaf in bottom of slow cooker.

2. Place chicken on top of vegetables.

3. Combine soup, water, thyme, salt, and pepper. Pour over chicken and vegetables.

4. Cover. Cook on Low 8–9 hours, or on High 4–4 1/2 hours.

5. Remove chicken from slow cooker. Cool slightly. Remove from bones, cut into bite-sized pieces, and return to slow cooker.

6. Remove and discard bay leaf.

7. Stir peas into mixture in slow cooker. Allow to cook for 5–10 more minutes.

8. Pour over cooked noodles. Toss gently to combine.

9. Serve with crusty bread and a salad.

Exchange List Values: Starch 2.0, Carbohydrate 0.5, Vegetable 2.0, Meat, lean 2.0

Basic Nutritional Values: Calories 357 (Calories from Fat 71), Total Fat 8 gm (Saturated Fat 2.4 gm, Polyunsat Fat 2.3 gm, Monounsat Fat 2.3 gm, Cholesterol 87 mg), Sodium 614 mg, Total Carbohydrate 48 gm, Dietary Fiber 5 gm, Sugars 9 gm, Protein 22 gm

Chicken in Mushroom Gravy

Rosemarie Fitzgerald • Gibsonia, PA / Audrey L. Kneer • Williamsfield, IL

Makes 6 servings (Ideal slow cooker size: 4-quart)

6 (5 ozs. each) boneless, skinless chicken breast halves

salt to taste

pepper to taste

1/4 cup dry white wine, or chicken broth

10 3/4-oz. can 98%-fat-free, reduced-sodium cream of mushroom soup

4-oz. can sliced mushrooms, drained

1. Place chicken in slow cooker. Season with salt and pepper.

2. Combine wine and soup. Pour over chicken. Top with mushrooms.

3. Cover. Cook on Low 7–9 hours.

Exchange List Values: Carbohydrate 0.5, Meat, very lean 4.0, Fat 0.5

Basic Nutritional Values: Calories 204 (Calories from Fat 40), Total Fat 4 gm (Saturated Fat 1.4 gm, Polyunsat Fat 1.0 gm, Monounsat Fat 1.3 gm, Cholesterol 85 mg), Sodium 320 mg, Total Carbohydrate 6 gm, Dietary Fiber 1 gm, Sugars 1 gm, Protein 34 gm

Mushroom Chicken in Sour Cream Sauce

Lavina Hochstedler • Grand Blanc, MI /
Joyce Shackelford • Green Bay, WI

Makes 6 servings (Ideal slow cooker size: 4-quart)

¼ tsp. salt

¼ tsp. pepper

½ tsp. paprika

¼ tsp. lemon pepper

1 tsp. garlic powder

6 bone-in, skinless chicken breast halves

10¾-oz. can 98%-fat-free, reduced-sodium
cream of mushroom soup

8-oz. container fat-free sour cream

½ cup dry white wine, or chicken broth

½ lb. fresh mushrooms, sliced

1. Combine salt, pepper, paprika, lemon
   pepper, and garlic powder. Rub over
   chicken. Place in slow cooker.

2. Combine soup, sour cream, and wine or
   broth. Stir in mushrooms. Pour over
   chicken.

3. Cover. Cook on Low 6–8 hours, or High
   5 hours.

4. Serve over potatoes, rice, or couscous.
   Delicious accompanied with broccoli-
   cauliflower salad and applesauce.

**Exchange List Values: Carbohydrate 1.0,
Meat, very lean 4.0**

Basic Nutritional Values: Calories 217 (Calories
from Fat 37), Total Fat 4 gm (Saturated Fat 1.2 gm,
Polyunsat Fat 0.9 gm, Monounsat Fat 1.2 gm,
Cholesterol 76 mg), Sodium 407 mg, Total
Carbohydrate 12 gm, Dietary Fiber 1 gm, Sugars
4 gm, Protein 30 gm

Chicken Azteca

Katrine Rose • Woodbridge, VA

**Makes 10–12 servings (Ideal slow cooker size:
5–6-quart)**

2 15-oz. cans black beans, drained

4 cups frozen corn kernels

2 cloves garlic, minced

¾ tsp. ground cumin

2 cups chunky salsa, divided

10 boneless, skinless chicken breast halves

12 ozs. fat-free cream cheese, cubed

1. Combine beans, corn, garlic, cumin, and
   half of salsa in slow cooker.

2. Arrange chicken breasts over top. Pour
   remaining salsa over top.

3. Cover. Cook on High 2–3 hours, or on
   Low 4–6 hours.

4. Remove chicken and cut into bite-sized
   pieces. Return to cooker.

5. Stir in cream cheese. Cook on High until
   cream cheese melts.

6. Spoon chicken and sauce over cooked
   rice. Top with shredded cheddar cheese if
   you wish.

**Exchange List Values: Starch 1.5, Meat,
very lean 4.0**

Basic Nutritional Values: Calories 252 (Calories
from Fat 27), Total Fat 3 gm (Saturated Fat 0.8 gm,
Polyunsat Fat 0.8 gm, Monounsat Fat 0.9 gm,
Cholesterol 64 mg), Sodium 366 mg, Total
Carbohydrate 24 gm, Dietary Fiber 5 gm, Sugars
4 gm, Protein 33 gm

*Did you know that people
who eat a lot of whole grains have
fewer heart attacks?*

Tamale Chicken

Jeanne Allen • Rye, CO

Makes 8 servings (Ideal slow cooker size: 4–5-quart)

1 medium onion, chopped

4-oz. can chopped green chilies

1 Tbsp. canola oil

10¾-oz. can 98%-fat-free, reduced-sodium cream of chicken soup

1 cup fat-free sour cream

1 cup sliced ripe olives

1 cup chopped no-salt-added stewed tomatoes

1¼ cups shredded fat-free cheddar cheese, divided

8 chicken breast halves, cooked and chopped

16-oz. can beef tamales, chopped

1 tsp. chili powder

1 tsp. garlic powder

1 tsp. pepper

1. Saute onion and chilies in oil in skillet.

2. Combine all ingredients except ¼ cup shredded cheese. Pour into slow cooker.

3. Top with remaining cheese.

4. Cover. Cook on High 3–4 hours.

5. Pass chopped fresh tomatoes, shredded lettuce, sour cream, salsa, and/or guacamole so guests can top their Tamale Chicken with these condiments.

Exchange List Values: Starch 0.5, Carbohydrate 0.5, Vegetable 1.0, Meat, lean 4.0, Fat 0.5

Basic Nutritional Values: Calories 341 (Calories from Fat 98), Total Fat 11 gm (Saturated Fat 2.7 gm, Polyunsat Fat 2.1 gm, Monounsat Fat 4.9 gm, Cholesterol 87 mg), Sodium 848 mg, Total Carbohydrate 21 gm, Dietary Fiber 3 gm, Sugars 5 gm, Protein 37 gm

Tex-Mex Chicken and Rice

Kelly Evenson • Pittsboro, NC

Makes 8 servings (Ideal slow cooker size: 4–5-quart)

1 cup converted white rice, uncooked

28-oz. can diced, peeled tomatoes

6-oz. can tomato paste

3 cups hot water

1 pkg. dry taco seasoning mix

4 whole boneless, skinless chicken breasts, uncooked and cut into ½" cubes

2 medium onions, chopped

1 green pepper, chopped

4-oz. can diced green chilies

1 tsp. garlic powder

½ tsp. pepper

1. Combine all ingredients except chilies, garlic powder, and pepper in large slow cooker.

2. Cover. Cook on Low 4–4½ hours, or until rice is tender and chicken is cooked.

3. Stir in green chilies and reserved seasonings.

4. Serve with mixed green leafy salad and refried beans.

Exchange List Values: Starch 1.5, Vegetable 3.0, Meat, very lean 3.0

Basic Nutritional Values: Calories 300 (Calories from Fat 32), Total Fat 4 gm (Saturated Fat 0.8 gm, Polyunsat Fat 0.9 gm, Monounsat Fat 1.1 gm, Cholesterol 73 mg), Sodium 656 mg, Total Carbohydrate 34 gm, Dietary Fiber 4 gm, Sugars 7 gm, Protein 32 gm

Wanda's Chicken and Rice Casserole

Wanda Roth • Napoleon, OH

Makes 6–8 servings (Ideal slow cooker size: 4–5-quart)

1 cup long-grain rice, uncooked

3 cups water

2 tsp. chicken bouillon granules

10¾-oz can 98%-fat-free, reduced-sodium cream of chicken soup

16-oz. bag frozen broccoli

2 cups chopped cooked chicken

½ tsp. garlic powder

¼ tsp. onion salt

1 cup grated fat-free cheddar cheese

1. Combine all ingredients in slow cooker.

2. Cook on High 3–4 hours.

Exchange List Values: Starch 1.5, Vegetable 1.0, Meat, lean 1.0

Basic Nutritional Values: Calories 214 (Calories from Fat 33), Total Fat 4 gm (Saturated Fat 1.0 gm, Polyunsat Fat 1.0 gm, Monounsat Fat 1.1 gm, Cholesterol 36 mg), Sodium 559 mg, Total Carbohydrate 26 gm, Dietary Fiber 2 gm, Sugars 3 gm, Protein 19 gm

Note: If casserole is too runny, remove lid from slow cooker for 15 minutes while continuing to cook on High.

Sharon's Chicken and Rice Casserole

Sharon Anders • Alburtis, PA

Makes 4 servings (Ideal slow cooker size: 3–4-quart)

10¾-oz. can cream of celery soup

2-oz. can sliced mushrooms, drained

½ cup long-grain rice, uncooked

4 chicken breast halves, boned and skinned

1 Tbsp. Sodium-Free Onion Soup Mix (see recipe on page 334)

1. Combine soup, mushrooms, and rice in greased slow cooker. Mix well.

2. Layer chicken breasts on top of mixture. Sprinkle with onion soup mix.

3. Cover. Cook on Low 4–6 hours.

Exchange List Values: Starch 2.0, Meat, very lean 4.0, Fat 1.0

Basic Nutritional Values: Calories 330 (Calories from Fat 71), Total Fat 8 gm (Saturated Fat 2.4 gm, Polyunsat Fat 2.5 gm, Monounsat Fat 2.0 gm, Cholesterol 86 mg), Sodium 677 mg, Total Carbohydrate 26 gm, Dietary Fiber 2 gm, Sugars 2 gm, Protein 35 gm

Buy a pedometer and seek out ways to take more steps today— shoot for 10,000 a day.

Scalloped Potatoes and Chicken

Carol Sommers • Millersburg, OH

Makes 6-8 servings (Ideal slow cooker size: 4-quart)

¼ cup chopped green peppers

½ cup chopped onions

1½ cups diced Velveeta Light cheese

7 medium potatoes, unpeeled, sliced

salt to taste

3 (about 10 ozs. each) whole boneless, skinless chicken breasts

10¾-oz. can cream of celery soup

1 soup can fat-free milk

1. Place layers of green peppers, onions, cheese, and potatoes in slow cooker.

2. Sprinkle salt over chicken breasts and lay on top of potatoes.

3. Combine soup and milk and pour into slow cooker, pushing meat down into liquid.

4. Cover. Cook on High 1½ hours. Reduce temperature to Low and cook 3–4 hours. Test that potatoes are soft. If not, continue cooking on Low another hour and test again, continuing to cook until potatoes are finished.

Exchange List Values: Starch 1.5, Carbohydrate 0.5, Meat, very lean 4.0, Fat 1.0

Basic Nutritional Values: Calories 336 (Calories from Fat 63), Total Fat 7 gm (Saturated Fat 3.0 gm, Polyunsat Fat 1.6 gm, Monounsat Fat 2.0 gm, Cholesterol 73 mg), Sodium 677 mg, Total Carbohydrate 34 gm, Dietary Fiber 3 gm, Sugars 8 gm, Protein 34 gm

Scalloped Chicken

Carolyn W. Carmichael • Berkeley Heights, NJ

Makes 4 servings (Ideal slow cooker size: 4-quart)

5-oz. pkg. scalloped potatoes

scalloped potatoes dry seasoning pack

2 chicken breast halves

2 chicken legs

10-oz. pkg. frozen peas

2 cups water

1. Put potatoes, seasoning pack, chicken, and peas in slow cooker. Pour water over all.

2. Cover. Cook on Low 8–10 hours, or on High 4 hours.

Exchange List Values: Starch 2.0, Meat, lean 3.0

Basic Nutritional Values: Calories 336 (Calories from Fat 64), Total Fat 7 gm (Saturated Fat 2.0 gm, Polyunsat Fat 2.1 gm, Monounsat Fat 2.1 gm, Cholesterol 87 mg), Sodium 861 mg, Total Carbohydrate 34 gm, Dietary Fiber 5 gm, Sugars 5 gm, Protein 35 gm

Even if you have limited mobility, you should still try to work some activity into your daily schedule. Many senior centers often offer armchair aerobics or yoga, for instance.

Chicken and Vegetables

Jeanne Heyerly • Chenoa, IL

Makes 2 servings (Ideal slow cooker size: 4-quart)

2 medium potatoes, quartered

2-3 carrots, sliced

5 ozs. frozen chicken breasts

1 frozen drumstick and thigh, split

salt to taste

pepper to taste

1 medium onion, chopped

2 cloves garlic, minced

1 cup shredded cabbage

2 tsp. sodium-free bouillon powder

2 cups water

1. Place potatoes and carrots in slow cooker. Layer chicken on top. Sprinkle with salt, pepper, onion, and garlic. Top with cabbage. Carefully pour chicken bouillon combined with water around edges.

2. Cover. Cook on Low 8–9 hours.

Exchange List Values: Starch 2.0, Vegetable 3.0, Meat, lean 2.0

Basic Nutritional Values: Calories 335 (Calories from Fat 30), Total Fat 3 gm (Saturated Fat 0.8 gm, Polyunsat Fat 1.0 gm, Monounsat Fat 1.0 gm, Cholesterol 62 mg), Sodium 129 mg, Total Carbohydrate 48 gm, Dietary Fiber 8 gm, Sugars 14 gm, Protein 28 gm

California Chicken

Shirley Sears • Tiskilwa, IL

Makes 4–6 servings (Ideal slow cooker size: 4-quart)

3-lb. chicken, quartered, skin removed, trimmed of visible fat

1 cup orange juice

1/3 cup chili sauce

2 Tbsp. light soy sauce

1 Tbsp. molasses

1 tsp. dry mustard

1/4 tsp. garlic powder

1/4 tsp. onion powder

2 Tbsp. chopped green peppers

3 medium oranges, peeled and separated into slices, or 13 1/2-oz. can mandarin oranges

1. Arrange chicken in slow cooker.

2. In separate bowl, combine juice, chili sauce, soy sauce, molasses, mustard, garlic powder, and onion powder. Pour over chicken.

3. Cover. Cook on Low 8–9 hours.

4. Stir in green peppers and oranges. Heat 30 minutes longer.

Exchange List Values: Fruit 1.0, Vegetable 1.0, Meat, lean 3.0

Basic Nutritional Values: Calories 224 (Calories from Fat 50), Total Fat 6 gm (Saturated Fat 1.5 gm, Polyunsat Fat 1.3 gm, Monounsat Fat 1.9 gm, Cholesterol 65 mg), Sodium 426 mg, Total Carbohydrate 20 gm, Dietary Fiber 2 gm, Sugars 15 gm, Protein 24 gm

VARIATION: Stir 1 tsp. curry powder in with sauces and seasonings. Stir 1 small can pineapple chunks and juice in with green peppers and oranges.

Dad's Spicy Chicken Curry

Tom and Sue Ruth • Lancaster, PA

Makes 8 servings (Ideal slow cooker size: 4-5-quart)

4 lbs. chicken pieces, with bones, trimmed of skin and fat

2 medium onions, diced

10-oz. pkg. frozen chopped spinach, thawed and squeezed dry

1 cup plain low-fat yogurt

2-3 diced red potatoes

1 tsp. salt

1 tsp. garlic powder

1 tsp. ground ginger

1 tsp. ground cumin

1 tsp. ground coriander

1 tsp. pepper

1 tsp. ground cloves

1 tsp. ground cardamom

1 tsp. ground cinnamon

½ tsp. chili powder

1 tsp. red pepper flakes

3 tsp. turmeric

1. Place chicken in large slow cooker. Cover with water.

2. Cover. Cook on High 2 hours, or until tender.

3. Drain chicken. Remove from slow cooker. Cool briefly and cut or shred into small pieces. Return to slow cooker.

4. Add remaining ingredients.

5. Cover. Cook on Low 4–6 hours, or until potatoes are tender.

6. Serve on rice. Accompany with fresh mango slices or mango chutney.

Exchange List Values: Carbohydrate 1.0, Meat, lean 3.0

Basic Nutritional Values: Calories 221 (Calories from Fat 56), Total Fat 6 gm (Saturated Fat 1.8 gm, Polyunsat Fat 1.4 gm, Monounsat Fat 2.1 gm, Cholesterol 67 mg), Sodium 402 mg, Total Carbohydrate 16 gm, Dietary Fiber 3 gm, Sugars 4 gm, Protein 25 gm

VARIATION: Substitute 5 tsp. curry powder for the garlic, ginger, cumin, coriander, and pepper.

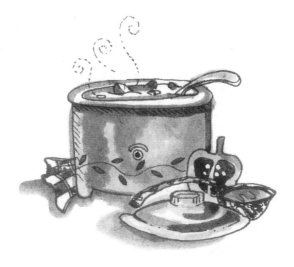

Orange Chicken Leg Quarters

Kimberly Jensen • Bailey, CO

Makes 5 servings (Ideal slow cooker size: 4-quart)

4 chicken drumsticks, all visible fat removed

4 chicken thighs, all visible fat removed

1 cup strips of green and red bell peppers

½ cup canned chicken broth

½ cup prepared orange juice

½ cup no-salt-added ketchup

2 Tbsp. light soy sauce

1 Tbsp. light molasses

1 Tbsp. prepared mustard

¼ tsp. garlic powder

11-oz. can mandarin oranges

2 tsp. cornstarch

1 cup frozen peas

2 green onions, sliced

1. Place chicken in slow cooker. Top with pepper strips.

2. Combine broth, juice, ketchup, soy sauce, molasses, mustard, and garlic powder. Pour over chicken.

3. Cover. Cook on Low 6–7 hours.

4. Remove chicken and vegetables from slow cooker. Keep warm.

5. Measure out 1 cup of cooking sauce. Put in saucepan and bring to boil. Discard remaining cooking sauce.

6. Drain oranges, reserving 1 Tbsp. juice. Stir cornstarch into reserved juice. Add to boiling sauce in pan.

7. Add peas to sauce and cook, stirring for 2–3 minutes, until sauce thickens and peas are warm. Stir in oranges.

8. Arrange chicken pieces on platter of cooked white rice, fried cellophane noodles, or lo mein noodles. Pour orange sauce over chicken and rice or noodles. Top with sliced green onions.

Exchange List Values: Carbohydrate 1.5, Meat, lean 3.0

Basic Nutritional Values: Calories 285 (Calories from Fat 77), Total Fat 9 gm (Saturated Fat 2.3 gm, Polyunsat Fat 2.0 gm, Monounsat Fat 3.1 gm, Cholesterol 90 mg), Sodium 382 mg, Total Carbohydrate 21 gm, Dietary Fiber 3 gm, Sugars 14 gm, Protein 30 gm

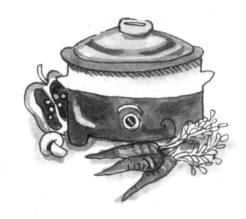

Creamy Nutmeg Chicken

Amber Swarey • Donalds, SC

Makes 6 servings (Ideal slow cooker size: 4-quart)

6 boneless chicken breast halves, skin and visible fat removed

1 Tbsp. canola oil

$1/4$ cup chopped onions

$1/4$ cup minced parsley

2 $10^3/4$-oz. cans 98%-fat-free, reduced-sodium cream of mushroom soup

$1/2$ cup fat-free sour cream

$1/2$ cup fat-free milk

1 Tbsp. ground nutmeg

$1/4$ tsp. sage

$1/4$ tsp. dried thyme

$1/4$ tsp. crushed rosemary

1. Brown chicken in skillet in oil. Reserve drippings and place chicken in slow cooker.

2. Saute onions and parsley in drippings until onions are tender.

3. Stir in remaining ingredients. Mix well. Pour over chicken.

4. Cover. Cook on Low 3 hours, or until juices run clear.

5. Serve over mashed or fried potatoes or rice.

Exchange List Values: Carbohydrate 1.0, Meat, very lean 4.0, Fat 1.0

Basic Nutritional Values: Calories 264 (Calories from Fat 69), Total Fat 8 gm (Saturated Fat 1.9 gm, Polyunsat Fat 2.1 gm, Monounsat Fat 2.8 gm, Cholesterol 83 mg), Sodium 495 mg, Total Carbohydrate 15 gm, Dietary Fiber 1 gm, Sugars 5 gm, Protein 31 gm

Orange Chicken and Sweet Potatoes

Kimberlee Greenawalt • Harrisonburg, VA

Makes 6 servings (Ideal slow cooker size: 4-quart)

2 ($5^1/2$ ozs. each) sweet potatoes, peeled and sliced

3 whole boneless, skinless chicken breasts, halved, all visible fat removed

$2/3$ cup flour

1 tsp. nutmeg

$1/2$ tsp. cinnamon

$10^3/4$-oz. can condensed, 98%-fat-free, reduced-sodium cream of chicken soup

4-oz. can sliced mushrooms, drained

$1/2$ cup orange juice

$1/2$ tsp. grated orange peel

2 tsp. brown sugar

3 Tbsp. flour

1. Place sweet potatoes in bottom of slow cooker.

2. Rinse chicken breasts and pat dry. Combine flour, nutmeg, and cinnamon. Thoroughly coat chicken in seasoned flour mixture. Place on top of sweet potatoes.

3. Combine soup with remaining ingredients. Stir well. Pour over chicken breasts.

4. Cover. Cook on Low 8–10 hours, or High 3–4 hours.

5. Serve over rice.

Exchange List Values: Starch 2.0, Carbohydrate 0.5, Meat, very lean 4.0

Basic Nutritional Values: Calories 337 (Calories from Fat 44), Total Fat 5 gm (Saturated Fat 1.4 gm, Polyunsat Fat 1.3 gm, Monounsat Fat 1.4 gm, Cholesterol 88 mg), Sodium 335 mg, Total Carbohydrate 34 gm, Dietary Fiber 3 gm, Sugars 8 gm, Protein 36 gm

Chicken with Applesauce

Kelly Evenson • Pittsboro, NC

Makes 4 servings (Ideal slow cooker size: 4-quart)

4 boneless, skinless chicken breast halves

salt to taste

pepper to taste

2 Tbsp. oil

2 cups applesauce, unsweetened

1/4 cup barbecue sauce

1/2 tsp. poultry seasoning

2 tsp. honey

1/2 tsp. lemon juice

1. Season chicken with salt and pepper. Brown in oil for 5 minutes per side.

2. Cut up chicken into 1" chunks and transfer to slow cooker.

3. Combine remaining ingredients. Pour over chicken and mix together well.

4. Cover. Cook on High 2–3 hours, or until chicken is tender.

5. Serve over rice or noodles.

Exchange List Values: Fruit 1.0, Meat, very lean 4.0, Fat 2.0

Basic Nutritional Values: Calories 301 (Calories from Fat 94), Total Fat 10 gm (Saturated Fat 1.5 gm, Polyunsat Fat 2.9 gm, Monounsat Fat 5.3 gm, Cholesterol 84 mg), Sodium 199 mg, Total Carbohydrate 19 gm, Dietary Fiber 2 gm, Sugars 16 gm, Protein 32 gm

Quitting smoking is not easy—
it often takes several tries. This time
may just be the one that works!

Maui Chicken

John D. Allen • Rye, CO

Makes 6 servings (Ideal slow cooker size: 4-quart)

6 boneless chicken breast halves, trimmed of skin and fat

2 Tbsp. oil

14 1/2-oz. can chicken broth

20-oz. can pineapple chunks

1/4 cup vinegar

2 Tbsp. brown sugar

2 tsp. soy sauce

1 clove garlic, minced

1 medium green bell pepper, chopped

3 Tbsp. cornstarch

1/4 cup water

1. Brown chicken in oil. Transfer chicken to slow cooker.

2. Combine remaining ingredients. Pour over chicken.

3. Cover. Cook on High 4–6 hours.

4. Serve over rice.

Exchange List Values: Fruit 1.0, Carbohydrate 0.5, Meat, very lean 4.0, Fat 1.5

Basic Nutritional Values: Calories 305 (Calories from Fat 75), Total Fat 8 gm (Saturated Fat 1.4 gm, Polyunsat Fat 2.2 gm, Monounsat Fat 4.0 gm, Cholesterol 82 mg), Sodium 601 mg, Total Carbohydrate 25 gm, Dietary Fiber 1 gm, Sugars 19 gm, Protein 32 gm

Sweet and Sour Chicken

Bernice A. Esau • North Newton, KS

Makes 6 servings (Ideal slow cooker size: 4-quart)

1½ cups sliced carrots

1 large green pepper, chopped

1 medium onion, chopped

2 Tbsp. quick-cooking tapioca

2½ lbs. chicken, cut into serving-size pieces, skin removed, trimmed of fat

8-oz. can pineapple chunks in juice

3 Tbsp. brown sugar

brown sugar substitute to equal 1½ Tbsp.

⅓ cup vinegar

1 Tbsp. soy sauce

½ tsp. instant chicken bouillon

¼ tsp. garlic powder

¼ tsp. ground ginger, or ½ tsp. freshly grated ginger

⅛ tsp. salt

1. Place vegetables in bottom of slow cooker. Sprinkle with tapioca. Add chicken.

2. In separate bowl, combine pineapple, brown sugar, brown sugar substitute, vinegar, soy sauce, bouillon, garlic powder, ginger, and salt. Pour over chicken.

3. Cover. Cook on Low 8–10 hours.

4. Serve over cooked rice.

Exchange List Values: Fruit 0.5, Carbohydrate 0.5, Vegetable 1.0, Meat, lean 2.0

Basic Nutritional Values: Calories 208 (Calories from Fat 41), Total Fat 5 gm (Saturated Fat 1.2 gm, Polyunsat Fat 1.1 gm, Monounsat Fat 1.6 gm, Cholesterol 54 mg), Sodium 365 mg, Total Carbohydrate 23 gm, Dietary Fiber 2 gm, Sugars 16 gm, Protein 19 gm

Ann's Chicken Cacciatore

Ann Driscoll • Albuquerque, NM

Makes 6–8 servings (Ideal slow cooker size: 4-quart)

1 large onion, thinly sliced

3 lbs. chicken, cut up, skin removed, trimmed of fat

2 6-oz. cans tomato paste

4-oz. can sliced mushrooms, drained

1 tsp. salt

¼ cup dry white wine

¼ tsp. pepper

1-2 cloves garlic, minced

1-2 tsp. dried oregano

½ tsp. dried basil

½ tsp. celery seed, optional

1 bay leaf

1. Place onion in slow cooker. Add chicken.

2. Combine remaining ingredients. Pour over chicken.

3. Cover. Cook on Low 7–9 hours, or High 3–4 hours.

4. Serve over spaghetti.

Exchange List Values: Vegetable 3.0, Meat, lean 2.0

Basic Nutritional Values: Calories 161 (Calories from Fat 40), Total Fat 4 gm (Saturated Fat 1.1 gm, Polyunsat Fat 1.1 gm, Monounsat Fat 1.5 gm, Cholesterol 49 mg), Sodium 405 mg, Total Carbohydrate 12 gm, Dietary Fiber 3 gm, Sugars 3 gm, Protein 19 gm

Coq au Vin

Kimberlee Greenawalt • Harrisonburg, VA

Makes 6 servings (Ideal slow cooker size: 4-quart)

2 cups frozen pearl onions, thawed

4 thick slices bacon, fried, drained, patted dry, and crumbled

1 cup sliced button mushrooms

1 clove garlic, minced

1 tsp. dried thyme leaves

1/8 tsp. black pepper

6 (5 ozs. each) boneless, skinless chicken breast halves, trimmed of fat

1/2 cup dry red wine

3/4 cup chicken broth

1/4 cup tomato paste

3 Tbsp. flour

1. Layer ingredients in slow cooker in the following order: onions, bacon, mushrooms, garlic, thyme, pepper, chicken, wine, broth.

2. Cover. Cook on Low 6–8 hours.

3. Remove chicken and vegetables. Cover and keep warm.

4. Ladle 1/2 cup cooking liquid into small bowl. Cool slightly. Turn slow cooker to High. Cover. Mix reserved liquid, tomato paste, and flour until smooth. Return mixture to slow cooker, cover, and cook 15 minutes, or until thickened.

5. Serve chicken, vegetables, and sauce over noodles.

Exchange List Values: Vegetable 2.0, Meat, very lean 4.0, Fat 1.5

Basic Nutritional Values: Calories 258 (Calories from Fat 66), Total Fat 7 gm (Saturated Fat 2.2 gm, Polyunsat Fat 1.2 gm, Monounsat Fat 2.9 gm, Cholesterol 91 mg), Sodium 388 mg, Total Carbohydrate 10 gm, Dietary Fiber 2 gm, Sugars 4 gm, Protein 36 gm

Lemon Garlic Chicken

Cindy Krestynick • Glen Lyon, PA

Makes 6 servings (Ideal slow cooker size: 4-quart)

1 tsp. dried oregano

1/2 tsp. seasoned salt

1/4 tsp. pepper

6 (5 ozs. each) chicken breast halves, skinned and rinsed

2 Tbsp. canola oil

1/4 cup water

3 Tbsp. lemon juice

2 cloves garlic, minced

1 tsp. chicken bouillon granules

1 tsp. minced fresh parsley

1. Combine oregano, salt, and pepper. Rub all of mixture into chicken. Brown chicken in canola oil in skillet. Transfer to slow cooker.

2. Place water, lemon juice, garlic, and bouillon cubes in skillet. Bring to boil, loosening browned bits from skillet. Pour over chicken.

3. Cover. Cook on High 2–2 1/2 hours, or Low 4–5 hours.

4. Add parsley and baste chicken. Cover. Cook on High 15–30 minutes, until chicken is tender.

Exchange List Values: Meat, very lean 4.0, Fat 1.5

Basic Nutritional Values: Calories 210 (Calories from Fat 71), Total Fat 8 gm (Saturated Fat 1.2 gm, Polyunsat Fat 2.1 gm, Monounsat Fat 3.8 gm, Cholesterol 84 mg), Sodium 283 mg, Total Carbohydrate 1 gm, Dietary Fiber 0 gm, Sugars 1 gm, Protein 32 gm

Melanie's Chicken Cordon Bleu

Melanie Thrower • McPherson, KS

Makes 6 servings (Ideal slow cooker size: 4-quart)

3 (1½ lbs.) whole boneless, skinless chicken breasts

6 (½ oz. per slice) pieces thinly sliced ham

6 (½ oz. per slice) thin slices reduced-fat Swiss cheese

salt to taste

pepper to taste

6 slices bacon, gently browned but not crispy, drained, and patted dry

¼ cup water

1 tsp. sodium-free chicken bouillon powder

½ cup white cooking wine

1 tsp. cornstarch

¼ cup cold water

1. Flatten chicken to ⅛"–¼" thickness. Place a slice of ham and a slice of cheese on top of each flattened breast. Sprinkle with salt and pepper. Roll up and wrap with strip of bacon. Secure with toothpick. Place in slow cooker.

2. Combine ¼ cup water, bouillon, and wine. Pour into slow cooker.

3. Cover. Cook on High 4 hours.

4. Combine cornstarch and ¼ cup cold water. Add to slow cooker. Cook until sauce thickens.

Exchange List Values: Meat, very lean 5.0, Fat 1.0

Basic Nutritional Values: Calories 231 (Calories from Fat 77), Total Fat 9 gm (Saturated Fat 3.1 gm, Polyunsat Fat 1.1 gm, Monounsat Fat 3.3 gm, Cholesterol 86 mg), Sodium 424 mg, Total Carbohydrate 1 gm, Dietary Fiber 0 gm, Sugars 0 gm, Protein 35 gm

Marcy's Barbecued Chicken

Marcy Engle • Harrisonburg, VA

Makes 6 servings (Ideal slow cooker size: 4-quart)

2 lbs. chicken pieces, skin and all visible fat removed

¼ cup flour

1 cup ketchup

2 cups water

⅓ cup Worcestershire sauce

1 tsp. chili powder

½ tsp. salt

½ tsp. pepper

2 drops Tabasco sauce

¼ tsp. garlic salt

¼ tsp. onion salt

1. Dust chicken with flour. Transfer to slow cooker.

2. Combine remaining ingredients. Pour over chicken.

3. Cover. Cook on Low 5 hours.

Exchange List Values: Carbohydrate 1.5, Meat, lean 2.0

Basic Nutritional Values: Calories 219 (Calories from Fat 37), Total Fat 4 gm (Saturated Fat 1.1 gm, Polyunsat Fat 0.9 gm, Monounsat Fat 1.4 gm, Cholesterol 66 mg), Sodium 348 mg, Total Carbohydrate 20 gm, Dietary Fiber 1 gm, Sugars 14 gm, Protein 24 gm

If you think you are having a heart attack (or someone you care about is), don't wait until you're "sure." Call 911 right away.

Levi's Sesame Chicken Wings

Shirley Unternahrer Hinh • Wayland, IA

Recipe photo appears in color section.

Makes 16 appetizer servings (Ideal slow cooker size: 4-quart)

3 lbs. chicken wings

salt to taste

pepper to taste

1 cup honey

sugar substitute to equal 6 Tbsp.

¾ cup light soy sauce

½ cup no-salt-added ketchup

2 Tbsp. canola oil

2 Tbsp. sesame oil

2 cloves garlic, minced

toasted sesame seeds

1. Rinse wings. Cut at joint. Sprinkle with salt and pepper. Place on broiler pan.

2. Broil 5" from broiler, 10 minutes on each side. Place chicken in slow cooker.

3. Combine remaining ingredients except sesame seeds. Pour over chicken.

4. Cover. Cook on Low 5 hours, or High 2½ hours.

5. Sprinkle sesame seeds over top just before serving.

6. Serve as appetizer, or with white or brown rice and shredded lettuce to turn this appetizer into a meal.

Exchange List Values: Carbohydrate 1.5, Meat, high fat 1.0

Basic Nutritional Values: Calories 192 (Calories from Fat 77), Total Fat 9 gm (Saturated Fat 1.8 gm, Polyunsat Fat 2.3 gm, Monounsat Fat 3.7 gm, Cholesterol 22 mg), Sodium 453 mg, Total Carbohydrate 21 gm, Dietary Fiber 0 gm, Sugars 21 gm, Protein 9 gm

Note: My husband and his co-workers have a "potluck lunch" at work. I think this is a nice way to break the monotony of the week or month. And it gives them a chance to share. What better way to keep it ready than in a slow cooker!

Tracy's Barbecued Chicken Wings

Tracy Supcoe • Barclay, MD

Makes 8 full-sized servings (Ideal slow cooker size: 4-quart)

4 lbs. chicken wings, skin removed

2 large onions, chopped

2 6-oz. cans tomato paste

2 large cloves garlic, minced

¼ cup Worcestershire sauce

¼ cup cider vinegar

¼ cup brown sugar

brown sugar substitute to equal 2 Tbsp.

½ cup sweet pickle relish

½ cup red, or white, wine

¼ tsp. salt

2 tsp. dry mustard

1. Cut off wing tips. Cut wings at joint. Place in slow cooker.

2. Combine remaining ingredients. Add to slow cooker. Stir.

3. Cover. Cook on Low 5–6 hours.

Exchange List Values: Carbohydrate 0.5, Vegetable 3.0, Meat, lean 2.0

Basic Nutritional Values: Calories 226 (Calories from Fat 45), Total Fat 5 gm (Saturated Fat 1.2 gm, Polyunsat Fat 1.1 gm, Monounsat Fat 1.5 gm, Cholesterol 44 mg), Sodium 369 mg, Total Carbohydrate 27 gm, Dietary Fiber 3 gm, Sugars 19 gm, Protein 19 gm

Chicken and Seafood Gumbo

Dianna Milhizer • Brighton, MI

Makes 12 servings (Ideal slow cooker size: 5–6-quart)

1 cup chopped celery

1 cup chopped onions

½ cup chopped green peppers

¼ cup olive oil

¼ cup, plus 1 Tbsp., flour

6 cups 100%-fat-free, 30–50% lower-sodium chicken broth

2 lbs. chicken, cut up, skin and visible fat removed

3 bay leaves

1½ cups sliced okra

12-oz. can diced tomatoes

1 tsp. Tabasco sauce

salt to taste

pepper to taste

1 lb. ready-to-eat shrimp

½ cup snipped fresh parsley

1. Saute celery, onions, and peppers in oil. Blend in flour and chicken broth until smooth. Cook 5 minutes. Pour into slow cooker.

2. Add remaining ingredients except seafood and parsley.

3. Cover. Cook on Low 10–12 hours.

4. One hour before serving, add shrimp and parsley.

5. Remove bay leaves before serving.

6. Serve with white rice.

Exchange List Values: Vegetable 2.0, Meat, lean 2.0

Basic Nutritional Values: Calories 162 (Calories from Fat 61), Total Fat 7 gm (Saturated Fat 1.2 gm, Polyunsat Fat 1.0 gm, Monounsat Fat 4.0 gm, Cholesterol 95 mg), Sodium 424 mg, Total Carbohydrate 7 gm, Dietary Fiber 1 gm, Sugars 3 gm, Protein 17 gm

Eat 3 vegetables and 2 fruits today—fresh or frozen is best.

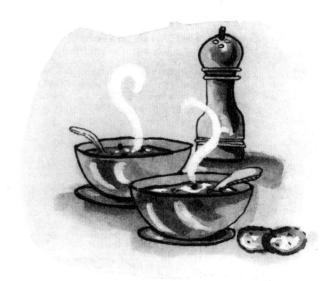

Szechwan-Style Chicken and Broccoli

Jane Meiser • Harrisonburg, VA

Makes 4 servings (Ideal slow cooker size: 4-quart)

2 whole boneless, skinless chicken or turkey breasts

1 Tbsp. canola oil

½ cup picante sauce

2 Tbsp. light soy sauce

½ tsp. sugar

½ Tbsp. quick-cooking tapioca

1 medium onion, chopped

2 cloves garlic, minced

½ tsp. ground ginger

2 cups broccoli florets

1 medium red pepper, cut into pieces

1. Cut meat into 1" cubes and brown lightly in oil in skillet. Place in slow cooker.

2. Stir in remaining ingredients.

3. Cover. Cook on High 1–1½ hours, or on Low 2–3 hours.

Exchange List Values: Vegetable 2.0, Meat, very lean 4.0, Fat 1.0

Basic Nutritional Values: Calories 254 (Calories from Fat 64), Total Fat 7 gm (Saturated Fat 1.2 gm, Polyunsat Fat 1.9 gm, Monounsat Fat 3.2 gm, Cholesterol 84 mg), Sodium 619 mg, Total Carbohydrate 12 gm, Dietary Fiber 3 gm, Sugars 7 gm, Protein 35 gm

Greek Chicken

Judy Govotsus • Monrovia, MD

Makes 4–6 servings (Ideal slow cooker size: 4-quart)

4 potatoes, unpeeled, quartered

2 lbs. chicken pieces, trimmed of skin and fat

2 large onions, quartered

1 whole bulb garlic, minced

3 tsp. dried oregano

¾ tsp. salt

½ tsp. pepper

1 Tbsp. olive oil

1. Place potatoes in bottom of slow cooker. Add chicken, onions, and garlic. Sprinkle with seasonings. Top with oil.

2. Cover. Cook on High 5–6 hours, or on Low 9–10 hours.

Exchange List Values: Starch 1.5, Vegetable 2.0, Meat, lean 2.0

Basic Nutritional Values: Calories 278 (Calories from Fat 56), Total Fat 6 gm (Saturated Fat 1.3 gm, Polyunsat Fat 1.1 gm, Monounsat Fat 3.0 gm, Cholesterol 65 mg), Sodium 358 mg, Total Carbohydrate 29 gm, Dietary Fiber 4 gm, Sugars 9 gm, Protein 27 gm

Chicken Casablanca

Joyce Kaut • Rochester, NY

Makes 6-8 servings (Ideal slow cooker size: 4-5-quart)

2 large onions, sliced

1 tsp. ground ginger

3 cloves garlic, minced

2 Tbsp. canola oil

3 large carrots, diced

2 large potatoes, unpeeled, diced

3 lbs. skinless chicken pieces

1/2 tsp. ground cumin

1/2 tsp. salt

1/2 tsp. pepper

1/4 tsp. cinnamon

2 Tbsp. raisins

14 1/2-oz. can chopped tomatoes

3 small zucchini, sliced

15-oz. can garbanzo beans, drained

2 Tbsp. chopped parsley

1. Saute onions, ginger, and garlic in oil in skillet. (Reserve oil.) Transfer to slow cooker. Add carrots and potatoes. Transfer to slow cooker, reserving oil.

2. Brown chicken over medium heat in reserved oil. Transfer to slow cooker. Mix gently with vegetables.

3. Combine seasonings in separate bowl. Sprinkle over chicken and vegetables. Add raisins and tomatoes.

4. Cover. Cook on High 4-6 hours.

5. Add sliced zucchini, beans, and parsley 30 minutes before serving.

6. Serve over cooked rice or couscous.

Exchange List Values: Starch 2.0, Vegetable 2.0, Meat, lean 3.0, Fat 0.5

Basic Nutritional Values: Calories 395 (Calories from Fat 93), Total Fat 10 gm (Saturated Fat 1.9 gm, Polyunsat Fat 2.9 gm, Monounsat Fat 4.3 gm, Cholesterol 87 mg), Sodium 390 mg, Total Carbohydrate 40 gm, Dietary Fiber 8 gm, Sugars 12 gm, Protein 36 gm

VARIATION: Add 1/2 tsp. turmeric and 1/4 tsp. cayenne pepper to Step 3.

Michelle Mann • Mt. Joy, PA

You can cut back on the number of calories you get each day and still eat your favorite foods—just reduce how much of them you eat. Control your portion sizes to control your weight!

Cathy's Chicken Creole

Cathy Boshart • Lebanon, PA

Makes 6 servings (Ideal slow cooker size: 4-quart)

2 Tbsp. canola oil

half a medium green pepper, chopped

2 medium onions, chopped

1/2 cup chopped celery

1-lb., 4-oz. can tomatoes

1/2 tsp. pepper, or your choice of dried herbs

1/8 tsp. red pepper

3/4 tsp. salt, or your choice of dried herbs

1 cup water

2 Tbsp. cornstarch

1 tsp. sugar

1 1/2 Tbsp. cold water

2 cups cooked and cubed chicken

6 green, or black, olives, sliced

1/2 cup sliced mushrooms

1. Place oil in slow cooker. Add green pepper, onions, and celery. Heat.

2. Add tomatoes, peppers, salt, and 1 cup water.

3. Cover. Cook on High while preparing remaining ingredients.

4. Combine cornstarch and sugar. Add 1 1/2 Tbsp. cold water and make a smooth paste. Stir into mixture in slow cooker. Add chicken, olives, and mushrooms.

5. Cover. Cook on Low 2–3 hours.

Exchange List Values: Vegetable 2.0, Meat, lean 2.0, Fat 0.5

Basic Nutritional Values: Calories 190 (Calories from Fat 79), Total Fat 9 gm (Saturated Fat 1.3 gm, Polyunsat Fat 2.3 gm, Monounsat Fat 4.3 gm, Cholesterol 42 mg), Sodium 521 mg, Total Carbohydrate 13 gm, Dietary Fiber 3 gm, Sugars 7 gm, Protein 15 gm

Mulligan Stew

Carol Ambrose • Ripon, CA

Makes 8 servings (Ideal slow cooker size: 4–5-quart)

3 lbs. stewing chicken, cut up, trimmed of skin and fat

1/2 tsp. salt

1 oz. salt pork, or bacon, cut in 1" squares

4 cups tomatoes, peeled and sliced

2 cups fresh corn, or 1-lb. pkg. frozen corn

1 cup coarsely chopped potatoes

10-oz. pkg. lima beans, frozen

1/2 cup chopped onions

1 tsp. salt

1/4 tsp. pepper

dash cayenne pepper

1. Place chicken in very large slow cooker. Add water to cover. Add 1/2 tsp. salt.

2. Cover. Cook on Low 2 hours. Add more water if needed.

3. Add remaining ingredients. (If you don't have a large cooker, divide the stew between 2 average-sized ones.) Simmer on Low 5 hours longer.

Exchange List Values: Starch 1.0, Vegetable 1.0, Meat, lean 2.0, Fat 0.5

Basic Nutritional Values: Calories 241 (Calories from Fat 68), Total Fat 8 gm (Saturated Fat 2.2 gm, Polyunsat Fat 1.5 gm, Monounsat Fat 3.0 gm, Cholesterol 52 mg), Sodium 563 mg, Total Carbohydrate 24 gm, Dietary Fiber 5 gm, Sugars 5 gm, Protein 21 gm

Notes:

1. Flavor improves if stew is refrigerated and reheated the next day. May also be made in advance and frozen.

2. You can debone the chicken after Step 2. Add the pieces back into cooker and continue with directions.

Marsha's Chicken Enchilada Casserole

Marsha Sabus • Falibrook, CA

Makes 4–6 servings (Ideal slow cooker size: 4–5-quart)

1 onion, chopped

1 clove garlic, minced

1 Tbsp. oil

10-oz. can enchilada sauce

8-oz. can no-salt-added tomato sauce

salt to taste

pepper to taste

8 corn tortillas

3 boneless chicken breast halves, cooked and cubed

15-oz. can ranch-style beans, drained

11-oz. can Mexicorn, drained

4 ozs. reduced-fat cheddar cheese, grated

2¼-oz. can sliced black olives, drained

1. Saute onion and garlic in oil in saucepan. Stir in enchilada sauce and tomato sauce. Season with salt and pepper.

2. Place two tortillas in bottom of slow cooker. Layer one-third of chicken on top. Top with one-third sauce mixture, one-third beans, one-third corn, one-third cheese, and one-third black olives. Repeat layers 2 more times. Top with 2 tortillas.

3. Cover. Cook on Low 6–8 hours.

Exchange List Values: Starch 2.5, Vegetable 1.0, Meat, lean 2.0, Fat 1.0

Basic Nutritional Values: Calories 370 (Calories from Fat 110), Total Fat 12 gm (Saturated Fat 3.3 gm, Polyunsat Fat 2.2 gm, Monounsat Fat 4.6 gm, Cholesterol 55 mg), Sodium 619 mg, Total Carbohydrate 43 gm, Dietary Fiber 8 gm, Sugars 7 gm, Protein 28 gm

VARIATION: Substitute 1 lb. cooked and drained hamburger for the chicken.

Cut the fat in at least one meal today.

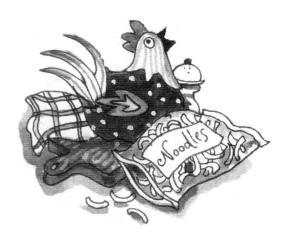

Gran's Big Potluck

Carol Ambrose • Ripon, CA

Makes 10 servings (Ideal slow cooker size: 5–6-quart)

2½-lb. stewing hen, cut into pieces, trimmed of skin and fat

½ lb. stewing beef, cubed, trimmed of skin and fat

½-lb. veal shoulder, or roast, trimmed of skin and fat, cubed

1½ qts. water

½ lb. small red potatoes, cubed

½ lb. small onions, cut in half

1 cup sliced carrots

1 cup chopped celery

1 medium green pepper, chopped

1-lb. pkg. frozen lima beans

1 cup okra, whole or diced, fresh or frozen

1 cup frozen whole-kernel corn

8-oz. can whole tomatoes with juice

15-oz. can tomato puree

1 tsp. salt

¼–½ tsp. pepper

1 tsp. dry mustard

½ tsp. chili powder

¼ cup chopped fresh parsley

1. Combine all ingredients except last 5 seasonings in one very large slow cooker, or divide between two medium-sized ones.

2. Cover. Cook on Low 10–12 hours. Add seasonings during last hour of cooking.

Exchange List Values: Starch 1.0, Vegetable 2.0, Meat, lean 2.0

Basic Nutritional Values: Calories 242 (Calories from Fat 42), Total Fat 5 gm (Saturated Fat 1.2 gm, Polyunsat Fat 0.9 gm, Monounsat Fat 1.6 gm, Cholesterol 63 mg), Sodium 535 mg, Total Carbohydrate 26 gm, Dietary Fiber 6 gm, Sugars 7 gm, Protein 25 gm

Note: You may want to debone the chicken and mix it back into the cooker before serving the meal.

Chicken and Stuffing

Janice Yoskovich • Carmichaels, PA /
Jo Ellen Moore • Pendleton, IN

Makes 14–16 side-dish servings (Ideal slow cooker size: 6-quart)

2½ tsp. sodium-free chicken bouillon powder

2½ cups water

¼ cup canola oil

½ cup chopped onions

½ cup chopped celery

4-oz. can mushrooms, stems and pieces, drained

¼ cup dried parsley flakes

1½ tsp. rubbed sage

1 tsp. poultry seasoning

½ tsp. salt

½ tsp. pepper

12 cups day-old bread cubes (½" pieces)

2 eggs

10¾-oz. can 98%-fat-free, reduced-sodium cream of chicken soup

5 cups cubed cooked chicken

1. Combine all ingredients except bread, eggs, soup, and chicken in large saucepan. Simmer for 10 minutes.

2. Place bread cubes in large bowl.

3. Combine eggs and soup. Stir into broth mixture until smooth. Pour over bread and toss well.

4. Layer half of stuffing and then half of chicken into very large slow cooker (or two medium-sized cookers). Repeat layers.

5. Cover. Cook on Low 4½–5 hours.

Exchange List Values: Starch 1.0, Meat, lean 2.0, Fat 0.5

Basic Nutritional Values: Calories 215 (Calories from Fat 78), Total Fat 9 gm (Saturated Fat 1.6 gm, Polyunsat Fat 2.5 gm, Monounsat Fat 3.7 gm, Cholesterol 67 mg), Sodium 362 mg, Total Carbohydrate 16 gm, Dietary Fiber 1 gm, Sugars 2 gm, Protein 16 gm

Joyce's Chicken Tetrazzini

Joyce Slaymaker • Strasburg, PA

Makes 4 servings (Ideal slow cooker size: 3–4-quart)

2 cups diced cooked chicken

2 tsp. sodium-free chicken bouillon powder

2 cups water

1 small onion, chopped

¼ cup sauterne, white wine, or milk

½ cup slivered almonds

2 4-oz. cans sliced mushrooms, drained

10¾-oz. can 98%-fat-free, reduced-sodium cream of mushroom soup

6 ozs. raw spaghetti, cooked

1. Combine all ingredients except spaghetti in slow cooker.

2. Cover. Cook on Low 6–8 hours.

3. Serve over spaghetti. Sprinkle with Parmesan cheese, if you wish.

Exchange List Values: Starch 2.0, Carbohydrate 1.0, Vegetable 1.0, Meat, lean 3.0, Fat 1.0

Basic Nutritional Values: Calories 469 (Calories from Fat 139), Total Fat 15 gm (Saturated Fat 2.8 gm, Polyunsat Fat 3.7 gm, Monounsat Fat 7.1 gm, Cholesterol 63 mg), Sodium 528 mg, Total Carbohydrate 48 gm, Dietary Fiber 6 gm, Sugars 6 gm, Protein 33 gm

VARIATIONS:

1. Place spaghetti in large baking dish. Pour sauce in center. Sprinkle with Parmesan cheese. Broil until lightly browned.

2. Add 10-oz. pkg. frozen peas to Step 1.

Darlene Raber • Wellman, IA

Chicken and Dumplings

Elva Ever • North English, IA

Recipe photo appears in color section.

Makes 8–10 servings (Ideal slow cooker size: 4-quart)

4 whole chicken breasts, or 1 small chicken

$3/4$ cup sliced carrots

$1/4$ cup chopped onions

$1/4$ cup chopped celery

$1\frac{1}{2}$ cups peas

4–6 Tbsp. flour

1 cup water

salt to taste

pepper to taste

1 cup buttermilk baking mix to make dumplings

paprika to taste

1. Cook chicken in water in soup pot. Cool, skin, and debone chicken. Return broth to boiling in soup pot.

2. Cook vegetables in microwave on High for 5 minutes.

3. Meanwhile, combine flour and water until smooth. Add to boiling chicken broth. Add enough extra water to make 4 cups broth, making sure gravy is fairly thick. Season with salt and pepper.

4. Combine chicken, vegetables, and gravy in slow cooker.

5. Mix dumplings as directed on baking mix box. Place dumplings on top of chicken in slow cooker. Sprinkle with paprika.

6. Cover. Cook on High 3 hours.

Exchange List Values: Starch 1.0, Meat, very lean 4.0

Basic Nutritional Values: Calories 222 (Calories from Fat 43), Total Fat 5 gm (Saturated Fat 0.8 gm, Polyunsat Fat 1.4 gm, Monounsat Fat 1.6 gm, Cholesterol 67 mg), Sodium 248 mg, Total Carbohydrate 15 gm, Dietary Fiber 2 gm, Sugars 3 gm, Protein 28 gm

Barbecue Chicken for Buns

Linda Sluiter • Schererville, IN

Makes 16–20 servings (Ideal slow cooker size: 4-quart)

6 cups diced cooked chicken

2 cups chopped celery

1 cup chopped onions

1 cup chopped green peppers

2 Tbsp. canola oil

2 cups ketchup

2 cups water

2 Tbsp. brown sugar

4 Tbsp. vinegar

2 tsp. dry mustard

1 tsp. pepper

$1/2$ tsp. salt

1. Combine all ingredients in slow cooker.

2. Cover. Cook on Low 8 hours.

3. Stir chicken until it shreds.

4. Pile into steak rolls and serve.

Exchange List Values: Carbohydrate 0.5, Meat, lean 2.0

Basic Nutritional Values: Calories 131 (Calories from Fat 43), Total Fat 5 gm (Saturated Fat 1.0 gm, Polyunsat Fat 1.1 gm, Monounsat Fat 1.9 gm, Cholesterol 37 mg), Sodium 391 mg, Total Carbohydrate 10 gm, Dietary Fiber 1 gm, Sugars 5 gm, Protein 13 gm

Chicken Reuben Bake

Gail Bush • Landenberg, PA

Makes 6 servings (Ideal slow cooker size: 4-quart)

4 boneless, skinless chicken breast halves

1-lb. bag sauerkraut, drained and rinsed

4–5 (1 oz. each) slices Swiss cheese

¾ cup fat-free Thousand Island salad dressing

2 Tbsp. chopped fresh parsley

1. Place chicken in slow cooker. Layer sauerkraut over chicken. Add cheese. Top with salad dressing. Sprinkle with parsley.

2. Cover. Cook on Low 6–8 hours.

Exchange List Values: Carbohydrate 1.0, Meat, very lean 4.0

Basic Nutritional Values: Calories 217 (Calories from Fat 41), Total Fat 5 gm (Saturated Fat 2.0 gm, Polyunsat Fat 0.6 gm, Monounsat Fat 1.4 gm, Cholesterol 63 mg), Sodium 693 mg, Total Carbohydrate 13 gm, Dietary Fiber 2 gm, Sugars 6 gm, Protein 28 gm

Order a vegetarian meal the next time you fly—they're tasty and usually low in cholesterol and saturated fat.

Turkey in a Pot

Dorothy M. Pittman • Pickens, SC

Makes 10–12 servings (Ideal slow cooker size: 6-quart)

4–5-lb. turkey breast, skin removed (if frozen, it doesn't have to be thawed)

1 medium onion, chopped

1 rib celery, chopped

¼ cup melted margarine

1½ cups chicken broth

1. Wash turkey breast. Pat dry. Place in greased slow cooker. Put onion and celery in cavity.

2. Pour margarine over turkey. Pour broth around turkey.

3. Cover. Cook on High 6 hours. Let stand 10 minutes before carving.

Exchange List Values: Meat, very lean 4.0, Fat 0.5

Basic Nutritional Values: Calories 160 (Calories from Fat 45), Total Fat 5 gm (Saturated Fat 0.8 gm, Polyunsat Fat 1.3 gm, Monounsat Fat 1.8 gm, Cholesterol 70 mg), Sodium 287 mg, Total Carbohydrate 1 gm, Dietary Fiber 0 gm, Sugars 1 gm, Protein 26 gm

Note: You may wish to season the turkey with salt and lemon-pepper seasoning to taste.

Slow Cooker Turkey Breast

Liz Ann Yoder • Hartville, OH

Makes 12 servings (Ideal slow cooker size: 6–7-quart)

6-lb. turkey breast, skin and visible fat removed

2 tsp. oil

salt to taste

pepper to taste

1 medium onion, quartered

4 cloves garlic, peeled

1. Rinse turkey and pat dry with paper towels.

2. Rub oil over turkey. Sprinkle with salt and pepper. Place, meaty side up, in large slow cooker.

3. Place onion and garlic around sides of cooker.

4. Cover. Cook on Low 9–10 hours, or until meat thermometer stuck in meaty part of breast registers 170°.

5. Remove from slow cooker and let stand 10 minutes before slicing.

6. Serve with mashed potatoes, cranberry salad, and corn or green beans.

Exchange List Values: Meat, very lean 5.0

Basic Nutritional Values: Calories 187 (Calories from Fat 16), Total Fat 2 gm (Saturated Fat 0.4 gm, Polyunsat Fat 0.5 gm, Monounsat Fat 0.6 gm, Cholesterol 107 mg), Sodium 68 mg, Total Carbohydrate 1 gm, Dietary Fiber 0 gm, Sugars 1 gm, Protein 39 gm

VARIATIONS:

1. Add carrot chunks and chopped celery to Step 3 to add more flavor to the turkey broth.

2. Reserve broth for soups, or thicken with flour-water paste and serve as gravy over sliced turkey.

3. Freeze broth in pint-sized containers for future use.

4. Debone turkey and freeze in pint-sized containers for future use. Or freeze any leftover turkey after serving the meal described above.

Easy and Delicious Turkey Breast

Gail Bush • Landenberg, PA

Makes 12 servings (Ideal slow cooker size: 6-quart)

5-lb. turkey breast, bone in, skin removed

15-oz. can whole berry cranberry sauce

1 envelope dry onion soup mix

½ cup orange juice

½ tsp. salt

¼ tsp. pepper

1. Place turkey in slow cooker.

2. Combine remaining ingredients. Pour over turkey.

3. Cover. Cook on Low 6–8 hours.

Exchange List Values: Carbohydrate 1.0, Meat, very lean 4.0

Basic Nutritional Values: Calories 210 (Calories from Fat 12), Total Fat 1 gm (Saturated Fat 0 gm, Polyunsat Fat 0.1 gm, Monounsat Fat 0.1 gm, Cholesterol 87 mg), Sodium 391 mg, Total Carbohydrate 16 gm, Dietary Fiber 1 gm, Sugars 15 gm, Protein 33 gm

Turkey Breast

Barbara Katrine Rose • Woodbridge, VA

Makes 6–8 servings (Ideal slow cooker size: 6-quart)

1 large (4½ lbs.) boneless turkey breast, skin removed

¼ cup apple cider, or juice

1 tsp. salt

¼ tsp. pepper

1. Put turkey breast in slow cooker. Drizzle apple cider over turkey. Sprinkle on both sides with salt and pepper.

2. Cover. Cook on High 3–4 hours.

3. Remove turkey breast. Let stand for 15 minutes before slicing.

Exchange List Values: Meat, very lean 4.0

Basic Nutritional Values: Calories 150 (Calories from Fat 10), Total Fat 1 gm (Saturated Fat 0 gm, Polyunsat Fat 0 gm, Monounsat Fat 0 gm, Cholesterol 89 mg), Sodium 252 mg, Total Carbohydrate 1 gm, Dietary Fiber 0 gm, Sugars 1 gm, Protein 33 gm

Turkey Breast with Orange Sauce

Jean Butzer • Batavia, NY

Makes 4–6 servings (Ideal slow cooker size: 4–5-quart)

1 large onion, chopped

3 cloves garlic, minced

1 tsp. dried rosemary

½ tsp. pepper

2-lb. boneless, skinless turkey breast

1½ cups orange juice

1. Place onions in slow cooker.

2. Combine garlic, rosemary, and pepper.

3. Make gashes in turkey, about ¾ of the way through at 2" intervals. Stuff with herb mixture. Place turkey in slow cooker.

4. Pour juice over turkey.

5. Cover. Cook on Low 7–8 hours, or until turkey is no longer pink in center.

Exchange List Values: Fruit 0.5, Meat, very lean 4.0

Basic Nutritional Values: Calories 178 (Calories from Fat 8), Total Fat 1 gm (Saturated Fat 0.3 gm, Polyunsat Fat 0.3 gm, Monounsat Fat 0.2 gm, Cholesterol 81 mg), Sodium 53 mg, Total Carbohydrate 10 gm, Dietary Fiber 1 gm, Sugars 9 gm, Protein 30 gm

This very easy, impressive-looking and tasting recipe is perfect for company.

Stuffed Turkey Breast

Jean Butzer • Batavia, NY

Recipe photo appears in color section.

Makes 12 servings (Ideal slow cooker size: 5–6-quart)

¼ cup margarine, melted

1 small onion, finely chopped

½ cup finely chopped celery

2½-oz. pkg. croutons with real bacon bits

1 cup chicken broth

2 Tbsp. fresh minced parsley

½ tsp. poultry seasoning

1 whole uncooked turkey breast, or 2 halves (about 5 lbs.), skin and visible fat removed

salt to taste

pepper to taste

24" x 26" piece of cheesecloth for each breast half

dry white wine

1. Combine margarine, onion, celery, croutons, broth, parsley, and poultry seasoning.

2. Cut turkey breast in thick slices from breastbone to rib cage, leaving slices attached to bone (crosswise across breast).

3. Sprinkle turkey with salt and pepper.

4. Soak cheesecloth in wine. Place turkey on cheesecloth. Stuff bread mixture into slits between turkey slices. Fold one end of cheesecloth over the other to cover meat. Place on metal rack or trivet in 5- or 6-qt. slow cooker.

5. Cover. Cook on Low 7–9 hours, or until tender. Pour additional wine over turkey during cooking.

6. Remove from pot and remove cheesecloth immediately. If you prefer the breast to be browner, remove from pot and brown in 400° oven for 15–20 minutes. Let stand 10 minutes before slicing through and serving.

Exchange List Values: Starch 0.5, Meat, very lean 5.0, Fat 0.5

Basic Nutritional Values: Calories 216 (Calories from Fat 57), Total Fat 6 gm (Saturated Fat 1.0 gm, Polyunsat Fat 1.4 gm, Monounsat Fat 2.4 gm, Cholesterol 89 mg), Sodium 341 mg, Total Carbohydrate 5 gm, Dietary Fiber 1 gm, Sugars 1 gm, Protein 34 gm

VARIATION: Thicken the drippings, if you wish, for gravy. Mix together 3 Tbsp. cornstarch and ¼ cup cold water. When smooth, stir into broth (with turkey removed from cooker). Turn cooker to High and stir until cornstarch paste is dissolved. Allow to cook for about 10 minutes, until broth is thickened and smooth.

Slow Cooker Turkey and Dressing

Carol Sherwood • Batavia, NY

Makes 8 servings (Ideal slow cooker size: 5-6-quart)

8-oz. pkg. herb-flavored stuffing mix

½ cup hot water

2 Tbsp. butter, softened

1 onion, chopped

½ cup chopped celery

¼ cup sweetened, dried cranberries

3-lb. boneless turkey breast

¼ tsp. dried basil

½ tsp. pepper

1. Spread dry stuffing mix in greased slow cooker.

2. Add water, butter, onion, celery, and cranberries. Mix well.

3. Sprinkle turkey breast with basil and pepper. Place over stuffing mixture.

4. Cover. Cook on Low 5–6 hours, or until turkey is done but not dry.

5. Remove turkey. Slice and set aside.

6. Gently stir stuffing and allow to sit for 5 minutes before serving.

7. Place stuffing on platter, topped with sliced turkey.

Exchange List Values: Starch 2.0, Meat, very lean 4.0

Basic Nutritional Values: Calories 307 (Calories from Fat 34), Total Fat 4 gm (Saturated Fat 2.1 gm, Polyunsat Fat 0.3 gm, Monounsat Fat 1.0 gm, Cholesterol 99 mg), Sodium 488 mg, Total Carbohydrate 26 gm, Dietary Fiber 3 gm, Sugars 5 gm, Protein 37 gm

Zucchini and Turkey Dish

Dolores Kratz • Souderton, PA

Makes 6 servings (Ideal slow cooker size: 3-4-quart)

3 cups zucchini, sliced

1 small onion, chopped

¼ tsp. salt

1 cup cubed cooked turkey

2 fresh tomatoes, sliced, or 14½-oz. can diced tomatoes

½ tsp. dried oregano

1 tsp. dried basil

¼ cup freshly grated Parmesan cheese

6 Tbsp. shredded provolone cheese

¾ cup Pepperidge Farms stuffing

1. Combine zucchini, onion, salt, turkey, tomatoes, oregano, and basil in slow cooker. Mix well.

2. Top with cheeses and stuffing.

3. Cover. Cook on Low 8–9 hours.

Exchange List Values: Starch 0.5, Vegetable 1.0, Meat, lean 1.0

Basic Nutritional Values: Calories 128 (Calories from Fat 39), Total Fat 4 gm (Saturated Fat 2.3 gm, Polyunsat Fat 0.5 gm, Monounsat Fat 1.2 gm, Cholesterol 23 mg), Sodium 312 mg, Total Carbohydrate 12 gm, Dietary Fiber 2 gm, Sugars 4 gm, Protein 11 gm

Slow-Cooked Turkey Dinner

Miriam Nolt • New Holland, PA

Makes 6 servings (Ideal slow cooker size: 4-5-quart)

1 onion, diced

6 (1 lb. total) small red potatoes, quartered

2 cups sliced carrots

1½ lbs. boneless, skinless turkey thighs

¼ cup flour

2 Tbsp. Sodium-Free Onion Soup Mix (see recipe on page 334)

10¾-oz. can 98%-fat-free, reduced-sodium cream of mushroom soup

⅔ cup fat-free, reduced-sodium chicken broth

1. Place vegetables in bottom of slow cooker.

2. Place turkey thighs over vegetables.

3. Combine remaining ingredients. Pour over turkey.

4. Cover. Cook on High 30 minutes. Reduce heat to Low and cook 7 hours.

Exchange List Values: Starch 1.5, Vegetable 1.0, Meat, lean 2.0

Basic Nutritional Values: Calories 274 (Calories from Fat 58), Total Fat 6 gm (Saturated Fat 2.2 gm, Polyunsat Fat 1.9 gm, Monounsat Fat 1.4 gm, Cholesterol 61 mg), Sodium 571 mg, Total Carbohydrate 29 gm, Dietary Fiber 4 gm, Sugars 6 gm, Protein 25 gm

Barbecued Turkey Legs

Barbara Walker • Sturgis, SC

Makes 4-6 servings (Ideal slow cooker size: 4-5-quart)

4 small skinless turkey drumsticks

¼-½ tsp. pepper

¼ cup molasses

¼ cup vinegar

½ cup ketchup

3 Tbsp. Worcestershire sauce

¾ tsp. hickory smoke

2 Tbsp. instant minced onion

1. Sprinkle turkey with pepper. Place in slow cooker.

2. Combine remaining ingredients. Pour over turkey.

3. Cover. Cook on Low 5-7 hours.

Exchange List Values: Carbohydrate 1.0, Meat, lean 4.0

Basic Nutritional Values: Calories 319 (Calories from Fat 87), Total Fat 10 gm (Saturated Fat 3.2 gm, Polyunsat Fat 2.9 gm, Monounsat Fat 2.2 gm, Cholesterol 112 mg), Sodium 445 mg, Total Carbohydrate 18 gm, Dietary Fiber 0 gm, Sugars 13 gm, Protein 38 gm

Barbecued Turkey Cutlets

Maricarol Magill • Freehold, NJ

Makes 6–8 servings (Ideal slow cooker size: 4-quart)

6–8 (2 lbs.) turkey cutlets

$\frac{1}{4}$ cup molasses

$\frac{1}{4}$ cup cider vinegar

$\frac{1}{4}$ cup ketchup

3 Tbsp. Worcestershire sauce

1 tsp. garlic salt

3 Tbsp. chopped onion

2 Tbsp. brown sugar

$\frac{1}{4}$ tsp. pepper

1. Place turkey cutlets in slow cooker.

2. Combine remaining ingredients. Pour over turkey.

3. Cover. Cook on Low 4 hours.

4. Serve over white or brown rice.

Exchange List Values: Carbohydrate 1.0, Meat, very lean 3.0

Basic Nutritional Values: Calories 155 (Calories from Fat 5), Total Fat 1 gm (Saturated Fat 0.2 gm, Polyunsat Fat 0.2 gm, Monounsat Fat 0.1 gm, Cholesterol 61 mg), Sodium 365 mg, Total Carbohydrate 14 gm, Dietary Fiber 0 gm, Sugars 12 gm, Protein 22 gm

Turkey and Sweet Potato Casserole

Michele Ruvola • Selden, NY

Makes 4 servings (Ideal slow cooker size: 4-quart)

3 medium ($6\frac{1}{4}$–$6\frac{1}{2}$ ozs. each) sweet potatoes, peeled and cut into 2" pieces

10-oz. pkg. frozen cut green beans

$1\frac{1}{2}$ lbs. turkey cutlets

12-oz. jar home-style turkey gravy

2 Tbsp. flour

1 tsp. parsley flakes

$\frac{1}{4}$–$\frac{1}{2}$ tsp. dried rosemary leaves, crumbled

$\frac{1}{8}$ tsp. pepper

1. Layer sweet potatoes, green beans, and turkey in slow cooker.

2. Combine remaining ingredients until smooth. Pour over mixture in slow cooker.

3. Cover. Cook on Low 8–10 hours.

4. Remove turkey and vegetables and keep warm. Stir sauce. Serve with sauce over meat and vegetables, or with sauce in a gravy boat.

5. Serve with biscuits and cranberry sauce.

Exchange List Values: Starch 2.0, Vegetable 1.0, Meat, very lean 4.0

Basic Nutritional Values: Calories 318 (Calories from Fat 24), Total Fat 3 gm (Saturated Fat 0.3 gm, Polyunsat Fat 0.7 gm, Monounsat Fat 0.9 gm, Cholesterol 93 mg), Sodium 473 mg, Total Carbohydrate 35 gm, Dietary Fiber 4 gm, Sugars 7 gm, Protein 37 gm

Savory Turkey Meatballs in Italian Sauce

Marla Folkerts • Holland, OH

Makes 8 servings (Ideal slow cooker size: 4-quart)

28-oz. can crushed tomatoes

1 Tbsp. red wine vinegar

1 medium onion, finely chopped

2 cloves garlic, minced

¼ tsp. Italian herb seasoning

1 tsp. dried basil

1 lb. ground turkey

⅛ tsp. garlic powder

⅛ tsp. black pepper

⅓ cup dried parsley

2 egg whites

¼ tsp. dried minced onion

⅓ cup quick oats

¼ cup grated Parmesan cheese

¼ cup flour

2 Tbsp. canola oil

1. Combine tomatoes, vinegar, onions, garlic, Italian seasonings, and basil in slow cooker. Turn to Low.

2. Combine remaining ingredients, except flour and oil. Form into 1" balls. Dredge each ball in flour. Brown in oil in skillet over medium heat. Drain. Transfer to slow cooker. Stir into sauce.

3. Cover. Cook on Low 6–8 hours.

4. Serve over pasta or rice.

Exchange List Values: Starch 0.5, Vegetable 2.0, Meat, lean 2.0, Fat 0.5

Basic Nutritional Values: Calories 226 (Calories from Fat 94), Total Fat 10 gm (Saturated Fat 2.4 gm, Polyunsat Fat 2.5 gm, Monounsat Fat 4.5 gm, Cholesterol 46 mg), Sodium 402 mg, Total Carbohydrate 16 gm, Dietary Fiber 3 gm, Sugars 7 gm, Protein 17 gm

Note: The meatballs and sauce freeze well.

People with diabetes should see their doctor at least twice a year.

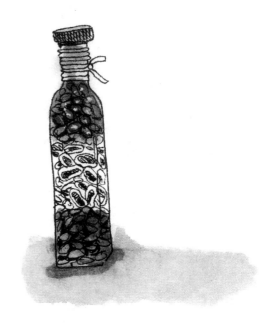

Turkey Sloppy Joes

Marla Folkerts • Holland, OH

Makes 6 servings (Ideal slow cooker size: 4-quart)

1 red onion, chopped

1 sweet pepper, chopped

1½ lbs. boneless cooked turkey, finely chopped

1 cup no-salt-added ketchup

½ tsp. salt

1 clove garlic, minced

1 tsp. Dijon-style mustard

⅛ tsp. pepper

6 (1½ ozs. each) multigrain sandwich rolls

1. Place onion, sweet pepper, and turkey in slow cooker.

2. Combine ketchup, salt, garlic, mustard, and pepper. Pour over turkey mixture. Mix well.

3. Cover. Cook on Low 4½–6 hours.

4. Serve on sandwich rolls.

Exchange List Values: Starch 1.5, Vegetable 3.0, Meat, lean 1.0, Fat 0.5

Basic Nutritional Values: Calories 271 (Calories from Fat 49), Total Fat 5 gm (Saturated Fat 1.6 gm, Polyunsat Fat 1.3 gm, Monounsat Fat 1.8 gm, Cholesterol 40 mg), Sodium 457 mg, Total Carbohydrate 36 gm, Dietary Fiber 3 gm, Sugars 16 gm, Protein 21 gm

Tricia's Cranberry Turkey Meatballs

Shirley Unternahrer Hinh • Wayland, IA

Makes 12 servings (Ideal slow cooker size: 4-quart)

16-oz. can jellied cranberry sauce

½ cup ketchup or barbecue sauce

1 egg

1 lb. ground turkey

half a small onion, chopped

1 tsp. salt

¼ tsp. black pepper

1–2 tsp. grated orange peel, optional

1. Combine cranberry sauce and ketchup in slow cooker.

2. Cover. Cook on High until sauce is mixed.

3. Combine remaining ingredients. Shape into 24 balls.

4. Cook over medium heat in skillet for 8–10 minutes, or just until browned. Add to sauce in slow cooker.

5. Cover. Cook on Low 3 hours.

6. Serve with rice and a steamed vegetable.

Exchange List Values: Carbohydrate 1.0, Meat, lean 1.0

Basic Nutritional Values: Calories 134 (Calories from Fat 34), Total Fat 4 gm (Saturated Fat 0.9 gm, Polyunsat Fat 0.9 gm, Monounsat Fat 1.4 gm, Cholesterol 28 mg), Sodium 353 mg, Total Carbohydrate 18 gm, Dietary Fiber 1 gm, Sugars 15 gm, Protein 8 gm

Turkey Meatballs and Gravy

Betty Sue Good • Broadway, VA

Makes 10 servings (Ideal slow cooker size: 4-quart)

2 eggs, beaten

$3/4$ cup bread crumbs

$1/2$ cup finely chopped onions

$1/2$ cup finely chopped celery

2 Tbsp. chopped fresh parsley

$1/4$ tsp. pepper

$1/8$ tsp. garlic powder

$1\frac{1}{2}$ lbs. ground turkey

$1\frac{1}{2}$ Tbsp. canola oil

$10\frac{3}{4}$-oz. can 99%-fat-free, reduced-sodium cream of mushroom soup

1 cup water

$7/8$-oz. pkg. turkey gravy mix

$1/2$ tsp. dried thyme

2 bay leaves

1. Combine eggs, bread crumbs, onions, celery, parsley, pepper, garlic powder, and meat. Shape into $3/4$" balls.

2. Brown meatballs in oil in skillet. Drain meatballs and pat dry. Transfer to slow cooker.

3. Combine soup, water, dry gravy mix, thyme, and bay leaves. Pour over meatballs.

4. Cover. Cook on Low 6–8 hours, or High 3–4 hours. Discard bay leaves before serving.

5. Serve over mashed potatoes or buttered noodles.

Exchange List Values: Starch 0.5, Carbohydrate 0.5, Meat, lean 2.0, Fat 0.5

Basic Nutritional Values: Calories 212 (Calories from Fat 97), Total Fat 11 gm (Saturated Fat 2.5 gm, Polyunsat Fat 2.7 gm, Monounsat Fat 4.4 gm, Cholesterol 94 mg), Sodium 365 mg, Total Carbohydrate 11 gm, Dietary Fiber 1 gm, Sugars 2 gm, Protein 17 gm

Oils are good for your heart. The solid fats—butter, margarine, shortening, and lard—are bad for your heart.

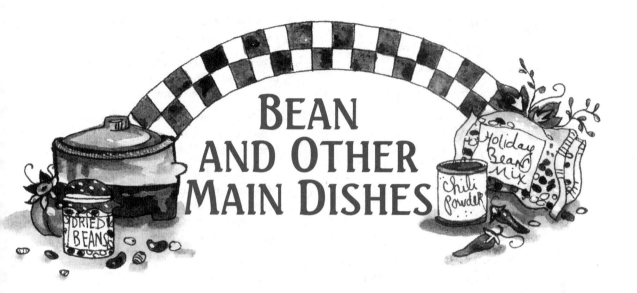

BEAN AND OTHER MAIN DISHES

New England Baked Beans

Mary Wheatley • Mashpee, MA /
Jean Butzer • Batavia, NY

Makes 8 servings (Ideal slow cooker size: 4-quart)

1 lb. dried beans—Great Northern, pea beans,
    or navy beans

2 ozs. salt pork, sliced or diced

1 qt. water

1 tsp. salt

1 Tbsp. brown sugar

½ cup molasses

½ tsp. dry mustard

½ tsp. baking soda

1 onion, coarsely chopped

5 cups water

1. Wash beans and remove any stones or
   shriveled beans.

2. Meanwhile, simmer salt pork in 1 qt.
   water in saucepan for 10 minutes. Drain.
   Do not reserve liquid.

3. Combine all ingredients in slow cooker.

4. Cook on High until contents come to
   boil. Turn to Low. Cook 14–16 hours, or
   until beans are tender.

**Exchange List Values: Starch 2.0,
Carbohydrate 1.0**

Basic Nutritional Values: Calories 269 (Calories
from Fat 41), Total Fat 5 gm (Saturated Fat 1.6 gm,
Polyunsat Fat 0.7 gm, Monounsat Fat 1.9 gm,
Cholesterol 4 mg), Sodium 444 mg, Total
Carbohydrate 47 gm, Dietary Fiber 10 gm, Sugars
18 gm, Protein 12 gm

VARIATIONS:

1. Add ½ tsp. pepper to Step 3.

Rachel Kauffman • Alton, MI

2. Add ¼ cup ketchup to Step 3.

Cheri Jantzen • Houston, TX

*To keep yourself motivated
once you start a weight-loss program,
reward yourself by buying a new CD,
getting a new exercise outfit,
or going to the movies.*

Deb's Baked Beans

Deborah Swartz • Grottoes, VA

Makes 8 servings (Ideal slow cooker size: 4-quart)

4 slices bacon, fried and drained

2 Tbsp. reserved drippings

½ cup chopped onions

2 15-oz. cans pork and beans

½ tsp. salt, optional

2 Tbsp. brown sugar

1 Tbsp. Worcestershire sauce

1 tsp. prepared mustard

1. Fry bacon in skillet until crisp. Reserve 2 Tbsp. drippings. Crumble bacon.

2. Cook onions in bacon drippings.

3. Combine all ingredients in slow cooker.

4. Cover. Cook on High 1½–2 hours.

Exchange List Values: Starch 1.5, Fat 1.0

Basic Nutritional Values: Calories 158 (Calories from Fat 43), Total Fat 5 gm (Saturated Fat 1.3 gm, Polyunsat Fat 0.7 gm, Monounsat Fat 2.1 gm, Cholesterol 8 mg), Sodium 549 mg, Total Carbohydrate 24 gm, Dietary Fiber 5 gm, Sugars 11 gm, Protein 5 gm

Refried Beans with Bacon

Arlene Wengerd • Millersburg, OH

Makes 8 servings (Ideal slow cooker size: 4-quart)

2 cups dried red, or pinto, beans

6 cups water

2 cloves garlic, minced

1 large tomato, peeled, seeded, and chopped

1 tsp. salt

2 ozs. bacon

1. Combine beans, water, garlic, tomato, and salt in slow cooker.

2. Cover. Cook on High 5 hours, stirring occasionally. When the beans become soft, drain off some liquid.

3. While the beans cook, brown bacon in skillet. Drain, reserving drippings. Crumble bacon. Add half of bacon and 1½ Tbsp. drippings to beans. Stir.

4. Mash or puree beans with a food processor. Fry the mashed bean mixture in the remaining bacon drippings. Add more salt to taste.

5. To serve, sprinkle the remaining bacon on top of beans.

Exchange List Values: Starch 1.5, Meat, very lean 1.0, Fat 0.5

Basic Nutritional Values: Calories 171 (Calories from Fat 34), Total Fat 4 gm (Saturated Fat 1.2 gm, Polyunsat Fat 0.6 gm, Monounsat Fat 1.5 gm, Cholesterol 5 mg), Sodium 354 mg, Total Carbohydrate 26 gm, Dietary Fiber 9 gm, Sugars 3 gm, Protein 9 gm

VARIATIONS:

1. Instead of draining off liquid, add ⅓ cup dry minute rice and continue cooking about 20 minutes. Add a dash of hot sauce and a dollop of sour cream to individual servings.

2. Instead of frying the mashed bean mixture, place several spoonfuls on flour tortillas, roll up, and serve.

Susan McClure • Dayton, VA

If you sometimes forget to take your pills, an inexpensive pill organizer may help you keep track.

"Famous" Baked Beans

Katrine Rose • Woodbridge, VA

Makes 15 servings (Ideal slow cooker size: 4–5-quart)

1 lb. ground beef

1/4 cup minced onions

1 cup no-salt-added ketchup

4 15-oz. cans pork and beans

1/3 cup brown sugar

brown sugar substitute to equal 1/4 cup

2 Tbsp. liquid smoke

1 Tbsp. Worcestershire sauce

1. Brown beef and onions in skillet. Drain. Spoon meat and onions into slow cooker.

2. Add remaining ingredients and stir well.

3. Cover. Cook on High 3 hours, or on Low 5–6 hours.

Exchange List Values: Starch 1.0, Carbohydrate 1.0, Meat, lean 1.0

Basic Nutritional Values: Calories 207 (Calories from Fat 44), Total Fat 5 gm (Saturated Fat 1.2 gm, Polyunsat Fat 0.5 gm, Monounsat Fat 2.0 gm, Cholesterol 22 mg), Sodium 539 mg, Total Carbohydrate 32 gm, Dietary Fiber 5 gm, Sugars 17 gm, Protein 10 gm

There are many worthy baked bean recipes, but these are both easy and absolutely delicious. The secret to this recipe is the liquid smoke. I get many requests for this recipe, and some friends have added the word "famous" to its name.

Barbecued Lima Beans

Hazel L. Propst • Oxford, PA

Makes 20 servings (Ideal slow cooker size: 4–5-quart)

1 1/2 lbs. dried lima beans

6 cups water

2 1/4 cups chopped onions

1/2 cup brown sugar

brown sugar substitute to equal 6 Tbsp.

1 1/2 cups ketchup

13 drops Tabasco sauce

1/2 cup dark corn syrup

1 tsp. salt

1/4 lb. bacon, diced

1. Soak washed beans in water overnight. Do not drain.

2. Add onions. Bring to boil. Simmer 30–60 minutes, or until beans are tender. Drain beans, reserving liquid.

3. Combine all ingredients except bean liquid in slow cooker. Mix well. Pour in enough liquid so that beans are barely covered.

4. Cover. Cook on Low 10 hours, or High 4–6 hours. Stir occasionally.

Exchange List Values: Starch 1.0, Carbohydrate 1.0, Vegetable 1.0, Fat 0.5

Basic Nutritional Values: Calories 195 (Calories from Fat 27), Total Fat 3 gm (Saturated Fat 0.9 gm, Polyunsat Fat 0.4 gm, Monounsat Fat 1.2 gm, Cholesterol 4 mg), Sodium 393 mg, Total Carbohydrate 36 gm, Dietary Fiber 7 gm, Sugars 15 gm, Protein 8 gm

Red Beans and Pasta

Naomi E. Fast • Hesston, KS

Makes 6-8 servings (Ideal slow cooker size: 4-5-quart)

3 14½-oz. cans 100%-fat-free, reduced-sodium chicken broth

½ tsp. ground cumin

1 Tbsp. chili powder

1 clove garlic, minced

8 ozs. uncooked spiral pasta

half a large green pepper, diced

half a large red pepper, diced

1 medium onion, diced

15-oz. can red beans, rinsed and drained

chopped fresh parsley

chopped fresh cilantro

1. Combine broth, cumin, chili powder, and garlic in slow cooker.

2. Cover. Cook on High until mixture comes to boil.

3. Add pasta, vegetables, and beans. Stir together well.

4. Cover. Cook on Low 3-4 hours.

5. Add parsley and cilantro before serving.

Exchange List Values: Starch 2.0, Vegetable 1.0

Basic Nutritional Values: Calories 180 (Calories from Fat 9), Total Fat 1 gm (Saturated Fat 0 gm, Polyunsat Fat 0.4 gm, Monounsat Fat 0.2 gm, Cholesterol 0 mg), Sodium 448 mg, Total Carbohydrate 34 gm, Dietary Fiber 4 gm, Sugars 4 gm, Protein 9 gm

Red Beans and Rice

Margaret A. Moffitt • Bartlett, TN

Makes 10 servings (Ideal slow cooker size: 4-5-quart)

1-lb. pkg. dried red beans

water

4 ozs. smoked sausage

½ tsp. salt

1 tsp. pepper

3-4 cups water

6-oz. can tomato paste

8-oz. can tomato sauce

4 cloves garlic, minced

1. Soak beans for 8 hours. Drain. Discard soaking water.

2. Mix together all ingredients in slow cooker.

3. Cover. Cook on Low 10-12 hours, or until beans are soft. Serve over rice.

Exchange List Values: Starch 1.5, Vegetable 1.0, Meat, lean 1.0

Basic Nutritional Values: Calories 198 (Calories from Fat 36), Total Fat 4 gm (Saturated Fat 1.2 gm, Polyunsat Fat 0.8 gm, Monounsat Fat 1.5 gm, Cholesterol 7 mg), Sodium 370 mg, Total Carbohydrate 30 gm, Dietary Fiber 8 gm, Sugars 4 gm, Protein 12 gm

VARIATION: Use canned red kidney beans. Cook 1 hour on High and then 3 hours on Low.

Note: These beans freeze well.

Party-Time Beans

Beatrice Martin • Goshen, IN

Makes 14 servings (Ideal slow cooker size: 6-quart)

1½ cups ketchup

1 onion, chopped

1 green pepper, chopped

1 sweet red pepper, chopped

½ cup water

¼ cup packed brown sugar

brown sugar substitute to equal 2 Tbsp.

2 bay leaves

2–3 tsp. cider vinegar

1 tsp. ground mustard

⅛ tsp. pepper

16-oz. can kidney beans, rinsed and drained

15½-oz. can Great Northern beans, rinsed and drained

15-oz. can lima beans, rinsed and drained

15-oz. can black beans, rinsed and drained

15½-oz. can black-eyed peas, rinsed and drained

1. Combine first 11 ingredients in slow cooker. Mix well.

2. Add remaining ingredients. Mix well.

3. Cover. Cook on Low 5–7 hours, or until onion and peppers are tender.

4. Remove bay leaves before serving.

5. Serve with grilled hamburgers, salad or veggie tray, chips, fruit, and cookies.

Exchange List Values: Starch 1.5, Carbohydrate 0.5

Basic Nutritional Values: Calories 172 (Calories from Fat 7), Total Fat 1 gm (Saturated Fat 0.1 gm, Polyunsat Fat 0.2 gm, Monounsat Fat 0 gm, Cholesterol 0 mg), Sodium 493 mg, Total Carbohydrate 35 gm, Dietary Fiber 8 gm, Sugars 11 gm, Protein 9 gm

New Mexico Pinto Beans

John D. Allen • Rye, CO

Makes 10 servings (Ideal slow cooker size: 4-quart)

2½ cups dried pinto beans

3 qts. water

½ cup ham, or salt pork, diced, or a small ham shank

2 cloves garlic, crushed

1 tsp. crushed red chili peppers, optional

1. Sort beans. Discard pebbles, shriveled beans, and floaters. Wash beans under running water. Place in saucepan, cover with 3 qts. water, and soak overnight.

2. Drain beans and discard soaking water. Pour beans into slow cooker. Cover with fresh water.

3. Add meat, garlic, and chili peppers. Cook on Low 6–10 hours, or until beans are soft.

Exchange List Values: Starch 1.5, Meat, very lean 1.0

Basic Nutritional Values: Calories 145 (Calories from Fat 8), Total Fat 1 gm (Saturated Fat 0.2 gm, Polyunsat Fat 0.2 gm, Monounsat Fat 0.3 gm, Cholesterol 4 mg), Sodium 95 mg, Total Carbohydrate 25 gm, Dietary Fiber 8 gm, Sugars 2 gm, Protein 10 gm

Scandinavian Beans

Virginia Bender • Dover, DE

Makes 8 servings (Ideal slow cooker size: 4–5-quart)

1 lb. dried pinto beans

6 cups water

1/4 lb. bacon, or 1 ham hock

1 onion, chopped

2-3 cloves garlic, minced

1/4 tsp. pepper

1/4 tsp. salt

2 Tbsp. molasses

1 cup ketchup

Tabasco to taste

1 tsp. Worcestershire sauce

1/4 cup brown sugar

brown sugar substitute to equal 1/4 cup

1/3 cup cider vinegar

1/4 tsp. dry mustard

1. Soak beans in water in soup pot for 8 hours. Bring beans to boil and cook 1 1/2–2 hours, or until soft. Drain, reserving liquid.

2. Combine all ingredients in slow cooker, using just enough bean liquid to cover everything. Cook on Low 5–6 hours.

Exchange List Values: Starch 2.0, Carbohydrate 1.0, Vegetable 1.0, Fat 0.5

Basic Nutritional Values: Calories 305 (Calories from Fat 65), Total Fat 7 gm (Saturated Fat 2.2 gm, Polyunsat Fat 0.9 gm, Monounsat Fat 3.0 gm, Cholesterol 10 mg), Sodium 564 mg, Total Carbohydrate 51 gm, Dietary Fiber 11 gm, Sugars 18 gm, Protein 12 gm

Calico Beans

Alice Miller • Stuarts Draft, VA

Makes 12 servings (Ideal slow cooker size: 6-quart)

1/2 lb. ground beef

1/4 lb. bacon, chopped

1/2 cup chopped onions

1/2 cup no-salt-added ketchup

1/3 cup brown sugar

brown sugar substitute to equal 3 Tbsp.

2 Tbsp. sugar

1 Tbsp. vinegar

1 tsp. dry mustard

16-oz. can pork and beans, undrained

16-oz. can red kidney beans, undrained

16-oz. can yellow limas, undrained

16-oz. can navy beans, undrained

1. Brown ground beef, bacon, and onions together in skillet. Drain. Spoon meat and onions into slow cooker.

2. Stir ketchup, brown sugar, sugar substitute, sugar, vinegar, and mustard. Mix together well. Add to slow cooker.

3. Pour beans into slow cooker and combine all ingredients thoroughly.

4. Cover. Cook on High 3–4 hours.

5. Serve over rice, or take to a picnic as is.

Exchange List Values: Starch 2.5, Meat, lean 1.0

Basic Nutritional Values: Calories 233 (Calories from Fat 39), Total Fat 4 gm (Saturated Fat 1.3 gm, Polyunsat Fat 0.5 gm, Monounsat Fat 1.7 gm, Cholesterol 15 mg), Sodium 620 mg, Total Carbohydrate 37 gm, Dietary Fiber 7 gm, Sugars 16 gm, Protein 12 gm

New Orleans Red Beans

Cheri Jantzen • Houston, TX

Makes 6 servings (Ideal slow cooker size: 4-quart)

2 cups dried kidney beans

5 cups water

8 ozs. low-fat smoked sausage, cut in small
pieces

2 medium onions, chopped

2 cloves garlic, minced

1/4 tsp. salt

1. Wash and sort beans. In saucepan, combine beans and water. Boil 2 minutes. Remove from heat. Soak 1 hour.

2. Brown sausage slowly in a skillet. (If needed, use non-fat cooking spray.) Add onions, garlic, and salt and saute until tender.

3. Combine all ingredients, including the bean water, in slow cooker.

4. Cover. Cook on Low 8–10 hours. During last 20 minutes of cooking, stir frequently and mash lightly with spoon.

5. Serve over hot white rice.

Exchange List Values: Starch 2.5, Vegetable 1.0, Meat, very lean 1.0

Basic Nutritional Values: Calories 260 (Calories from Fat 23), Total Fat 3 gm (Saturated Fat 0.8 gm, Polyunsat Fat 1.1 gm, Monounsat Fat 0.5 gm, Cholesterol 16 mg), Sodium 422 mg, Total Carbohydrate 42 gm, Dietary Fiber 10 gm, Sugars 8 gm, Protein 18 gm

*Instead of rice or potatoes,
try couscous or quinoa [KEEN-wa],
whole grains that cook fast,
are easy to make, and taste great!*

Pioneer Beans

Kay Magruder • Seminole, OK

Makes 8 servings (Ideal slow cooker size: 4-quart)

1 lb. dry lima beans

1 bunch green onions, chopped

3 tsp. sodium-free beef bouillon powder

6 cups water

1 lb. low-fat smoked sausage

1/2 tsp. garlic powder

3/4 tsp. Tabasco sauce

1. Combine all ingredients in slow cooker. Mix well.

2. Cover. Cook on High 8–9 hours, or until beans are soft but not mushy.

3. Serve with home-baked bread.

Exchange List Values: Starch 2.5, Meat, very lean 2.0

Basic Nutritional Values: Calories 252 (Calories from Fat 28), Total Fat 3 gm (Saturated Fat 1.1 gm, Polyunsat Fat 1.3 gm, Monounsat Fat 0.7 gm, Cholesterol 24 mg), Sodium 487 mg, Total Carbohydrate 38 gm, Dietary Fiber 10 gm, Sugars 7 gm, Protein 18 gm

Cowboy Beans

Sharon Timpe • Mequon, WI

Makes 12 servings (Ideal slow cooker size: 5–6-quart)

6 slices bacon, cut in pieces

$\frac{1}{2}$ cup onions, chopped

1 clove garlic, minced

16-oz. can baked beans

16-oz. can kidney beans, drained

15-oz. can butter beans, or pinto beans, drained

2 Tbsp. dill pickle relish, or chopped dill pickles

$\frac{1}{3}$ cup chili sauce, or ketchup

2 tsp. Worcestershire sauce

$\frac{1}{4}$ cup brown sugar

brown sugar substitute to equal 2 Tbsp.

$\frac{1}{8}$ tsp. hot pepper sauce, optional

1. Lightly brown bacon, onions, and garlic in skillet. Drain.

2. Combine all ingredients in slow cooker. Mix well.

3. Cover. Cook on Low 5–7 hours, or High 3–4 hours.

Exchange List Values: Starch 1.0, Carbohydrate 0.5, Fat 0.5

Basic Nutritional Values: Calories 138 (Calories from Fat 17), Total Fat 2 gm (Saturated Fat 0.6 gm, Polyunsat Fat 0.3 gm, Monounsat Fat 0.7 gm, Cholesterol 3 mg), Sodium 441 mg, Total Carbohydrate 25 gm, Dietary Fiber 5 gm, Sugars 9 gm, Protein 7 gm

Four Beans and Sausage

Mary Seielstad • Sparks, NV

Recipe photo appears in color section.

Makes 8 servings (Ideal slow cooker size: 5-quart)

15-oz. can Great Northern beans, drained

$15\frac{1}{2}$-oz. can black beans, rinsed and drained

16-oz. can red kidney beans, drained

15-oz. can butter beans, drained

$1\frac{1}{2}$ cups no-salt-added ketchup

$\frac{1}{2}$ cup chopped onions

1 medium green pepper, chopped

1 lb. low-fat smoked sausage, cooked and cut into $\frac{1}{2}$" slices

2 Tbsp. brown sugar

brown sugar substitute to equal 1 Tbsp.

2 cloves garlic, minced

1 tsp. Worcestershire sauce

$\frac{1}{2}$ tsp. dry mustard

$\frac{1}{2}$ tsp. Tabasco sauce

1. Combine all ingredients in slow cooker.

2. Cover. Cook on Low 9–10 hours, or High 4–5 hours.

Exchange List Values: Starch 2.0, Carbohydrate 1.5, Meat, lean 1.0

Basic Nutritional Values: Calories 328 (Calories from Fat 31), Total Fat 3 gm (Saturated Fat 1.2 gm, Polyunsat Fat 1.4 gm, Monounsat Fat 0.7 gm, Cholesterol 24 mg), Sodium 764 mg, Total Carbohydrate 56 gm, Dietary Fiber 11 gm, Sugars 22 gm, Protein 19 gm

Creole Black Beans

Joyce Kaut • Rochester, NY

Makes 8 servings (Ideal slow cooker size: 4-quart)

14 ozs. low-fat smoked sausage, sliced in
$\frac{1}{2}$" pieces, browned

3 15-oz. cans black beans, drained

$1\frac{1}{2}$ cups chopped onions

$1\frac{1}{2}$ cups chopped green peppers

$1\frac{1}{2}$ cups chopped celery

4 cloves garlic, minced

2 tsp. dried thyme

$1\frac{1}{2}$ tsp. dried oregano

$1\frac{1}{2}$ tsp. pepper

1 tsp. sodium-free chicken bouillon powder

3 bay leaves

8-oz. can no-salt-added tomato sauce

1 cup water

1. Combine all ingredients in slow cooker.

2. Cover. Cook on Low 8 hours, or on High 4 hours.

3. Remove bay leaves.

4. Serve over rice, with a salad and fresh fruit for dessert.

Exchange List Values: Starch 1.5, Vegetable 2.0, Meat, lean 1.0

Basic Nutritional Values: Calories 223 (Calories from Fat 27), Total Fat 3 gm (Saturated Fat 1.0 gm, Polyunsat Fat 1.2 gm, Monounsat Fat 0.6 gm, Cholesterol 21 mg), Sodium 566 mg, Total Carbohydrate 34 gm, Dietary Fiber 10 gm, Sugars 9 gm, Protein 15 gm

VARIATION: You may substitute a $14\frac{1}{2}$-oz. can of stewed tomatoes for the tomato sauce.

Cajun Sausage and Beans

Melanie Thrower • McPherson, KS

Makes 6 servings (Ideal slow cooker size: 4-quart)

1 lb. low-fat smoked sausage, sliced into
$\frac{1}{4}$" pieces

16-oz. can no-salt-added red kidney beans

16-oz. can crushed tomatoes with green chilies

1 cup chopped celery

half an onion, chopped

2 Tbsp. Italian seasoning

Tabasco sauce to taste

1. Combine all ingredients in slow cooker.

2. Cover. Cook on Low 8 hours.

3. Serve over rice or as a thick, zesty soup.

Exchange List Values: Starch 1.0, Vegetable 1.0, Meat, lean 1.0

Basic Nutritional Values: Calories 158 (Calories from Fat 22), Total Fat 2 gm (Saturated Fat 0.8 gm, Polyunsat Fat 1.0 gm, Monounsat Fat 0.5 gm, Cholesterol 18 mg), Sodium 588 mg, Total Carbohydrate 23 gm, Dietary Fiber 7 gm, Sugars 7 gm, Protein 11 gm

Pizza Beans

Kelly Evenson • Pittsboro, NC

Makes 6 servings (Ideal slow cooker size: 4-quart)

16-oz. can pinto beans, drained

16-oz. can kidney beans, drained

2¼-oz. can ripe olives, sliced, drained

28-oz. can no-salt-added stewed or
    whole tomatoes

¾ lb. bulk lean turkey Italian sausage

1 Tbsp. oil

1 green pepper, chopped

1 medium onion, chopped

1 clove garlic, minced

1 tsp. dried oregano

1 tsp. dried basil

1. Combine beans, olives, and tomatoes in
slow cooker.

2. Brown sausage in ½ Tbsp. oil in skillet.
Drain. Transfer sausage to slow cooker.

3. Saute green pepper in ½ Tbsp. oil for
1 minute, stirring constantly. Add onions
and continue stirring until onions start
to become translucent. Add garlic
and cook 1 more minute. Transfer to
slow cooker.

4. Stir in seasonings.

5. Cover. Cook on Low 7–9 hours.

6. To serve, sprinkle with Parmesan cheese,
if you wish.

**Exchange List Values: Starch 1.5,
Vegetable 3.0, Meat, lean 2.0, Fat 1.0**

Basic Nutritional Values: Calories 335 (Calories
from Fat 104), Total Fat 12 gm (Saturated Fat
2.2 gm, Polyunsat Fat 2.0 gm, Monounsat Fat
3.7 gm, Cholesterol 45 mg), Sodium 632 mg, Total
Carbohydrate 39 gm, Dietary Fiber 10 gm, Sugars
8 gm, Protein 23 gm

VARIATION: For a thicker soup, 20 minutes
before serving remove ¼ cup liquid from cooker
and add 1 Tbsp. cornstarch to it. Stir until
dissolved. Return to soup. Cook on High for
15 minutes, or until thickened.

*For many people, diabetes
still means you cannot eat sugar.
Be patient; it takes years for
new information to reach the general
public, and years to change old
ways of thinking.*

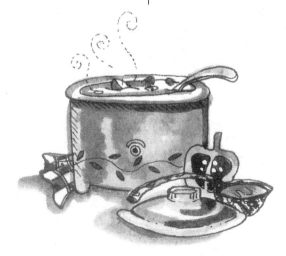

Beans with Rice

Miriam Christophel • Battle Creek, MI

Makes 8 servings (Ideal slow cooker size: 5-6-quart)

3 cups dried small red beans

8 cups water

3 cloves garlic, minced

1 large onion, chopped

8 cups fresh water

1 ham hock

½ cup ketchup

½ tsp. salt

pinch pepper

1½–2 tsp. ground cumin

1 Tbsp. parsley

1–2 bay leaves

1. Soak beans overnight in 8 cups water. Drain. Place soaked beans in slow cooker with garlic, onion, 8 cups fresh water, and ham hock.

2. Cover. Cook on High 12–14 hours.

3. Take ham hock out of cooker and allow to cool. Remove meat from bones. Remove and discard visible fat and skin. Cut up ham and return to slow cooker. Add remaining ingredients.

4. Cover. Cook on High 2–3 hours.

5. Serve over rice with dollop of sour cream, if you wish.

Exchange List Values: Starch 1.5, Fat 0.5

Basic Nutritional Values: Calories 148 (Calories from Fat 25), Total Fat 3 gm (Saturated Fat 0.8 gm, Polyunsat Fat 0.5 gm, Monounsat Fat 1.0 gm, Cholesterol 4 mg), Sodium 382 mg, Total Carbohydrate 24 gm, Dietary Fiber 6 gm, Sugars 5 gm, Protein 8 gm

Six-Bean Barbecued Beans

Gladys Longacre • Susquehanna, PA

Makes 24 (½ cup) servings (Ideal slow cooker size: 6-quart)

1-lb. can kidney beans, drained

1-lb. can pinto beans, drained

1-lb. can Great Northern beans, drained

1-lb. can butter beans, drained

1-lb. can navy beans, drained

1-lb. can pork and beans

¼ cup barbecue sauce

⅓ cup prepared mustard

⅓ cup ketchup

2 Tbsp. Worcestershire sauce

1 small onion, chopped

1 small bell pepper, chopped

2 Tbsp. molasses, or sorghum molasses

½ cup brown sugar

brown sugar substitute to equal ¼ cup

1. Mix together all ingredients in slow cooker.

2. Cook on Low 4–6 hours.

Exchange List Values: Starch 1.5

Basic Nutritional Values: Calories 122 (Calories from Fat 6), Total Fat 1 gm (Saturated Fat 0.1 gm, Polyunsat Fat 0.2 gm, Monounsat Fat 0.2 gm, Cholesterol 1 mg), Sodium 322 mg, Total Carbohydrate 24 gm, Dietary Fiber 6 gm, Sugars 7 gm, Protein 6 gm

Time and again, studies have shown that getting your blood sugars down to near-normal levels lowers your risk of developing diabetes complications.

Sweet and Sour Beans

Julette Leaman • Harrisonburg, VA

Makes 8 servings (Ideal slow cooker size: 4–5-quart)

5 slices bacon

4 medium onions, cut in rings

1/4 cup brown sugar

brown sugar substitute to equal 2 Tbsp.

1 tsp. dry mustard

1/2 tsp. salt

1/4 cup cider vinegar

1-lb. can green beans, drained

2 1-lb. cans butter beans, drained

2 14 1/2-oz. cans no-salt-added baked beans

1. Brown bacon in skillet and crumble. Drain all but 3 tsp. bacon drippings. Stir in onions, brown sugar, sugar substitute, mustard, salt, and vinegar. Simmer 20 minutes.

2. Combine all ingredients in slow cooker.

3. Cover. Cook on Low 3 hours.

Exchange List Values: Starch 2.0, Carbohydrate 1.0, Vegetable 1.0, Meat, lean 1.0

Basic Nutritional Values: Calories 289 (Calories from Fat 40), Total Fat 4 gm (Saturated Fat 1.5 gm, Polyunsat Fat 0.7 gm, Monounsat Fat 1.7 gm, Cholesterol 5 mg), Sodium 519 mg, Total Carbohydrate 51 gm, Dietary Fiber 13 gm, Sugars 22 gm, Protein 13 gm

Four-Bean Medley

Sharon Brubaker • Myerstown, PA

Makes 8 servings (Ideal slow cooker size: 4–5-quart)

8 bacon slices, diced and browned until crisp

2 medium onions, chopped

6 Tbsp. brown sugar

brown sugar substitute to equal 3 Tbsp.

1/2 cup vinegar

1 tsp. dry mustard

1/2 tsp. garlic powder

16-oz. can baked beans, undrained

16-oz. can kidney beans, drained

15 1/2-oz. can butter beans, drained

14 1/2-oz. can green beans, drained

2 Tbsp. ketchup

1. Mix together all ingredients. Pour into slow cooker.

2. Cover. Cook on Low 6–8 hours.

Exchange List Values: Starch 2.0, Carbohydrate 0.5, Vegetable 1.0, Fat 0.5

Basic Nutritional Values: Calories 242 (Calories from Fat 34), Total Fat 4 gm (Saturated Fat 1.1 gm, Polyunsat Fat 0.6 gm, Monounsat Fat 1.5 gm, Cholesterol 5 mg), Sodium 619 mg, Total Carbohydrate 44 gm, Dietary Fiber 9 gm, Sugars 19 gm, Protein 11 gm

VARIATION: Make this a main dish by adding 1 lb. hamburger to the bacon, browning it along with the bacon and chopped onions in a skillet, then adding that mixture to the rest of the ingredients before pouring into the slow cooker.

Main Dish Baked Beans

Sue Pennington • Bridgewater, VA

Makes 8 servings (Ideal slow cooker size: 4-quart)

1 lb. ground beef

28-oz. can baked beans

8-oz. can pineapple tidbits packed in juice, drained

4½-oz. can sliced mushrooms, drained

1 large onion, chopped

1 large green pepper, chopped

½ cup Phyllis's Homemade Barbecue Sauce (see recipe on page 334)

2 Tbsp. light soy sauce

1 clove garlic, minced

¼ tsp. pepper

1. Brown ground beef in skillet. Drain. Place in slow cooker.

2. Stir in remaining ingredients. Mix well.

3. Cover. Cook on Low 4–8 hours, or until bubbly. Serve in soup bowls.

Exchange List Values: Starch 1.0, Carbohydrate 0.5, Vegetable 1.0, Meat, lean 1.0, Fat 1.0

Basic Nutritional Values: Calories 238 (Calories from Fat 58), Total Fat 6 gm (Saturated Fat 2.4 gm, Polyunsat Fat 0.5 gm, Monounsat Fat 2.6 gm, Cholesterol 34 mg), Sodium 663 mg, Total Carbohydrate 31 gm, Dietary Fiber 7 gm, Sugars 13 gm, Protein 17 gm

Slow Cooker Kidney Beans

Jeanette Oberholtzer • Manheim, PA

Makes 12 servings (Ideal slow cooker size: 4-quart)

2 30-oz. cans kidney beans, rinsed and drained

28-oz. can no-salt-added diced tomatoes, drained

2 medium-sized red bell peppers, chopped

1 cup ketchup

¼ cup brown sugar

brown sugar substitute to equal 2 Tbsp.

2 Tbsp. honey

2 Tbsp. molasses

1 Tbsp. Worcestershire sauce

1 tsp. dry mustard

2 medium red apples, cored, cut into pieces

1. Combine all ingredients, except apples, in slow cooker.

2. Cover. Cook on Low 4–5 hours.

3. Stir in apples.

4. Cover. Cook 2 more hours on Low.

Exchange List Values: Starch 1.5, Carbohydrate 1.0, Vegetable 1.0

Basic Nutritional Values: Calories 216 (Calories from Fat 8), Total Fat 1 gm (Saturated Fat 0 gm, Polyunsat Fat 0.4 gm, Monounsat Fat 0.1 gm, Cholesterol 0 mg), Sodium 445 mg, Total Carbohydrate 46 gm, Dietary Fiber 9 gm, Sugars 20 gm, Protein 10 gm

One-Pot Dinner

Vicki Dinkel • Sharon Springs, KS

Makes 8 servings (Ideal slow cooker size: 4-quart)

½ lb. ground beef

¼ lb. bacon, cut in pieces

1 cup chopped onions

2 16-oz. cans pork and beans

16-oz. can kidney beans, drained

1 cup no-salt-added ketchup

16-oz. can butter beans, drained

2 Tbsp. brown sugar

brown sugar substitute to equal 1 Tbsp.

1 Tbsp. liquid smoke

2 Tbsp. white vinegar

dash pepper

1. Brown ground beef in skillet. Drain off drippings. Place beef in slow cooker.

2. Brown bacon and onions in skillet. Drain off drippings. Pat dry with absorbent towling. Add bacon and onions to slow cooker.

3. Stir remaining ingredients into cooker.

4. Cover. Cook on Low 5–9 hours, or High 3 hours.

Exchange List Values: Starch 2.5, Carbohydrate 1.0, Meat, lean 1.0

Basic Nutritional Values: Calories 338 (Calories from Fat 68), Total Fat 8 gm (Saturated Fat 2.1 gm, Polyunsat Fat 0.9 gm, Monounsat Fat 3.2 gm, Cholesterol 25 mg), Sodium 763 mg, Total Carbohydrate 52 gm, Dietary Fiber 11 gm, Sugars 22 gm, Protein 17 gm

Apple Bean Bake

Barbara A. Yoder • Goshen, IN

Makes 12 side dish servings (Ideal slow cooker size: 4–5-quart)

4 Tbsp. margarine

2 large Granny Smith apples, unpeeled, cubed

¼ cup brown sugar

2 Tbsp. sugar

brown sugar substitute to equal 2 Tbsp.

white sugar substitute to equal 1 Tbsp.

½ cup no-salt-added ketchup

1 tsp. cinnamon

1 Tbsp. molasses

24-oz. can Great Northern beans, undrained

24-oz. can pinto beans, undrained

1. Melt margarine in skillet. Add apples and cook until tender.

2. Stir in brown sugar, sugar, and sugar substitutes. Cook until they melt. Stir in ketchup, cinnamon, and molasses.

3. Add beans. Mix well. Pour into slow cooker.

4. Cover. Cook on High 2–4 hours.

Exchange List Values: Starch 1.0, Fruit 0.5, Carbohydrate 0.5, Fat 1.0

Basic Nutritional Values: Calories 195 (Calories from Fat 44), Total Fat 5 gm (Saturated Fat 0.8 gm, Polyunsat Fat 1.5 gm, Monounsat Fat 1.8 gm, Cholesterol 0 mg), Sodium 399 mg, Total Carbohydrate 32 gm, Dietary Fiber 6 gm, Sugars 17 gm, Protein 6 gm

Fruity Baked Bean Casserole

Elaine Unruh • Minneapolis, MN

Makes 8 servings (Ideal slow cooker size: 4–5-quart)

½ lb. bacon

3 medium onions, chopped

16-oz. can lima beans, drained

16-oz. can kidney beans, drained

16-oz. can baked beans

14½-oz. can no-salt-added baked beans

15½-oz. can pineapple chunks, canned in juice

2 Tbsp. brown sugar

brown sugar substitute to equal 2 Tbsp.

¼ cup cider vinegar

2 Tbsp. molasses

½ cup ketchup

2 Tbsp. prepared mustard

½ tsp. garlic powder

1 medium green pepper, chopped

1. Cook bacon in skillet. Crumble. Place bacon in slow cooker. Rinse skillet.

2. Saute onions in skillet with fat-free non-stick cooking spray until soft. Drain.

3. Add onions, beans, and pineapple to cooker. Mix well.

4. Combine brown sugar, sugar substitute, vinegar, molasses, ketchup, mustard, garlic powder, and green pepper. Mix well. Stir into mixture in slow cooker.

5. Cover. Cook on High 2–3 hours.

Exchange List Values: Starch 2.5, Fruit 0.5, Carbohydrate 1.0, Vegetable 1.0

Basic Nutritional Values: Calories 350 (Calories from Fat 46), Total Fat 5 gm (Saturated Fat 1.5 gm, Polyunsat Fat 0.9 gm, Monounsat Fat 2.0 gm, Cholesterol 7 mg), Sodium 577 mg, Total Carbohydrate 65 gm, Dietary Fiber 13 gm, Sugars 32 gm, Protein 15 gm

Ann's Boston Baked Beans

Ann Driscoll • Albuquerque, NM

Makes 20 side dish servings (Ideal slow cooker size: 4–5-quart)

1 cup raisins

2 small onions, diced

2 tart apples, unpeeled, diced

1 cup chili sauce

1 cup chopped extra-lean, reduced-sodium ham

1-lb. 15-oz. can baked beans

2 14½-oz. cans no-salt-added baked beans

3 tsp. dry mustard

½ cup sweet pickle relish

1. Mix together all ingredients.

2. Cover. Cook on Low 6–8 hours.

Exchange List Values: Starch 1.0, Fruit 0.5, Carbohydrate 0.5

Basic Nutritional Values: Calories 148 (Calories from Fat 6), Total Fat 1 gm (Saturated Fat 0.1 gm, Polyunsat Fat 0.2 gm, Monounsat Fat 0.1 gm, Cholesterol 3 mg), Sodium 443 mg, Total Carbohydrate 32 gm, Dietary Fiber 6 gm, Sugars 16 gm, Protein 6 gm

Swimming and water aerobics are just two activities that don't stress the joints. You'll be surprised at how much more energy you have!

Pheasant a la Elizabeth

Elizabeth L. Richards • Rapid City, SD

Makes 8 servings (Ideal slow cooker size: 4-quart)

6 (6½ ozs. each) boneless, skinless pheasant breast halves, cubed

¾ cup teriyaki sauce

⅓ cup flour

1½ tsp. garlic salt

pepper to taste

2 Tbsp. olive oil

1 large onion, sliced

12-oz. can beer

¾ cup fresh mushrooms, sliced

1. Marinate pheasant in teriyaki sauce for 2–4 hours. Remove breasts from teriyaki sauce (teriyaki sauce should be disposed of).

2. Combine flour, garlic salt, and pepper. Dredge pheasant in flour. Brown in olive oil in skillet. Add onion and saute for 3 minutes, stirring frequently. Transfer to slow cooker.

3. Add beer and mushrooms.

4. Cover. Cook on Low 6–8 hours.

Exchange List Values: Carbohydrate 0.5, Meat, lean 4.0

Basic Nutritional Values: Calories 260 (Calories from Fat 75), Total Fat 8 gm (Saturated Fat 0.5 gm, Polyunsat Fat 1.3 gm, Monounsat Fat 3.9 gm, Cholesterol 92 mg), Sodium 357 mg, Total Carbohydrate 10 gm, Dietary Fiber 1 gm, Sugars 5 gm, Protein 34 gm

VARIATION: Instead of pheasant, use chicken.

Pot-Roasted Rabbit

Donna Treloar • Gaston, IN

Makes 6 servings (Ideal slow cooker size: 4-quart)

2 onions, sliced

4-lb. roasting rabbit, skinned

1 clove garlic, sliced

2 bay leaves

1 whole clove

1 cup hot water

2 Tbsp. soy sauce

2 Tbsp. flour

½ cup cold water

1. Place onion in bottom of slow cooker.

2. Insert garlic in rabbit cavity. Place rabbit in slow cooker.

3. Add bay leaves, clove, hot water, and soy sauce to slow cooker.

4. Cover. Cook on Low 10–12 hours.

5. Remove rabbit and thicken gravy by stirring 2 Tbsp. flour blended into ½ cup water into simmering juices in cooker. Continue stirring until gravy thickens. Cut rabbit into serving-size pieces and serve with gravy.

Exchange List Values: Carbohydrate 0.5, Meat, lean 5.0

Basic Nutritional Values: Calories 294 (Calories from Fat 97), Total Fat 11 gm (Saturated Fat 3.2 gm, Polyunsat Fat 2.1 gm, Monounsat Fat 2.9 gm, Cholesterol 110 mg), Sodium 390 mg, Total Carbohydrate 7 gm, Dietary Fiber 1 gm, Sugars 4 gm, Protein 40 gm

Venison in Sauce

Anona M. Teel • Bangor, PA

Makes 12 sandwiches (Ideal slow cooker size: 5-quart)

¼ cup vinegar

2 cloves garlic, minced

¼ tsp. salt

3-4-lb. venison roast

cold water

2 Tbsp. oil

1 large onion, sliced

half a green pepper, sliced

2 ribs celery, sliced

1-2 cloves garlic, minced

1½-2 tsp. salt

¼ tsp. pepper

½ tsp. dried oregano

¼ cup ketchup

1 cup tomato juice

1. Combine vinegar, 2 garlic cloves, and ¼ tsp. salt. Pour over venison. Add cold water until meat is covered. Marinate 6–8 hours.

2. Cut meat into pieces. Brown in oil in skillet. Place in slow cooker.

3. Mix remaining ingredients together; then pour into cooker. Stir in meat.

4. Cover. Cook on Low 8–10 hours.

5. Using two forks, pull the meat apart and then stir it through the sauce.

6. Serve on sandwich rolls, or over rice or pasta.

Exchange List Values: Vegetable 1.0, Meat, very lean 3.0, Fat 1.0

Basic Nutritional Values: Calories 176 (Calories from Fat 46), Total Fat 5 gm (Saturated Fat 1.4 gm, Polyunsat Fat 1.3 gm, Monounsat Fat 2.0 gm, Cholesterol 96 mg), Sodium 429 mg, Total Carbohydrate 5 gm, Dietary Fiber 1 gm, Sugars 3 gm, Protein 26 gm

Eat some avocado, olives, almonds, or sesame seeds today. Small amounts give your body the good fat that it needs.

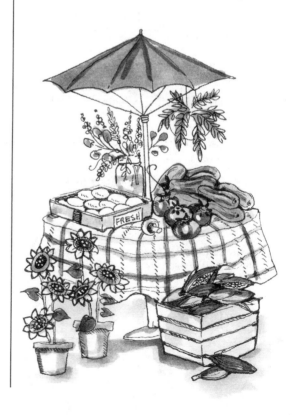

Beef-Venison Barbecue

Gladys Longacre • Susquehanna, PA

Makes 8 servings (Ideal slow cooker size: 4-quart)

1½ lbs. ground beef

½ lb. ground venison

1 medium onion, chopped

½ cup chopped green peppers

1 clove garlic, minced

¼ tsp. pepper

½ tsp. dried thyme

1 tsp. dried oregano

1 tsp. dried basil

¼ cup brown sugar

¼ cup vinegar

1 Tbsp. dry mustard

1 cup ketchup

½–1 Tbsp. hickory-smoked barbecue sauce

8 hamburger rolls

1. Brown meat in skillet. Place in slow cooker.

2. Add remaining ingredients except rolls. Mix well.

3. Cover. Cook on High 1 hour, or Low 2–3 hours.

4. Serve barbecue in hamburger rolls.

Exchange List Values: Starch 2.0, Carbohydrate 0.5, Meat, lean 3.0

Basic Nutritional Values: Calories 366 (Calories from Fat 111), Total Fat 12 gm (Saturated Fat 4.3 gm, Polyunsat Fat 0.9 gm, Monounsat Fat 5.2 gm, Cholesterol 76 mg), Sodium 634 mg, Total Carbohydrate 37 gm, Dietary Fiber 3 gm, Sugars 15 gm, Protein 27 gm

Note: This recipe can be made in larger quantities to freeze and then reheat when needed. This barbecue recipe was made in large quantities and served at the concession stand for our farm machinery sale in 1987. They used ice cream dippers to scoop the meat into the sandwich rolls.

Put on some classical music and conduct a pretend orchestra from your chair at home—it can be quite a workout!

Venison Roast

Colleen Heatwole • Burton, MI

Makes 10 servings (Ideal slow cooker size: 4–5-quart)

3-lb. venison roast

¼ cup vinegar

2 cloves garlic, minced

1 tsp. salt

½ cup chopped onions

15-oz. can no-salt-added tomato sauce

1 Tbsp. ground mustard

1 pkg. brown gravy mix

½ tsp. salt

¼ cup water

1. Place venison in deep bowl. Combine vinegar, garlic, and salt. Pour over venison. Add enough cold water to cover venison. Marinate for at least 8 hours in refrigerator.

2. Rinse and drain venison. Place in slow cooker.

3. Combine remaining ingredients and pour over venison.

4. Cover. Cook on Low 10–12 hours.

5. If you wish, serve with a green salad, potatoes, and rolls to make a complete meal.

Exchange List Values: Vegetable 1.0, Meat, very lean 4.0

Basic Nutritional Values: Calories 186 (Calories from Fat 31), Total Fat 3 gm (Saturated Fat 1.4 gm, Polyunsat Fat 0.7 gm, Monounsat Fat 0.7 gm, Cholesterol 115 mg), Sodium 530 mg, Total Carbohydrate 5 gm, Dietary Fiber 1 gm, Sugars 4 gm, Protein 31 gm

Note: The sauce on this roast works well for any meat.

This is an easy meal to have for a Saturday dinner with guests or extended family. There is usually a lot of sauce, so make plenty of potatoes, noodles, or rice.

Baked Lamb Shanks

Irma H. Schoen • Windsor, CT

Makes 6 servings (Ideal slow cooker size: 4-quart)

1 medium onion, thinly sliced

2 small carrots, cut in thin strips

1 rib celery, chopped

3 (1 lb. each) lamb shanks, cracked, trimmed of fat

1–2 cloves garlic, split

$\frac{1}{8}$ tsp. salt

$\frac{1}{4}$ tsp. pepper

1 tsp. dried oregano

1 tsp. dried thyme

2 bay leaves, crumbled

$\frac{1}{2}$ cup dry white wine

8-oz. can tomato sauce

1. Place onions, carrots, and celery in slow cooker.

2. Rub lamb with garlic and season with salt and pepper. Add to slow cooker.

3. Mix remaining ingredients together in separate bowl and add to meat and vegetables.

4. Cover. Cook on Low 8–10 hours, or High 4–6 hours.

Exchange List Values: Vegetable 1.0, Meat, very lean 4.0, Fat 0.5

Basic Nutritional Values: Calories 182 (Calories from Fat 44), Total Fat 5 gm (Saturated Fat 1.7 gm, Polyunsat Fat 0.3 gm, Monounsat Fat 2.1 gm, Cholesterol 83 mg), Sodium 386 mg, Total Carbohydrate 7 gm, Dietary Fiber 2 gm, Sugars 4 gm, Protein 26 gm

Lamb Stew

Dottie Schmidt • Kansas City, MO

Makes 6 servings (Ideal slow cooker size: 4-quart)

2 lbs. lamb, cubed

$\frac{1}{2}$ tsp. sugar

2 Tbsp. oil

2 tsp. salt

$\frac{1}{4}$ tsp. pepper

$\frac{1}{4}$ cup flour

2 cups water

$\frac{3}{4}$ cup red cooking wine

$\frac{1}{4}$ tsp. powdered garlic

2 tsp. Worcestershire sauce

6 medium carrots, sliced

4 small onions, quartered

4 ribs celery, sliced

3 medium potatoes, unpeeled, diced

1. Sprinkle lamb with sugar. Brown in oil in skillet.

2. Remove lamb and place in cooker, reserving drippings. Stir salt, pepper, and flour into drippings until smooth. Stir in water and wine until smooth, stirring until broth simmers and thickens.

3. Pour into cooker. Add remaining ingredients and stir until well mixed.

4. Cover. Cook on Low 8–10 hours.

5. Serve with crusty bread.

Exchange List Values: Starch 1.5, Vegetable 2.0, Meat, lean 4.0

Basic Nutritional Values: Calories 388 (Calories from Fat 116), Total Fat 13 gm (Saturated Fat 3.2 gm, Polyunsat Fat 2.3 gm, Monounsat Fat 5.9 gm, Cholesterol 98 mg), Sodium 943 mg, Total Carbohydrate 32 gm, Dietary Fiber 5 gm, Sugars 9 gm, Protein 35 gm

Lamb Chops

Shirley Sears • Tiskilwa, IL

Makes 6–8 servings (Ideal slow cooker size: 4-quart)

1 medium onion, sliced

1 tsp. dried oregano

$\frac{1}{2}$ tsp. dried thyme

$\frac{1}{2}$ tsp. garlic powder

$\frac{1}{4}$ tsp. salt

$\frac{1}{8}$ tsp. pepper

8 loin lamb chops ($1\frac{3}{4}$–2 lbs.), bone-in, trimmed of visible fat

2 cloves garlic, minced

$\frac{1}{4}$ cup water

1. Place onion in slow cooker.

2. Combine oregano, thyme, garlic powder, salt, and pepper. Rub over lamb chops. Place in slow cooker. Top with garlic. Pour water down along side of cooker, so as not to disturb the rub on the chops.

3. Cover. Cook on Low 4–6 hours.

Exchange List Values: Meat, lean 2.0

Basic Nutritional Values: Calories 117 (Calories from Fat 44), Total Fat 5 gm (Saturated Fat 1.7 gm, Polyunsat Fat 0.3 gm, Monounsat Fat 2.1 gm, Cholesterol 48 mg), Sodium 116 mg, Total Carbohydrate 2 gm, Dietary Fiber 0 gm, Sugars 1 gm, Protein 15 gm

Herb Potato-Fish Bake

Barbara Sparks • Glen Burnie, MD

Makes 4 servings (Ideal slow cooker size: 4-quart)

10¾-oz. can cream of celery soup

½ cup water

1-lb. perch fillet, fresh or thawed

2 cups cooked, diced potatoes, drained

¼ cup freshly grated Parmesan cheese

1 Tbsp. chopped parsley

½ tsp. dried basil

¼ tsp. dried oregano

1. Combine soup and water. Pour half in slow cooker. Spread fillet on top. Place potatoes on fillet. Pour remaining soup mix over top.

2. Combine cheese and herbs. Sprinkle over ingredients in slow cooker.

3. Cover. Cook on High 1–2 hours, being careful not to overcook fish.

Exchange List Values: Starch 1.0, Carbohydrate 0.5, Meat, lean 3.0

Basic Nutritional Values: Calories 269 (Calories from Fat 73), Total Fat 8 gm (Saturated Fat 2.8 gm, Polyunsat Fat 2.3 gm, Monounsat Fat 2.2 gm, Cholesterol 56 mg), Sodium 696 mg, Total Carbohydrate 22 gm, Dietary Fiber 2 gm, Sugars 2 gm, Protein 26 gm

Jambalaya

Doris M. Coyle-Zipp • South Ozone Park, NY

Makes 5–6 servings (Ideal slow cooker size: 4-quart)

3½–4-lb. roasting chicken, trimmed of skin and fat, cut up

3 onions, diced

1 carrot, sliced

3–4 cloves garlic, minced

1 tsp. dried oregano

1 tsp. dried basil

½ tsp. salt

⅛ tsp. white pepper

14-oz. can crushed tomatoes

1 lb. shelled raw shrimp

2 cups cooked rice

1. Combine all ingredients except shrimp and rice in slow cooker.

2. Cover. Cook on Low 2–3½ hours, or until chicken is tender.

3. Add shrimp and rice.

4. Cover. Cook on High 15–20 minutes, or until shrimp are done.

Exchange List Values: Starch 1.0, Vegetable 3.0, Meat, lean 4.0

Basic Nutritional Values: Calories 354 (Calories from Fat 65), Total Fat 7 gm (Saturated Fat 1.9 gm, Polyunsat Fat 1.8 gm, Monounsat Fat 2.4 gm, Cholesterol 192 mg), Sodium 589 mg, Total Carbohydrate 29 gm, Dietary Fiber 4 gm, Sugars 9 gm, Protein 41 gm

Shrimp Jambalaya

Karen Ashworth • Duenweg, MO

Recipe photo appears in color section.

Makes 8 servings (Ideal slow cooker size: 4-quart)

2 Tbsp. margarine

2 medium onions, chopped

2 green bell peppers, chopped

3 ribs celery, chopped

1 cup chopped extra-lean, reduced-sodium cooked ham

2 cloves garlic, chopped

1½ cups minute rice

1½ cups 99%-fat-free, reduced-sodium beef broth

28-oz. can chopped tomatoes

2 Tbsp. chopped parsley

1 tsp. dried basil

½ tsp. dried thyme

¼ tsp. pepper

⅛ tsp. cayenne pepper

1 lb. shelled, deveined, medium-size shrimp

1 Tbsp. chopped parsley for garnish

1. Melt margarine in slow cooker set on High. Add onions, peppers, celery, ham, and garlic. Cook 30 minutes.

2. Add rice. Cover and cook 15 minutes.

3. Add broth, tomatoes, 2 Tbsp. parsley, and remaining seasonings. Cover and cook on High 1 hour.

4. Add shrimp. Cook on High 30 minutes, or until liquid is absorbed.

5. Garnish with 1 Tbsp. parsley.

Exchange List Values: Starch 1.0, Vegetable 2.0, Meat, lean 1.0, Fat 0.5

Basic Nutritional Values: Calories 205 (Calories from Fat 36), Total Fat 4 gm (Saturated Fat 0.8 gm, Polyunsat Fat 1.3 gm, Monounsat Fat 1.5 gm, Cholesterol 95 mg), Sodium 529 mg, Total Carbohydrate 26 gm, Dietary Fiber 3 gm, Sugars 7 gm, Protein 16 gm

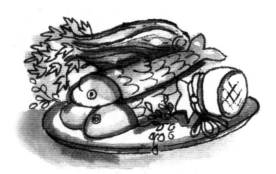

Shrimp Creole

Carol Findling • Princeton, IL

Makes 8–10 servings (Ideal slow cooker size: 4–5-quart)

1/4 cup canola oil

1/3 cup flour

1 3/4 cups sliced onions

1 cup diced green bell peppers

1 cup diced celery

1 1/2 large carrots, shredded

2 3/4-lb. can tomatoes

3/4 cup water

1/2 tsp. dried thyme

1 clove garlic, minced

pinch rosemary

1 Tbsp. sugar

3 bay leaves

1 Tbsp. Worcestershire sauce

3/4 tsp. salt

1/8 tsp. dried oregano

2 lbs. shelled shrimp, deveined

1. Combine canola oil and flour in a skillet. Brown, stirring constantly. Add onions, green peppers, celery, and carrots. Cook 5–10 minutes. Transfer to slow cooker.

2. Add remaining ingredients, except shrimp, and stir well.

3. Cover. Cook on Low 6–8 hours.

4. Add shrimp during last hour.

5. Serve over rice.

Exchange List Values: Vegetable 3.0, Meat, very lean 2.0, Fat 1.0

Basic Nutritional Values: Calories 187 (Calories from Fat 59), Total Fat 7 gm (Saturated Fat 0.6 gm, Polyunsat Fat 2.1 gm, Monounsat Fat 3.4 gm, Cholesterol 140 mg), Sodium 563 mg, Total Carbohydrate 15 gm, Dietary Fiber 3 gm, Sugars 8 gm, Protein 17 gm

Oriental Shrimp Casserole

Sharon Wantland • Menomonee Falls, WI

Makes 10 servings (Ideal slow cooker size: 4-quart)

4 cups cooked rice

2 cups cooked or canned shrimp

1 cup cooked or canned chicken

1-lb. can (2 cups) Chinese vegetables

10¾-oz. can cream of celery soup

½ cup milk

½ cup chopped green peppers

1 Tbsp. soy sauce

3-oz. can dried Chinese noodles

1. Combine all ingredients except noodles in slow cooker.

2. Cover. Cook on Low 45 minutes.

3. Top with noodles just before serving.

Exchange List Values: Starch 2.0, Meat, lean 1.0

Basic Nutritional Values: Calories 216 (Calories from Fat 54), Total Fat 6 gm (Saturated Fat 1.5 gm, Polyunsat Fat 2.5 gm, Monounsat Fat 1.5 gm, Cholesterol 58 mg), Sodium 452 mg, Total Carbohydrate 27 gm, Dietary Fiber 1 gm, Sugars 1 gm, Protein 12 gm

Talk positively to yourself; don't talk down. If your sugar level was high, think, "I was high, and I treated it," rather than "I was high; I failed."

Seafood Gumbo

Barbara Katrine Rose • Woodbridge, VA

Makes 6 servings (Ideal slow cooker size: 4-5-quart)

1 lb. okra, sliced

3 Tbsp. canola oil

¼ cup flour

1 bunch green onions, sliced

½ cup chopped celery

2 cloves garlic, minced

16-oz. can tomatoes and juice

1 bay leaf

1 Tbsp. chopped fresh parsley

1 fresh thyme sprig

½ tsp. salt

½-1 tsp. red pepper

3-5 cups water, depending upon the consistency you like

1 lb. peeled and deveined fresh shrimp

½ lb. fresh crabmeat

1. Saute okra in 1 Tbsp. canola oil until it is lightly browned. Transfer to slow cooker.

2. Combine 2 Tbsp. canola oil and flour in skillet. Cook over medium heat, stirring constantly until roux is the color of chocolate, 20-25 minutes. Stir in green onions, celery, and garlic. Cook until vegetables are tender. Add to slow cooker. Gently stir in remaining ingredients.

3. Cover. Cook on High 3-4 hours. Serve over hot rice.

Exchange List Values: Vegetable 3.0, Meat, very lean 2.0, Fat 1.5

Basic Nutritional Values: Calories 221 (Calories from Fat 75), Total Fat 8 gm (Saturated Fat 0.7 gm, Polyunsat Fat 2.6 gm, Monounsat Fat 4.3 gm, Cholesterol 148 mg), Sodium 548 mg, Total Carbohydrate 15 gm, Dietary Fiber 3 gm, Sugars 5 gm, Protein 22 gm

Curried Shrimp

Charlotte Shaffer • East Earl, PA

Makes 5 servings (Ideal slow cooker size: 3–4-quart)

1 small onion, chopped

2 cups cooked shrimp

1 tsp. curry powder

10¾-oz. can 98%-fat-free, reduced-sodium cream of mushroom soup

1 cup fat-free sour cream

1. Combine all ingredients except sour cream in slow cooker.

2. Cover. Cook on Low 4–6 hours.

3. Ten minutes before serving, stir in sour cream.

4. Serve over rice or puff pastry.

Exchange List Values: Starch 2.0, Meat, lean 1.0

Basic Nutritional Values: Calories 130 (Calories from Fat 16), Total Fat 2 gm (Saturated Fat 0.6 gm, Polyunsat Fat 0.5 gm, Monounsat Fat 0.4 gm, Cholesterol 92 mg), Sodium 390 mg, Total Carbohydrate 15 gm, Dietary Fiber 1 gm, Sugars 5 gm, Protein 12 gm

VARIATION: Add another ½ tsp. curry for some added flavor.

Company Seafood Pasta

Jennifer Yoder Sommers • Harrisonburg, VA

Recipe photo appears in color section.

Makes 8 servings (Ideal slow cooker size: 4-quart)

2 cups fat-free sour cream

5 ozs. (1¼ cups) shredded reduced-fat Monterey Jack cheese

1 Tbsp. light, soft tub margarine, melted

½ lb. fresh crabmeat

⅛ tsp. pepper

½ lb. bay scallops, lightly cooked

1 lb. medium shrimp, cooked and peeled

4 cups cooked linguine

1. Combine sour cream, cheese, and margarine in slow cooker.

2. Stir in remaining ingredients, except linguine.

3. Cover. Cook on Low 1–2 hours.

4. Serve immediately over linguine. Garnish with fresh parsley.

Exchange List Values: Starch 2.0, Meat, lean 3.0

Basic Nutritional Values: Calories 308 (Calories from Fat 59), Total Fat 7 gm (Saturated Fat 3.1 gm, Polyunsat Fat 1.1 gm, Monounsat Fat 2.1 gm, Cholesterol 127 mg), Sodium 449 mg, Total Carbohydrate 31 gm, Dietary Fiber 1 gm, Sugars 5 gm, Protein 29 gm

Seafood Medley

Susan Alexander • Baltimore, MD

Makes 12 servings (Ideal slow cooker size: 4-quart)

1 lb. peeled and deveined shrimp

1 lb. crabmeat

1 lb. bay scallops

2 10¾-oz. cans cream of celery soup

2 soup cans fat-free milk

3 tsp. margarine

1 tsp. Old Bay seasoning

¼ tsp. pepper

1. Layer shrimp, crab, and scallops in slow cooker.

2. Combine soup and milk. Pour over seafood.

3. Mix together margarine and spices and pour over top.

4. Cover. Cook on Low 3–4 hours.

5. Serve over rice or noodles.

Exchange List Values: Carbohydrate 0.5, Meat, very lean 3.0, Fat 0.5

Basic Nutritional Values: Calories 168 (Calories from Fat 51), Total Fat 6 gm (Saturated Fat 1.6 gm, Polyunsat Fat 2.1 gm, Monounsat Fat 1.5 gm, Cholesterol 106 mg), Sodium 679 mg, Total Carbohydrate 7 gm, Dietary Fiber 0 gm, Sugars 3 gm, Protein 20 gm

Salmon Cheese Casserole

Wanda S. Curtin • Bradenton, FL

Makes 6 servings (Ideal slow cooker size: 4-quart)

14¾-oz. can salmon, canned without salt, but with liquid

4-oz. can mushrooms, drained

1½ cups bread crumbs

2 eggs, beaten

½ cup grated reduced-fat cheddar cheese

1 Tbsp. lemon juice

1 Tbsp. minced onion

1. Flake fish in bowl, removing bones. Stir in remaining ingredients. Pour into lightly greased slow cooker.

2. Cover. Cook on Low 3–4 hours.

Exchange List Values: Starch 1.5, Meat, medium fat 2.0

Basic Nutritional Values: Calories 257 (Calories from Fat 85), Total Fat 9 gm (Saturated Fat 2.9 gm, Polyunsat Fat 2.2 gm, Monounsat Fat 3.0 gm, Cholesterol 116 mg), Sodium 442 mg, Total Carbohydrate 21 gm, Dietary Fiber 1 gm, Sugars 2 gm, Protein 23 gm

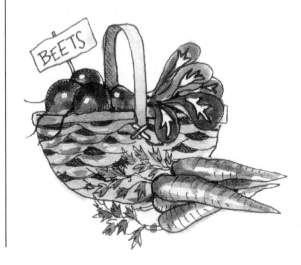

Tuna Barbecue

Esther Martin • Ephrata, PA

Makes 4 servings (Ideal slow cooker size: 3-4-quart)

12-oz. can tuna, packed in water, drained

2 cups no-salt-added tomato juice

1 medium green pepper, finely chopped

2 Tbsp. onion flakes

2 Tbsp. Worcestershire sauce

3 Tbsp. vinegar

2 Tbsp. sugar

1 Tbsp. prepared mustard

1 rib celery, chopped

dash chili powder

½ tsp. cinnamon

dash hot sauce, optional

1. Combine all ingredients in slow cooker.

2. Cover. Cook on Low 8–10 hours, or High 4–5 hours. If mixture becomes too dry while cooking, add ½ cup tomato juice.

3. Serve on buns.

Exchange List Values: Carbohydrate 0.5, Vegetable 2.0, Meat, very lean 2.0

Basic Nutritional Values: Calories 162 (Calories from Fat 8), Total Fat 1 gm (Saturated Fat 0.2 gm, Polyunsat Fat 0.3 gm, Monounsat Fat 0.3 gm, Cholesterol 23 mg), Sodium 423 mg, Total Carbohydrate 18 gm, Dietary Fiber 2 gm, Sugars 14 gm, Protein 21 gm

Tuna Noodle Casserole

Leona Miller • Millersburg, OH

Recipe photo appears in color section.

Makes 6 servings (Ideal slow cooker size: 4-quart)

2 6½-oz. cans water-packed tuna, drained

2 10½-oz. cans 98%-fat-free, reduced-sodium cream of mushroom soup

1 cup milk

2 Tbsp. dried parsley

10-oz. pkg. frozen mixed vegetables, thawed

8-oz. pkg. noodles, cooked and drained

½ cup toasted sliced almonds

1. Combine tuna, soup, milk, parsley, and vegetables. Fold in noodles. Pour into greased slow cooker. Top with almonds.

2. Cover. Cook on Low 7–9 hours, or High 3–4 hours.

Exchange List Values: Starch 2.0, Carbohydrate 1.0, Meat, lean 3.0

Basic Nutritional Values: Calories 395 (Calories from Fat 101), Total Fat 11 gm (Saturated Fat 1.9 gm, Polyunsat Fat 2.5 gm, Monounsat Fat 5.7 gm, Cholesterol 21 mg), Sodium 637 mg, Total Carbohydrate 46 gm, Dietary Fiber 5 gm, Sugars 8 gm, Protein 27 gm

Easy Stuffed Shells

Rebecca Plank Leichty • Harrisonburg, VA

Makes 7 servings (Ideal slow cooker size: 4-quart)

20-oz. bag frozen stuffed shells

15-oz. can marinara or spaghetti sauce

15-oz. can green beans, drained

1. Place shells around edge of greased slow cooker.

2. Cover with marinara sauce.

3. Pour green beans in center.

4. Cover. Cook on Low 8 hours, or on High 3 hours.

5. Serve with garlic toast and salad.

Exchange List Values: Starch 1.0, Vegetable 2.0, Fat 1.5

Basic Nutritional Values: Calories 221 (Calories from Fat 66), Total Fat 7 gm (Saturated Fat 3.2 gm, Polyunsat Fat 0.9 gm, Monounsat Fat 2.2 gm, Cholesterol 66 mg), Sodium 728 mg, Total Carbohydrate 27 gm, Dietary Fiber 3 gm, Sugars 7 gm, Protein 10 gm

VARIATION: Reverse Steps 2 and 3. Double the amount of marinara sauce and pour over both the shells and the beans.

Tempeh-Stuffed Peppers

Sara Harter Fredette • Williamsburg, MA

Makes 4 servings (Ideal slow cooker size: 6-quart oval, so the peppers can each sit on the bottom of slow cooker)

4 ozs. tempeh, cubed

1 clove garlic, minced

2 14½-oz. cans no-salt-added diced tomatoes

2 tsp. soy sauce

¼ cup chopped onions

1½ cups cooked rice

1 cup shredded fat-free cheddar cheese

Tabasco sauce, optional

4 green, red, or yellow bell peppers, tops removed and seeded

¼ cup shredded fat-free cheddar cheese

1. Steam tempeh 10 minutes in saucepan. Mash in bowl with garlic, half the tomatoes, and soy sauce.

2. Stir in onions, rice, 1 cup cheese, and Tabasco sauce. Stuff into peppers.

3. Place peppers in slow cooker. Pour remaining half of tomatoes over peppers.

4. Cover. Cook on Low 6–8 hours, or High 3–4 hours. Top with ¼ cup cheese in last 30 minutes.

Exchange List Values: Starch 2.0, Vegetable 3.0, Meat, lean 1.0

Basic Nutritional Values: Calories 266 (Calories from Fat 26), Total Fat 3 gm (Saturated Fat 0.1 gm, Polyunsat Fat 1.5 gm, Monounsat Fat 0.6 gm, Cholesterol 4 mg), Sodium 510 mg, Total Carbohydrate 42 gm, Dietary Fiber 6 gm, Sugars 17 gm, Protein 21 gm

Minestra di Ceci

Jeanette Oberholtzer • Manheim, PA

Makes 8 servings (Ideal slow cooker size: 4-quart)

1 lb. dry chickpeas

1 sprig fresh rosemary

10 leaves fresh sage

1 Tbsp. salt

1-2 large cloves garlic, minced

1 tsp. canola oil

1 cup small dry pasta, your choice of shape

1. Wash chickpeas. Place in slow cooker. Soak for 8 hours in full pot of water, along with rosemary, sage, and salt.

2. Drain water. Remove herbs.

3. Refill slow cooker with water to 1" above peas.

4. Cover. Cook on Low 5 hours.

5. Saute garlic in oil in skillet until clear.

6. Puree half of peas, along with several cups of broth from cooker, in blender. Return puree to slow cooker. Add garlic and oil.

7. Boil pasta in saucepan until al dente, about 5 minutes. Drain. Add to peas.

8. Cover. Cook on High 30-60 minutes, or until pasta is tender and heated through, but not mushy.

Exchange List Values: Starch 2.5, Meat, very lean 1.0

Basic Nutritional Values: Calories 236 (Calories from Fat 34), Total Fat 4 gm (Saturated Fat 0.4 gm, Polyunsat Fat 1.5 gm, Monounsat Fat 1.1 gm, Cholesterol 0 mg), Sodium 445 mg, Total Carbohydrate 40 gm, Dietary Fiber 9 gm, Sugars 7 gm, Protein 12 gm

VARIATION: Add ½ tsp. black pepper to Step 1, if you like.

Barbecued Lentils

Sue Hamilton • Minooka, IL

Makes 8 servings (Ideal slow cooker size: 4-quart)

2 cups Phyllis's Homemade Barbecue Sauce (see recipe on page 334)

3½ cups water

1 lb. dry lentils

9.7-oz. pkg. vegetarian hot dogs, sliced

1. Combine all ingredients in slow cooker.

2. Cover. Cook on Low 6-8 hours.

Exchange List Values: Starch 2.0, Vegetable 2.0, Meat, very lean 2.0

Basic Nutritional Values: Calories 270 (Calories from Fat 9), Total Fat 1 gm (Saturated Fat 0.1 gm, Polyunsat Fat 0.5 gm, Monounsat Fat 0.2 gm, Cholesterol 0 mg), Sodium 464 mg, Total Carbohydrate 43 gm, Dietary Fiber 15 gm, Sugars 12 gm, Protein 23 gm

Wear a medical alert bracelet or necklace that says "diabetes"— not to call attention to your condition, but to tell medical personnel to check your sugar level if an emergency happened.

Arroz con Queso

Nadine L. Martinitz • Salina, KS

Makes 6–8 servings (Ideal slow cooker size: 4-quart)

14½-oz. can whole tomatoes, mashed

15-oz. can Mexican style beans, undrained

1½ cups uncooked long-grain rice

3 ozs. grated reduced-fat Monterey Jack cheese

1 large onion, finely chopped

1 cup low-fat cottage cheese

4¼-oz. can chopped green chili peppers, drained

1 Tbsp. canola oil

3 cloves garlic, minced

3 ozs. grated reduced-fat Monterey Jack cheese

1. Combine all ingredients except final 3 ozs. of cheese. Pour into well-greased slow cooker.

2. Cover. Cook on Low 6–9 hours.

3. Sprinkle with remaining cheese before serving.

4. Serve with salsa.

Exchange List Values: Starch 2.5, Vegetable 1.0, Meat, medium fat 1.0

Basic Nutritional Values: Calories 294 (Calories from Fat 59), Total Fat 7 gm (Saturated Fat 3.3 gm, Polyunsat Fat 0.9 gm, Monounsat Fat 2.3 gm, Cholesterol 16 mg), Sodium 589 mg, Total Carbohydrate 42 gm, Dietary Fiber 4 gm, Sugars 6 gm, Protein 16 gm

Cheese Souffle Casserole

Vicki Dinkel • Sharon Spring, KS

Makes 8 servings (Ideal slow cooker size: 4-quart)

14 slices fresh bread, crusts removed, divided

5 ozs. (1¼ cups) grated reduced-fat sharp cheddar cheese, divided

1 Tbsp. light, soft tub margarine, melted, divided

3 eggs

4 egg whites

2 cups fat-free milk, scalded

1 cup fat-free half-and-half

2 tsp. Worcestershire sauce

paprika

1. Tear bread into small pieces. Place half in well-greased slow cooker. Add half the grated cheese and half the margarine. Repeat layers.

2. Beat together eggs and egg whites, milk, half-and-half, and Worcestershire sauce. Pour over bread and cheese. Sprinkle top with paprika.

3. Cover. Cook on Low 4–6 hours.

Exchange List Values: Starch 1.0, Milk, fat-free 0.5, Meat, medium fat 1.0

Basic Nutritional Values: Calories 205 (Calories from Fat 70), Total Fat 8 gm (Saturated Fat 3.4 gm, Polyunsat Fat 1.1 gm, Monounsat Fat 2.3 gm, Cholesterol 96 mg), Sodium 468 mg, Total Carbohydrate 23 gm, Dietary Fiber 1 gm, Sugars 7 gm, Protein 14 gm

Macaroni and Cheese

Sherry L. Lapp • Lancaster, PA

Makes 10 servings (Ideal slow cooker size: 4–5-quart)

8-oz. pkg. elbow macaroni, cooked al dente

12-oz. can fat-free evaporated milk

1 cup fat-free half-and-half

2 Tbsp. light, soft tub margarine, melted

2 large eggs, slightly beaten

6 ozs. (1½ cups) grated sharp reduced-fat cheddar cheese, divided

⅛ tsp. white pepper

¼ cup grated Parmesan cheese

1. In slow cooker, combine lightly cooked macaroni, evaporated milk, half-and-half, melted margarine, eggs, 1 cup cheddar cheese, and pepper.

2. Top with remaining cheddar and Parmesan cheeses.

3. Cover. Cook on Low 3 hours.

Exchange List Values: Starch 1.0, Milk, fat-free 0.5, Meat, lean 1.0, Fat 0.5

Basic Nutritional Values: Calories 200 (Calories from Fat 64), Total Fat 7 gm (Saturated Fat 3.3 gm, Polyunsat Fat 0.6 gm, Monounsat Fat 2.3 gm, Cholesterol 59 mg), Sodium 310 mg, Total Carbohydrate 24 gm, Dietary Fiber 1 gm, Sugars 6 gm, Protein 13 gm

Crockpot Macaroni

Lisa F. Good • Harrisonburg, VA

Makes 6 servings (Ideal slow cooker size: 4-quart)

1½ cups dry macaroni

1½ Tbsp. light, soft tub margarine

6 ozs. light Velveeta cheese, sliced

2 cups fat-free milk

1 cup fat-free half-and-half

1. Combine macaroni and margarine in a slow cooker.

2. Layer cheese over top.

3. Pour in milk and half-and-half.

4. Cover. Cook on High 3–4 hours, or until macaroni are soft.

Exchange List Values: Starch 1.0, Milk, fat-free 1.0, Fat 1.0

Basic Nutritional Values: Calories 208 (Calories from Fat 45), Total Fat 5 gm (Saturated Fat 2.5 gm, Polyunsat Fat 0.5 gm, Monounsat Fat 1.6 gm, Cholesterol 15 mg), Sodium 555 mg, Total Carbohydrate 27 gm, Dietary Fiber 0 gm, Sugars 12 gm, Protein 14 gm

Spaghetti Sauce

Doris Perkins • Mashpee, MA

Makes 20 servings (Ideal slow cooker size: 4–5-quart)

2 slices bacon, diced

1¼ lbs. ground beef

½ lb. ground pork

1 cup chopped onions

½ cup chopped green peppers

3 cloves garlic, minced

2 2-lb. 3-oz. cans Italian tomatoes

2 6-oz. cans tomato paste

1 cup dry red wine, or water

2½ tsp. dried oregano

2½ tsp. dried basil

1 bay leaf, crumbled

¾ cup water

¼ cup chopped fresh parsley

1 tsp. dried thyme

1 tsp. salt

¼ tsp. pepper

¼ cup dry red wine, or water

1. Brown bacon in skillet until crisp. Drain. Remove. Add ground beef and pork. Crumble and cook until brown. Stir in onions, green peppers, and garlic. Cook 10 minutes. Drain fat and pat dry with absorbent toweling.

2. Pour tomatoes into slow cooker and crush with back of spoon.

3. Add all other ingredients, except ¼ cup wine, in slow cooker.

4. Cover. Bring to boil on High. Reduce heat to Low for 3–4 hours.

5. During last 30 minutes, stir in wine or water.

Exchange List Values: Vegetable 2.0, Meat, medium fat 1.0

Basic Nutritional Values: Calories 115 (Calories from Fat 46), Total Fat 5 gm (Saturated Fat 1.8 gm, Polyunsat Fat 0.4 gm, Monounsat Fat 2.2 gm, Cholesterol 25 mg), Sodium 309 mg, Total Carbohydrate 9 gm, Dietary Fiber 2 gm, Sugars 4 gm, Protein 9 gm

Did you know that fat-free foods can sometimes be higher in calories and carbohydrates than the original version? Read the two labels and compare.

Chunky Spaghetti Sauce

Patti Boston • Newark, OH

Makes 12 cups (Ideal slow cooker size: 4-quart)

1 lb. ground beef, browned and drained

½ lb. bulk sausage, browned and drained

14½-oz. can no-salt-added Italian tomatoes with basil

15-oz. can Italian tomato sauce

1 medium onion, chopped

1 green pepper, chopped

8-oz. can sliced mushrooms

½ cup dry red wine

2 tsp. sugar

1 tsp. minced garlic

1½ tsp. dried basil

1. Combine all ingredients in slow cooker.

2. Cover. Cook on High 3½–4 hours, or Low 7–8 hours.

Exchange List Values: Vegetable 2.0, Meat, medium fat 1.0

Basic Nutritional Values: Calories 134 (Calories from Fat 61), Total Fat 7 gm (Saturated Fat 2.5 gm, Polyunsat Fat 0.5 gm, Monounsat Fat 2.9 gm, Cholesterol 30 mg), Sodium 397 mg, Total Carbohydrate 8 gm, Dietary Fiber 2 gm, Sugars 4 gm, Protein 11 gm

VARIATIONS:

1. For added texture and zest, add 3 fresh, medium-sized tomatoes, chopped, and 4 large fresh basil leaves, torn. Stir in 1 tsp. salt and ½ tsp. pepper.

2. To any leftover sauce, add chickpeas or kidney beans and serve chili!

Sausage-Beef Spaghetti Sauce

Jeannine Janzen • Elbing, KS

Makes 16–20 servings (Ideal slow cooker size: 4-quart)

1 lb. ground beef

1 lb. Italian sausage, sliced

2 28-oz. cans crushed tomatoes

¾ can (28-oz. tomato can) water

2 tsp. garlic powder

1 tsp. pepper

2 Tbsp. or more parsley

2 Tbsp. dried oregano

2 12-oz. cans tomato paste

2 12-oz. cans tomato puree

1. Brown ground beef and sausage in skillet. Drain. Transfer to large slow cooker.

2. Add crushed tomatoes, water, garlic powder, pepper, parsley, and oregano.

3. Cover. Cook on High 30 minutes. Add tomato paste and tomato puree. Cook on Low 6 hours.

Exchange List Values: Vegetable 3.0, Meat, high fat 1.0

Basic Nutritional Values: Calories 176 (Calories from Fat 71), Total Fat 8 gm (Saturated Fat 2.7 gm, Polyunsat Fat 0.8 gm, Monounsat Fat 3.1 gm, Cholesterol 27 mg), Sodium 408 mg, Total Carbohydrate 17 gm, Dietary Fiber 4 gm, Sugars 6 gm, Protein 10 gm

Note: Leftovers freeze well.

Mom's Meatballs

Mary C. Casey • Scranton, PA

Makes 8-10 servings (Ideal slow cooker size: 4-5-quart)

SAUCE:

¼-½ cup chopped onions

3 cloves garlic, minced

2 Tbsp. canola oil

29-oz. can tomato puree

29-oz. can water

12-oz. can tomato paste

12-oz. can water

1 Tbsp. sugar

2 tsp. dried oregano

¼ tsp. Italian seasoning

½ tsp. dried basil

⅛ tsp. pepper

¼ cup diced green peppers

MEATBALLS:

1 lb. 85%-lean ground beef

1 egg

2 Tbsp. water

¾ cup Italian bread crumbs

⅛ tsp. black pepper

⅛ tsp. salt

1 Tbsp. canola oil

1. Saute onions and garlic in oil in saucepan.

2. Combine all sauce ingredients in slow cooker.

3. Cover. Cook on Low while making meatballs.

4. Mix together all meatball ingredients except oil. Form into small meatballs, then brown on all sides in oil in saucepan. Drain on paper towels. Add to sauce.

5. Cover. Cook on Low 4–5 hours.

Exchange List Values: Starch 0.5, Vegetable 3.0, Meat, medium fat 1.0, Fat 1.0

Basic Nutritional Values: Calories 221 (Calories from Fat 91), Total Fat 10 gm (Saturated Fat 2.4 gm, Polyunsat Fat 1.7 gm, Monounsat Fat 4.9 gm, Cholesterol 48 mg), Sodium 540 mg, Total Carbohydrate 22 gm, Dietary Fiber 4 gm, Sugars 7 gm, Protein 13 gm

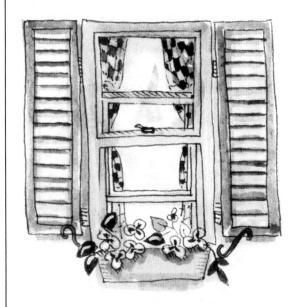

Easy-Does-It Spaghetti

Rachel Kauffman • Alto, MI / Lois Stoltzfus • Honey Brook, PA / Deb Unternahrer • Wayland, IA

Makes 12 servings (Ideal slow cooker size: 4-quart)

2 lbs. 85%-lean ground chuck, browned and drained

1 cup chopped onions

2 cloves garlic, minced

2 15-oz. cans no-salt-added tomato sauce

3 tsp. Italian seasoning

1/4 tsp. pepper

2 4-oz. cans sliced mushrooms, drained

6 cups tomato juice

16 ozs. dry spaghetti, broken into 4"-5" pieces

1. Combine all ingredients except spaghetti in slow cooker.

2. Cover. Cook on Low 6–8 hours, or High 3–5 hours. Turn to High during last 30 minutes and stir in dry spaghetti. (If spaghetti is not fully cooked, continue cooking another 10 minutes, checking to make sure it is not becoming overcooked.)

3. Sprinkle individual servings with Parmesan cheese, if diets permit.

Exchange List Values: Starch 2.0, Vegetable 2.0, Meat, lean 2.0

Basic Nutritional Values: Calories 328 (Calories from Fat 78), Total Fat 9 gm (Saturated Fat 3.0 gm, Polyunsat Fat 0.6 gm, Monounsat Fat 3.5 gm, Cholesterol 45 mg), Sodium 547 mg, Total Carbohydrate 42 gm, Dietary Fiber 3 gm, Sugars 10 gm, Protein 22 gm

VARIATION: Add 1 tsp. dry mustard and 1/2 tsp. allspice in Step 1.

Kathy Hertzler • Lancaster, PA

Nancy's Spaghetti Sauce

Nancy Graves • Manhattan, KS

Makes 4–6 servings (Ideal slow cooker size: 4-quart)

1/4 cup minced onion

garlic powder to taste

3 cups chopped fresh tomatoes

6-oz. can tomato paste

1/2 tsp. salt

dash pepper

1 basil leaf

1 chopped green pepper

1 lb. ground beef, browned and drained

4-oz. can sliced mushrooms, undrained

1. Combine all ingredients in slow cooker.

2. Cover. Cook on Low 3 hours.

Exchange List Values: Vegetable 2.0, Meat, lean 2.0, Fat 0.5

Basic Nutritional Values: Calories 186 (Calories from Fat 75), Total Fat 8 gm (Saturated Fat 3.0 gm, Polyunsat Fat 0.5 gm, Monounsat Fat 3.4 gm, Cholesterol 45 mg), Sodium 372 mg, Total Carbohydrate 12 gm, Dietary Fiber 3 gm, Sugars 4 gm, Protein 17 gm

Take a walk after dinner instead of watching TV.

Spaghetti with Meat Sauce

Esther Lehman • Croghan, NY

Makes 8-10 servings (Ideal slow cooker size: 4-5-quart)

1 lb. ground beef, browned

2 28-oz. cans tomatoes

2 medium onions, quartered

2 medium carrots, cut into chunks

2 cloves garlic, minced

6-oz. can tomato paste

2 Tbsp. chopped fresh parsley

1 bay leaf

1 Tbsp. sugar

1 tsp. dried basil

½ tsp. salt

½ tsp. dried oregano

dash pepper

2 Tbsp. cold water

2 Tbsp. cornstarch

1. Place meat in slow cooker.

2. In blender, combine 1 can tomatoes, onions, carrots, and garlic. Cover and blend until finely chopped. Stir into meat.

3. Cut up the remaining can of tomatoes. Stir into meat mixture. Add tomato paste, parsley, bay leaf, sugar, basil, salt, oregano, and pepper. Mix well.

4. Cover. Cook on Low 8-10 hours.

5. To serve, turn to High. Remove bay leaf. Cover and heat until bubbly, about 10 minutes.

6. Combine water and cornstarch. Stir into tomato mixture. Cook 10 minutes longer.

7. Serve with spaghetti and Parmesan cheese.

Exchange List Values: Vegetable 3.0, Meat, lean 1.0, Fat 0.5

Basic Nutritional Values: Calories 151 (Calories from Fat 46), Total Fat 5 gm (Saturated Fat 1.8 gm, Polyunsat Fat 0.4 gm, Monounsat Fat 2.1 gm, Cholesterol 27 mg), Sodium 403 mg, Total Carbohydrate 17 gm, Dietary Fiber 3 gm, Sugars 8 gm, Protein 11 gm

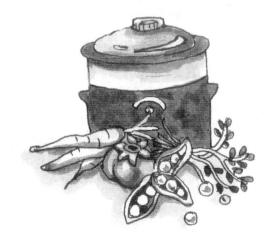

Pasta Sauce with Meat and Veggies

Maria Foikerts • Holland, OH

Makes 6 servings (Ideal slow cooker size: 4-quart)

1/2 lb. ground turkey, browned and drained

1/2 lb. ground beef, browned and drained

1 rib celery, chopped

2 medium carrots, chopped

1 clove garlic, minced

1 medium onion, chopped

28-oz. can diced tomatoes with juice

1/4 tsp. salt

1/4 tsp. dried thyme

6-oz. can tomato paste

1/8 tsp. pepper

1. Combine turkey, beef, celery, carrots, garlic, and onion in slow cooker.

2. Add remaining ingredients. Mix well.

3. Cover. Cook on Low 7–8 hours.

4. Serve over pasta or rice.

Exchange List Values: Vegetable 3.0, Meat, lean 2.0, Fat 0.5

Basic Nutritional Values: Calories 200 (Calories from Fat 72), Total Fat 8 gm (Saturated Fat 2.4 gm, Polyunsat Fat 1.3 gm, Monounsat Fat 3.1 gm, Cholesterol 50 mg), Sodium 391 mg, Total Carbohydrate 16 gm, Dietary Fiber 4 gm, Sugars 7 gm, Protein 17 gm

Katelyn's Spaghetti Sauce

Katelyn Bailey • Mechanicsburg, PA

Makes 10–12 servings (Ideal slow cooker size: 4–5-quart)

1 lb. ground beef, browned and drained

3/4 cup chopped onions

1 clove garlic, minced

3 Tbsp. oil

2 6-oz. cans tomato paste

1 Tbsp. sugar

1 1/2 tsp. salt

1–1 1/2 tsp. dried oregano

1/2 tsp. pepper

1 bay leaf

2 qts. fresh tomatoes, or tomato sauce

1. Combine all ingredients in slow cooker.

2. Cover. Cook on Low 8–10 hours. Remove bay leaf before serving.

Exchange List Values: Vegetable 3.0, Meat, lean 1.0, Fat 0.5

Basic Nutritional Values: Calories 151 (Calories from Fat 71), Total Fat 8 gm (Saturated Fat 1.7 gm, Polyunsat Fat 1.4 gm, Monounsat Fat 3.8 gm, Cholesterol 22 mg), Sodium 342 mg, Total Carbohydrate 13 gm, Dietary Fiber 3 gm, Sugars 6 gm, Protein 9 gm

Note: This sauce freezes well.

Italian Vegetable Pasta Sauce

Sherril Bieberly • Sauna, KS

Makes 20 1/2-cup servings (Ideal slow cooker size: 4–5-quart)

3 Tbsp. olive oil

1 cup packed chopped fresh parsley

3 ribs celery, chopped

1 medium onion, chopped

2 cloves garlic, minced

2" sprig fresh rosemary, or 1/2 tsp. dried rosemary

2 small fresh sage leaves, or 1/2 tsp. dried sage

32-oz. can tomato sauce

32-oz. can chopped tomatoes

1 small dried hot chili pepper

1/4 lb. fresh mushrooms, sliced, or 8-oz. can sliced mushrooms, drained

1/2 tsp. salt

1. Heat oil in skillet. Add parsley, celery, onion, garlic, rosemary, and sage. Saute until vegetables are tender. Place in slow cooker.

2. Add sauce, tomatoes, chili pepper, mushrooms, and salt.

3. Cover. Cook on Low 12–18 hours, or on High 5–6 hours.

Exchange List Values: Vegetable 1.0, Fat 0.5

Basic Nutritional Values: Calories 49 (Calories from Fat 20), Total Fat 2 gm (Saturated Fat 0.3 gm, Polyunsat Fat 0.3 gm, Monounsat Fat 1.5 gm, Cholesterol 0 mg), Sodium 402 mg, Total Carbohydrate 7 gm, Dietary Fiber 2 gm, Sugars 4 gm, Protein 1 gm

VARIATION: Add 2 lbs. browned ground beef to olive oil and sauteed vegetables. Continue with recipe.

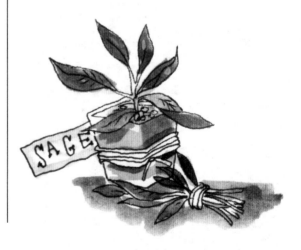

Creamy Spaghetti

Dale Peterson • Rapid City, SD

Makes 8 servings (Ideal slow cooker size: 5-quart)

1 cup chopped onions

1 cup chopped green peppers

1 Tbsp. olive oil

28-oz. can tomatoes with juice

4-oz. can mushrooms, chopped and drained

2¼-oz. can sliced ripe olives, drained

2 tsp. dried oregano

1 lb. ground beef, browned and drained

12 ozs. spaghetti, cooked and drained

10¾-oz. can 98%-fat-free, reduced-sodium cream of mushroom soup

½ cup water

1½ cups (6 ozs.) shredded fat-free cheddar cheese

¼ cup freshly grated Parmesan cheese

1. Saute onions and green peppers in olive oil in skillet until tender. Add tomatoes, mushrooms, olives, oregano, and beef. Simmer for 10 minutes. Transfer to slow cooker.

2. Add spaghetti. Mix well.

3. Combine soup and water. Pour over casserole. Sprinkle with cheeses.

4. Cover. Cook on Low 4–6 hours.

Exchange List Values: Starch 2.5, Vegetable 2.0, Meat, medium fat 2.0

Basic Nutritional Values: Calories 390 (Calories from Fat 103), Total Fat 11 gm (Saturated Fat 3.5 gm, Polyunsat Fat 1.1 gm, Monounsat Fat 5.2 gm, Cholesterol 39 mg), Sodium 607 mg, Total Carbohydrate 45 gm, Dietary Fiber 4 gm, Sugars 7 gm, Protein 26 gm

Louise's Vegetable Spaghetti Sauce

Louise Stackhouse • Benton, PA

Makes 4–6 servings (Ideal slow cooker size: 4-quart)

6 fresh medium tomatoes, peeled and crushed

1 medium onion, chopped

2 medium green peppers, chopped

2 cloves garlic, minced

½ tsp. dried basil

½ tsp. dried oregano

¼ tsp. salt

2 Tbsp. sugar

sweetener substitute to equal 1 Tbsp. sugar

1. Combine all ingredients in slow cooker.

2. Cover. Cook on Low 8–10 hours. If the sauce is too watery for your liking, stir in a 6-oz. can of tomato paste during the last hour of cooking.

3. Serve over cooked spaghetti or other pasta.

Exchange List Values: Vegetable 3.0

Basic Nutritional Values: Calories 69 (Calories from Fat 6), Total Fat 1 gm (Saturated Fat 0 gm, Polyunsat Fat 0.2 gm, Monounsat Fat 0.1 gm, Cholesterol 0 mg), Sodium 113 mg, Total Carbohydrate 16 gm, Dietary Fiber 3 gm, Sugars 11 gm, Protein 2 gm

Eat salmon—it has a type of fat that's great for your heart.

Pizza in a Pot

Marianne J. Troyer • Millersburg, OH

Makes 6–8 servings (Ideal slow cooker size: 4-quart)

1 lb. bulk lean sweet Italian turkey sausage, browned and drained

28-oz. can crushed tomatoes

15½-oz. can chili beans

2¼-oz. can sliced black olives, drained

1 medium onion, chopped

1 small green pepper, chopped

2 cloves garlic, minced

¼ cup grated Parmesan cheese

1 Tbsp. quick-cooking tapioca

1 Tbsp. dried basil

1 bay leaf

1. Combine all ingredients in slow cooker.

2. Cover. Cook on Low 8–9 hours.

3. Discard bay leaf. Stir well.

4. Serve over pasta. Top with mozzarella cheese.

Exchange List Values: Starch 1.0, Vegetable 2.0, Meat, lean 2.0, Fat 0.5

Basic Nutritional Values: Calories 251 (Calories from Fat 87), Total Fat 10 gm (Saturated Fat 2.8 gm, Polyunsat Fat 1.1 gm, Monounsat Fat 2.3 gm, Cholesterol 49 mg), Sodium 937 mg, Total Carbohydrate 23 gm, Dietary Fiber 7 gm, Sugars 8 gm, Protein 18 gm

Pizza Rice

Sue Hamilton • Minooka, IL

Makes 14 servings (Idea slow cooker size: 3-4-quart)

2 cups white or brown rice, uncooked

2 cups chunky pizza sauce

3½ cups water

7-oz. can mushrooms, drained and rinsed

3 ozs. turkey pepperoni, sliced

1 cup grated reduced-fat cheddar cheese

1. Combine rice, sauce, water, mushrooms, and pepperoni in slow cooker. Stir.

2. Cover. Cook on Low 4–6 hours, or on High 3–5 hours.

3. Sprinkle with cheese before serving.

Exchange List Values: Starch 1.5, Fat 0.5

Basic Nutritional Values: Calories 151 (Calories from Fat 30), Total Fat 3 gm (Saturated Fat 1.4 gm, Polyunsat Fat 0.5 gm, Monounsat Fat 0.9 gm, Cholesterol 14 mg), Sodium 365 mg, Total Carbohydrate 24 gm, Dietary Fiber 1 gm, Sugars 2 gm, Protein 7 gm

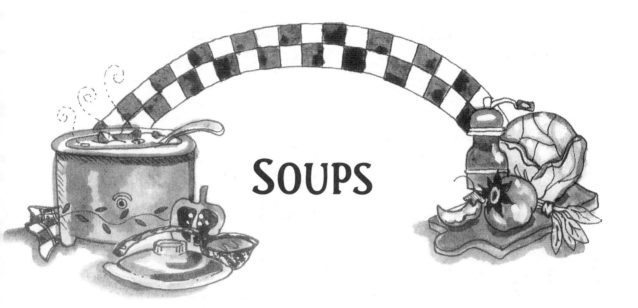

SOUPS

Frances's Hearty Vegetable Soup

Frances Schrag • Newton, KS

Makes 10 servings (Ideal slow cooker size: 6-quart)

1-lb. round steak, cut into ½" pieces

14½-oz. can diced tomatoes

3 cups water

2 potatoes, peeled and cubed

2 onions, sliced

3 ribs celery, sliced

2 carrots, sliced

3 beef bouillon cubes

½ tsp. dried basil

½ tsp. dried oregano

¼ tsp. pepper

1½ cups frozen mixed vegetables, or your choice of frozen vegetables

1. Combine first 3 ingredients in slow cooker.

2. Cover. Cook on High 6 hours.

3. Add remaining ingredients. Cover and cook on High 2 hours more, or until meat and vegetables are tender.

Exchange List Values: Starch 0.5, Vegetable 1.0, Meat, lean 1.0

Basic Nutritional Values: Calories 117 (Calories from Fat 20), Total Fat 2 gm (Saturated Fat 0.7 gm, Polyunsat Fat 0.2 gm, Monounsat Fat 0.9 gm, Cholesterol 26 mg), Sodium 405 mg, Total Carbohydrate 14 gm, Dietary Fiber 3 gm, Sugars 5 gm, Protein 11 gm

VARIATION: Increase dried basil to 1 tsp. and dried oregano to 1 tsp.

Tracy Clark • Mt. Crawford, VA

If you tend to develop nighttime lows, set your alarm and check your blood sugar level at 3:00 a.m. each night.

Nancy's Vegetable Beef Soup

Nancy Graves • Manhattan, KS

Makes 6–8 servings (Ideal slow cooker size: 5–6-quart)

2-lb. roast cut into bite-sized pieces, or 2 lbs. stewing meat

15-oz. can corn

15-oz. can green beans

1-lb. bag frozen peas

40-oz. can no-salt-added stewed tomatoes

5 tsp. sodium-free beef bouillon powder

Tabasco to taste

½ tsp. salt

1. Combine all ingredients in slow cooker. Do not drain vegetables.

2. Add water to fill slow cooker to within 3" of top.

3. Cover. Cook on Low 8 hours, or until meat is tender and vegetables are soft.

Exchange List Values: Starch 1.0, Vegetable 2.0, Meat, lean 2.0

Basic Nutritional Values: Calories 229 (Calories from Fat 46), Total Fat 5 gm (Saturated Fat 1.4 gm, Polyunsat Fat 0.5 gm, Monounsat Fat 2.2 gm, Cholesterol 56 mg), Sodium 545 mg, Total Carbohydrate 24 gm, Dietary Fiber 6 gm, Sugars 10 gm, Protein 23 gm

VARIATION: Add 1 large onion, sliced, 2 cups sliced carrots, and ¾ cup pearl barley to mixture before cooking.

Anona's Beef Vegetable Soup

Anona M. Teel • Bangor, PA

Makes 6 servings (Ideal slow cooker size: 4-quart)

1–1½-lb. soup bone

1 lb. stewing beef cubes

1½ qts. cold water

½ tsp. salt

¾ cup diced celery

¾ cup diced carrots

¾ cup diced potatoes

¾ cup diced onion

1 cup frozen mixed vegetables of your choice

1-lb. can tomatoes

⅛ tsp. pepper

1 Tbsp. chopped dried parsley

1. Put all ingredients in slow cooker.

2. Cover. Cook on Low 8–10 hours. Remove bone before serving.

Exchange List Values: Starch 0.5, Vegetable 1.0, Meat, lean 1.0

Basic Nutritional Values: Calories 134 (Calories from Fat 28), Total Fat 3 gm (Saturated Fat 0.9 gm, Polyunsat Fat 0.3 gm, Monounsat Fat 1.4 gm, Cholesterol 38 mg), Sodium 407 mg, Total Carbohydrate 13 gm, Dietary Fiber 3 gm, Sugars 6 gm, Protein 14 gm

"Absent Cook" Stew

Kathy Hertzler • Lancaster, PA

Makes 5–6 servings (Ideal slow cooker size: 4-quart)

2 lbs. stewing beef, cubed

2–3 carrots, sliced

1 onion, chopped

3 large potatoes, cubed

3 ribs celery, sliced

10¾-oz. can tomato soup

1 soup can water

⅛ tsp. salt

dash pepper

2 Tbsp. vinegar

1. Combine all ingredients in slow cooker.

2. Cover. Cook on Low 10–12 hours.

Exchange List Values: Starch 2.0, Vegetable 1.0, Meat, lean 2.0

Basic Nutritional Values: Calories 314 (Calories from Fat 59), Total Fat 7 gm (Saturated Fat 2.0 gm, Polyunsat Fat 0.8 gm, Monounsat Fat 2.9 gm, Cholesterol 75 mg), Sodium 427 mg, Total Carbohydrate 35 gm, Dietary Fiber 5 gm, Sugars 9 gm, Protein 28 gm

Lilli's Vegetable Beef Soup

Lilli Peters • Dodge City, KS

Makes 10–12 servings (Ideal slow cooker size: 4–5-quart)

3 lbs. stewing meat, cut in 1" pieces

2 Tbsp. canola oil

4 potatoes, cubed

4 carrots, sliced

3 ribs celery, sliced

14-oz. can diced tomatoes

14-oz. can Italian tomatoes, crushed

2 medium onions, chopped

2 wedges cabbage, sliced thin

2 tsp. sodium-free beef bouillon powder

2 Tbsp. fresh parsley

1 tsp. seasoned salt

1 tsp. garlic salt

½ tsp. pepper

water

1. Brown meat in oil in skillet. Drain.

2. Combine all ingredients except water in large slow cooker. Cover with water.

3. Cover. Cook on Low 8–10 hours.

Exchange List Values: Starch 0.5, Vegetable 2.0, Meat, lean 2.0, Fat 0.5

Basic Nutritional Values: Calories 223 (Calories from Fat 61), Total Fat 7 gm (Saturated Fat 1.5 gm, Polyunsat Fat 1.0 gm, Monounsat Fat 3.4 gm, Cholesterol 56 mg), Sodium 465 mg, Total Carbohydrate 20 gm, Dietary Fiber 4 gm, Sugars 7 gm, Protein 21 gm

Jeanne's Vegetable Beef Borscht

Jeanne Heyerly • Chenoa, IL

Makes 8 servings (Ideal slow cooker size: 5-quart)

1-lb. beef roast, cooked and cubed

half a head of cabbage, sliced thin

3 medium potatoes, diced

4 carrots, sliced

1 large onion, diced

1 cup tomatoes, diced

1 cup corn

1 cup green beans

2 cups 98%-fat-free, lower-sodium beef broth

2 cups tomato juice

1/4 tsp. garlic powder

1/4 tsp. dill seed

1/2 tsp. pepper

water

sour cream

1. Mix together all ingredients except water and sour cream. Add water to fill slow cooker three-quarters full.

2. Cover. Cook on Low 8–10 hours.

3. Top individual servings with sour cream.

Exchange List Values: Starch 1.0, Vegetable 3.0, Meat, lean 1.0

Basic Nutritional Values: Calories 185 (Calories from Fat 25), Total Fat 3 gm (Saturated Fat 0.7 gm, Polyunsat Fat 0.4 gm, Monounsat Fat 1.1 gm, Cholesterol 28 mg), Sodium 434 mg, Total Carbohydrate 29 gm, Dietary Fiber 6 gm, Sugars 10 gm, Protein 14 gm

VARIATION: Add 1 cup diced cooked red beets during the last half hour of cooking.

Beef Dumpling Soup

Barbara Walker • Sturgis, SD

Makes 6 servings (Ideal slow cooker size: 4-quart)

1 lb. beef stewing meat, trimmed of visible fat, cubed

Sodium-Free Onion Soup Mix (see recipe on page 334)

6 cups hot water

2 carrots, peeled and shredded

1 rib celery, finely chopped

1 tomato, peeled and chopped

2 cloves garlic

1/2 tsp. dried basil

1/4 tsp. dill weed

1 cup buttermilk biscuit mix

1 Tbsp. finely chopped parsley

6 Tbsp. fat-free milk

1. Place meat in slow cooker. Sprinkle with onion soup mix. Pour water over meat.

2. Add carrots, celery, tomato, garlic, basil, and dill weed.

3. Cover. Cook on Low 4–6 hours, or until meat is tender.

4. Combine biscuit mix and parsley. Stir in milk with fork until moistened. Drop dumplings by teaspoonfuls into pot.

5. Cover. Cook on High 30 minutes.

Exchange List Values: Starch 1.0, Vegetable 1.0, Meat, lean 1.0, Fat 0.5

Basic Nutritional Values: Calories 206 (Calories from Fat 57), Total Fat 6 gm (Saturated Fat 0.9 gm, Polyunsat Fat 1.4 gm, Monounsat Fat 2.6 gm, Cholesterol 38 mg), Sodium 329 mg, Total Carbohydrate 22 gm, Dietary Fiber 2 gm, Sugars 6 gm, Protein 15 gm

Southwestern Bean Soup with Cornmeal Dumplings

Melba Eshleman • Manheim, PA

Recipe photo appears in color section.

Makes 8 servings (Ideal slow cooker size: 4–5-quart)

15½-oz. can red kidney beans, rinsed and drained

15½-oz. can black beans, pinto beans, or Great Northern beans, rinsed and drained

3 cups water

14½-oz. can Mexican-style stewed tomatoes

10-oz. pkg. frozen whole-kernel corn, thawed

1 cup sliced carrots

1 cup chopped onions

4-oz. can chopped green chilies

3 tsp. sodium-free instant bouillon powder (any flavor)

1–2 tsp. chili powder

2 cloves garlic, minced

DUMPLINGS:

⅓ cup flour

¼ cup yellow cornmeal

1 tsp. baking powder

dash salt

dash pepper

1 egg white, beaten

2 Tbsp. milk

1 Tbsp. oil

1. Combine all soup ingredients in slow cooker.

2. Cover. Cook on Low 10–12 hours, or High 4–5 hours.

3. Make dumplings by mixing together flour, cornmeal, baking powder, salt, and pepper.

4. Combine egg white, milk, and oil. Add to flour mixture. Stir with fork until just combined.

5. At the end of the soup's cooking time, turn slow cooker to High. Drop dumpling mixture by rounded teaspoonfuls to make 8 mounds atop the soup.

6. Cover. Cook for 30 minutes (do not lift lid).

Exchange List Values: Starch 2.0, Vegetable 2.0

Basic Nutritional Values: Calories 197 (Calories from Fat 13), Total Fat 1 gm (Saturated Fat 0.2 gm, Polyunsat Fat 0.6 gm, Monounsat Fat 0.5 gm, Cholesterol 0 mg), Sodium 367 mg, Total Carbohydrate 39 gm, Dietary Fiber 8 gm, Sugars 6 gm, Protein 9 gm

Instead of getting frustrated looking for the closest parking spot at the mall, park farther away and walk.

Winter's Night Beef Soup

Kimberly Jensen • Bailey, CO

Makes 12 servings (Ideal slow cooker size: 5-quart)

1-lb. boneless chuck, cut in ½" cubes

1–2 Tbsp. oil

28-oz. can tomatoes

2 carrots, sliced

2 ribs celery, sliced

2 tsp. garlic powder

4 cups water

½ cup red wine

1 small onion, coarsely chopped

4 beef bouillon cubes

1 tsp. pepper

1 tsp. dry oregano

½ tsp. dry thyme

1 bay leaf

¼-½ cup couscous

1. Brown beef cubes in oil in skillet.

2. Place vegetables in bottom of slow cooker. Add beef.

3. Combine all other ingredients except couscous in separate bowl. Pour over ingredients in slow cooker.

4. Cover. Cook on Low 6 hours. Stir in couscous. Cover and cook 30 minutes.

Exchange List Values: Vegetable 2.0, Meat, lean 1.0

Basic Nutritional Values: Calories 88 (Calories from Fat 25), Total Fat 3 gm (Saturated Fat 0.5 gm, Polyunsat Fat 0.5 gm, Monounsat Fat 1.4 gm, Cholesterol 19 mg), Sodium 461 mg, Total Carbohydrate 9 gm, Dietary Fiber 2 gm, Sugars 4 gm, Protein 8 gm

VARIATION: Add zucchini or mushrooms to the rest of the vegetables before cooking.

Old-Fashioned Vegetable Beef Soup

Pam Hochstedler • Kalona, IA

Makes 8-10 servings (Ideal slow cooker size: 4-quart)

1 lb. beef short ribs, trimmed of all visible fat

2 qts. water

1 tsp. salt

½ tsp. celery salt

1 small onion, chopped

1 cup diced carrots

½ cup diced celery

2 cups diced potatoes

1-lb. can whole-kernel corn, undrained

1-lb. can diced tomatoes and juice

1. Combine meat, water, salt, celery salt, onion, carrots, and celery in slow cooker.

2. Cover. Cook on Low 4–6 hours.

3. Debone meat, cut into bite-sized pieces, and return to pot.

4. Add potatoes, corn, and tomatoes.

5. Cover and cook on High 2–3 hours.

Exchange List Values: Starch 0.5, Vegetable 1.0, Fat 0.5

Basic Nutritional Values: Calories 99 (Calories from Fat 24), Total Fat 3 gm (Saturated Fat 1.0 gm, Polyunsat Fat 0.3 gm, Monounsat Fat 1.0 gm, Cholesterol 11 mg), Sodium 413 mg, Total Carbohydrate 13 gm, Dietary Fiber 3 gm, Sugars 6 gm, Protein 6 gm

Lifting light weights (start with 1 to 5 pounds) builds muscle and strength, whether you're age 9 or age 95.

Green Chili Corn Chowder

Kelly Evenson • Pittsboro, NC

Makes 8 servings (Ideal slow cooker size: 4-quart)

16-oz. can cream-style corn

3 potatoes, peeled and diced

2 Tbsp. chopped fresh chives

4-oz. can diced green chilies, drained

2-oz. jar chopped pimentos, drained

½ cup chopped cooked ham

2 10½-oz. cans 100%-fat-free, lower-sodium chicken broth

salt to taste

pepper to taste

Tabasco sauce to taste

1 cup milk

1. Combine all ingredients except milk in slow cooker.

2. Cover. Cook on Low 7–8 hours, or until potatoes are tender.

3. Stir in milk. Heat until hot.

4. Serve with homemade bread.

Exchange List Values: Starch 1.5

Basic Nutritional Values: Calories 124 (Calories from Fat 16), Total Fat 2 gm (Saturated Fat 0.5 gm, Polyunsat Fat 0.3 gm, Monounsat Fat 0.7 gm, Cholesterol 7 mg), Sodium 563 mg, Total Carbohydrate 21 gm, Dietary Fiber 2 gm, Sugars 7 gm, Protein 6 gm

Three-Bean Chili

Chris Kaczynski • Schenectady, NY

Makes 12 servings (Ideal slow cooker size: 6-quart)

2 lbs. ground beef

2 medium onions, diced

16-oz. jar medium salsa

2 pkgs. dry chili seasoning

2 16-oz. cans red kidney beans, drained

2 16-oz. cans black beans, drained

2 16-oz. cans white kidney, or garbanzo, beans, drained

28-oz. can crushed tomatoes

16-oz. can diced tomatoes

2 tsp. sugar

1. Brown beef and onions in skillet.

2. Combine all ingredients in 6-qt. slow cooker, or in 2 4- or 5-qt. cookers.

3. Cover. Cook on Low 8–10 hours.

4. Serve with chopped raw onions.

Exchange List Values: Starch 2.5, Vegetable 2.0, Meat, lean 2.0, Fat 0.5

Basic Nutritional Values: Calories 381 (Calories from Fat 80), Total Fat 9 gm (Saturated Fat 3.1 gm, Polyunsat Fat 0.7 gm, Monounsat Fat 3.4 gm, Cholesterol 45 mg), Sodium 717 mg, Total Carbohydrate 47 gm, Dietary Fiber 14 gm, Sugars 9 gm, Protein 29 gm

Note: This recipe can be cut in half without injuring the flavor, if you don't have a cooker large enough to handle the full amount.

Make exercise fun!

Country Auction Chili Soup

Clara Newswanger • Gordonville, PA

Makes 20 servings (Ideal slow cooker size: 6-quart)

1½ lbs. ground beef

¼ cup chopped onions

½ cup flour

1 Tbsp. chili powder

1 tsp. salt

6 cups water

2 cups ketchup

⅓ cup brown sugar

3 15½-oz. cans kidney beans, undrained

1. Brown ground beef and onions in skillet. Drain. Spoon meat mixture into slow cooker.

2. Stir flour into meat and onions. Add seasonings.

3. Slowly stir in water. Add ketchup, brown sugar, and beans.

4. Cover. Cook on High 4 hours, or on Low 8 hours.

Exchange List Values: Starch 1.0, Vegetable 1.0, Meat, lean 1.0

Basic Nutritional Values: Calories 163 (Calories from Fat 35), Total Fat 4 gm (Saturated Fat 1.4 gm, Polyunsat Fat 0.3 gm, Monounsat Fat 1.5 gm, Cholesterol 20 mg), Sodium 655 mg, Total Carbohydrate 23 gm, Dietary Fiber 3 gm, Sugars 8 gm, Protein 10 gm

Texican Chili

Becky Oswald • Broadway, VA

Makes 15 servings (Ideal slow cooker size: 5–6-quart)

8 bacon strips, diced

2½ lbs. beef stewing meat, cubed

28-oz. can stewed tomatoes

14½-oz. can stewed tomatoes

8-oz. can tomato sauce

8-oz. can no-salt-added tomato sauce

16-oz. can kidney beans, rinsed and drained

2 cups sliced carrots

1 medium onion, chopped

1 cup chopped celery

½ cup chopped green pepper

¼ cup minced fresh parsley

1 Tbsp. chili powder

½ tsp. ground cumin

¼ tsp. pepper

1. Cook bacon in skillet until crisp. Drain on paper towel.

2. Brown beef in bacon drippings in skillet.

3. Combine all ingredients in slow cooker.

4. Cover. Cook on Low 9–10 hours, or until meat is tender. Stir occasionally.

Exchange List Values: Starch 0.5, Vegetable 2.0, Meat, lean 1.0, Fat 0.5

Basic Nutritional Values: Calories 165 (Calories from Fat 44), Total Fat 5 gm (Saturated Fat 1.5 gm, Polyunsat Fat 0.5 gm, Monounsat Fat 2.2 gm, Cholesterol 40 mg), Sodium 434 mg, Total Carbohydrate 15 gm, Dietary Fiber 3 gm, Sugars 6 gm, Protein 16 gm

Spicy Chili

Deborah Swartz • Grottoes, VA

Makes 4–6 servings (Ideal slow cooker size: 3–4-quart)

½ lb. sausage, either cut in thin slices or removed from casings

½ lb. ground beef

½ cup chopped onions

½ lb. fresh mushrooms, sliced

⅛ cup chopped celery

⅛ cup chopped green peppers

1 cup salsa

16-oz. can low-sodium tomato juice

6-oz. can tomato paste

½ tsp. sugar

¼ tsp. salt

½ tsp. dried oregano

½ tsp. Worcestershire sauce

¼ tsp. dried basil

¼ tsp. pepper

1. Brown sausage, ground beef, and onion in deep skillet. During last 3 minutes of browning, add mushrooms, celery, and green peppers. Continue cooking; then drain.

2. Add remaining ingredients. Pour into slow cooker.

3. Cover. Cook on High 2–3 hours.

Exchange List Values: Vegetable 3.0, Meat, medium fat 1.0, Fat 1.0

Basic Nutritional Values: Calories 195 (Calories from Fat 89), Total Fat 10 gm (Saturated Fat 3.5 gm, Polyunsat Fat 1.1 gm, Monounsat Fat 4.2 gm, Cholesterol 37 mg), Sodium 499 mg, Total Carbohydrate 15 gm, Dietary Fiber 3 gm, Sugars 6 gm, Protein 14 gm

VARIATIONS: Add any or all of the following to Step 2:

1 tsp. chili powder

1 tsp. ground cumin

15-oz. can black beans, undrained

15-oz. can whole-kernel corn, undrained

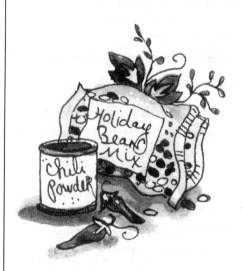

Cassoulet Chowder

Miriam Friesen • Staunton, VA

Makes 8-10 servings (Ideal slow cooker size: 4-5-quart)

1¼ cups dry pinto beans

4 cups water

8-oz. pkg. brown-and-serve sausage links, cooked and drained

2 cups cubed cooked chicken

2 cups cubed extra-lean, lower-sodium cooked ham

1½ cups sliced carrots

8-oz. can tomato sauce

¾ cup dry red wine

½ cup chopped onions

½ tsp. garlic powder

1 bay leaf

1. Combine beans and water in large saucepan. Bring to boil. Reduce heat and simmer 1½ hours. Refrigerate beans and liquid 4–8 hours.

2. Combine all ingredients in slow cooker.

3. Cover. Cook on Low 8–10 hours, or on High 4 hours. If the chowder seems too thin, remove lid during last 30 minutes of cooking time to allow it to thicken.

4. Remove bay leaf before serving.

Exchange List Values: Starch 1.0, Meat, lean 3.0

Basic Nutritional Values: Calories 249 (Calories from Fat 90), Total Fat 10 gm (Saturated Fat 3.4 gm, Polyunsat Fat 1.6 gm, Monounsat Fat 3.8 gm, Cholesterol 46 mg), Sodium 554 mg, Total Carbohydrate 18 gm, Dietary Fiber 5 gm, Sugars 5 gm, Protein 21 gm

Forgotten Minestrone

Phyllis Attig • Reynolds, IL

Recipe photo appears in color section.

Makes 8 servings (Ideal slow cooker size: 4-5-quart)

1 lb. beef stewing meat, all visible fat removed

6 cups water

28-oz. can tomatoes, diced, undrained

1 beef bouillon cube

1 medium onion, chopped

2 Tbsp. minced dried parsley

¼ tsp. salt

1½ tsp. dried thyme

½ tsp. pepper

1 medium zucchini, thinly sliced

2 cups finely chopped cabbage

16-oz. can garbanzo beans, drained

1 cup uncooked small elbow, or shell, macaroni

3 Tbsp. freshly grated Parmesan cheese

1. Combine beef, water, tomatoes, bouillon, onion, parsley, salt, thyme, and pepper.

2. Cover. Cook on Low 7–9 hours, or until meat is tender.

3. Stir in zucchini, cabbage, beans, and macaroni. Cover and cook on High 30–45 minutes, or until vegetables are tender.

4. Sprinkle individual servings with Parmesan cheese.

Exchange List Values: Starch 1.0, Vegetable 2.0, Meat, lean 2.0

Basic Nutritional Values: Calories 235 (Calories from Fat 47), Total Fat 5 gm (Saturated Fat 1.5 gm, Polyunsat Fat 0.8 gm, Monounsat Fat 2.0 gm, Cholesterol 44 mg), Sodium 489 mg, Total Carbohydrate 27 gm, Dietary Fiber 5 gm, Sugars 8 gm, Protein 20 gm

Slow Cooker Minestrone

Dorothy Shank • Sterling, IL

Makes 8 servings (Ideal slow cooker size: 4-quart)

3 cups water

1½ lbs. stewing meat, cut into bite-sized pieces, all visible fat removed

1 medium onion, diced

4 carrots, diced

14½-oz. can tomatoes

¾ tsp. salt

10-oz. pkg. frozen mixed vegetables, or your choice of frozen vegetables

1 Tbsp. dried basil

½ cup dry vermicelli

1 tsp. dried oregano

grated Parmesan cheese

1. Combine all ingredients except cheese in slow cooker. Stir well.

2. Cover. Cook on Low 10–12 hours, or on High 4–5 hours.

3. Top individual servings with Parmesan cheese.

Exchange List Values: Starch 1.0, Vegetable 2.0, Meat, lean 1.0

Basic Nutritional Values: Calories 183 (Calories from Fat 33), Total Fat 4 gm (Saturated Fat 1.0 gm, Polyunsat Fat 0.4 gm, Monounsat Fat 1.6 gm, Cholesterol 42 mg), Sodium 413 mg, Total Carbohydrate 21 gm, Dietary Fiber 4 gm, Sugars 7 gm, Protein 17 gm

Stretching keeps the body younger. As people age, they lose flexibility and balance. Stretching gives them back.

Hamburger Vegetable Soup

Donna Conto • Saylorsburg, PA

Makes 8 servings (Ideal slow cooker size: 4-quart)

½ lb. ground beef, browned, drained, and patted dry with paper toweling

1 beef bouillon cube, crushed

5 tsp. sodium-free beef bouillon powder

16-oz. can tomatoes

1 large onion, diced

¾ cup sliced celery

1 medium carrot, diced

1 clove garlic, minced

1 bay leaf

½ tsp. salt

⅛ tsp. pepper

1–2 cups water (depending upon how much liquid you like soup to have)

10-oz. pkg. frozen peas

3 Tbsp. chopped parsley

1. Combine all ingredients except peas and parsley in slow cooker.

2. Cover. Cook on Low 5 hours.

3. Stir in peas during last hour.

4. Garnish with parsley before serving.

Exchange List Values: Vegetable 2.0, Meat, lean 1.0

Basic Nutritional Values: Calories 107 (Calories from Fat 28), Total Fat 3 gm (Saturated Fat 1.1 gm, Polyunsat Fat 0.2 gm, Monounsat Fat 1.3 gm, Cholesterol 17 mg), Sodium 431 mg, Total Carbohydrate 12 gm, Dietary Fiber 3 gm, Sugars 7 gm, Protein 8 gm

Hearty Alphabet Soup

Maryann Markano • Wilmington, DE

Makes 6 servings (Ideal slow cooker size: 4-quart)

½ lb. beef stewing meat or round steak,
    all visible fat removed, cubed

14½-oz. can stewed tomatoes

8-oz. can tomato sauce

1 cup water

Sodium-Free Onion Soup Mix (see recipe on
    page 334)

10-oz. pkg. frozen vegetables, partially thawed

½ cup uncooked alphabet noodles

1. Combine meat, tomatoes, tomato sauce,
   water, and soup mix in slow cooker.

2. Cover. Cook on Low 6–8 hours. Turn
   to High.

3. Stir in vegetables and noodles. Add more
   water if mixture is too dry and thick.

4. Cover. Cook on High 30 minutes, or until
   vegetables are tender.

**Exchange List Values: Starch 1.0,
Vegetable 2.0, Meat, lean 1.0**

Basic Nutritional Values: Calories 165 (Calories
from Fat 17), Total Fat 2 gm (Saturated Fat 0.5 gm,
Polyunsat Fat 0.3 gm, Monounsat Fat 0.8 gm,
Cholesterol 19 mg), Sodium 443 mg, Total
Carbohydrate 28 gm, Dietary Fiber 3 gm, Sugars
8 gm, Protein 10 gm

Quick and Easy Italian Vegetable Beef Soup

Lisa Warren • Parkesburg, PA

**Makes 10 servings (Ideal slow cooker size:
4-quart)**

¾ lb. 85%-lean ground beef, or turkey, browned
    and drained

3 carrots, sliced

4 potatoes, peeled and cubed

1 small onion, diced

1 tsp. garlic powder

1 tsp. Italian seasoning

½ tsp. salt

¼ tsp. pepper

15-oz. can diced Italian tomatoes, or 2 fresh
    tomatoes, chopped

6-oz. can Italian-flavored tomato paste

4½ cups water

1 quart 99%-fat-free, lower-sodium beef broth

1. Combine all ingredients in slow cooker.

2. Cover. Cook on High 6–8 hours, or until
   potatoes and carrots are tender.

**Exchange List Values: Starch 0.5,
Vegetable 2.0, Meat, lean 1.0**

Basic Nutritional Values: Calories 138 (Calories
from Fat 34), Total Fat 4 gm (Saturated Fat 1.4 gm,
Polyunsat Fat 0.3 gm, Monounsat Fat 1.5 gm,
Cholesterol 20 mg), Sodium 423 mg, Total
Carbohydrate 17 gm, Dietary Fiber 3 gm, Sugars
4 gm, Protein 9 gm

Spicy Beef Vegetable Stew

Melissa Raber • Millersburg, OH

Makes 12 servings (Ideal slow cooker size: 4-quart)

3/4 lb. ground beef

1 cup chopped onions

30-oz. jar meatless spaghetti sauce

3 1/2 cups water

1 lb. frozen mixed vegetables

10-oz. can diced tomatoes with green chilies

1 cup sliced celery

1 tsp. sodium-free beef bouillon powder

1 tsp. pepper

1. Cook beef and onions in skillet until meat is no longer pink. Drain. Transfer to slow cooker.

2. Stir in remaining ingredients.

3. Cover. Cook on Low 8 hours.

Exchange List Values: Starch 0.5, Vegetable 2.0, Meat, lean 1.0

Basic Nutritional Values: Calories 150 (Calories from Fat 44), Total Fat 5 gm (Saturated Fat 1.4 gm, Polyunsat Fat 0.7 gm, Monounsat Fat 1.9 gm, Cholesterol 17 mg), Sodium 489 mg, Total Carbohydrate 17 gm, Dietary Fiber 3 gm, Sugars 10 gm, Protein 8 gm

Hearty Beef and Cabbage Soup

Carolyn Mathias • Williamsville, NY

Makes 8 servings (Ideal slow cooker size: 4-quart)

2/3 lb. (about 11 ozs.) ground beef

1 medium onion, chopped

40-oz. can tomatoes

2 cups water

15-oz. can kidney beans

1/2 tsp. pepper

1 Tbsp. chili powder

1/2 cup chopped celery

2 cups thinly sliced cabbage

1. Saute beef in skillet. Drain.

2. Combine all ingredients except cabbage in slow cooker.

3. Cover. Cook on Low 3 hours. Add cabbage. Cook on High 30–60 minutes longer.

Exchange List Values: Starch 0.5, Vegetable 2.0, Meat, lean 1.0

Basic Nutritional Values: Calories 150 (Calories from Fat 40), Total Fat 4 gm (Saturated Fat 1.5 gm, Polyunsat Fat 0.4 gm, Monounsat Fat 1.7 gm, Cholesterol 22 mg), Sodium 507 mg, Total Carbohydrate 18 gm, Dietary Fiber 5 gm, Sugars 8 gm, Protein 12 gm

Hamburger Soup
with Barley

Becky Oswald • Broadway, VA

Makes 10 servings (Ideal slow cooker size: 4-quart)

¾ lb. 85%-lean ground beef

1 medium onion, chopped

2 14½-oz. cans beef consommé

1¾ cups water

2 tsp. sodium-free beef bouillon powder

28-oz. can no-salt-added diced, or crushed, tomatoes

3 carrots, sliced

3 ribs celery, sliced

8 Tbsp. barley

1 bay leaf

1 tsp. dried thyme

1 Tbsp. dried parsley

½ tsp. pepper

1. Brown beef and onion in skillet. Drain.

2. Combine all ingredients in slow cooker.

3. Cover. Cook on High 3 hours, or Low 6–8 hours.

Exchange List Values: Starch 1.0, Vegetable 1.0, Meat, lean 1.0

Basic Nutritional Values: Calories 154 (Calories from Fat 34), Total Fat 4 gm (Saturated Fat 1.4 gm, Polyunsat Fat 0.3 gm, Monounsat Fat 1.5 gm, Cholesterol 22 mg), Sodium 623 mg, Total Carbohydrate 20 gm, Dietary Fiber 4 gm, Sugars 6 gm, Protein 11 gm

Vegetable Soup
with Potatoes

Annabelle Unternahrer • Shipshewana, IN

Makes 8 servings (Ideal slow cooker size: 4-quart)

⅔ lb. 85%-lean ground beef, browned and drained

2 15-oz. cans diced tomatoes

2 carrots, sliced or cubed

2 onions, sliced or cubed

2 potatoes, diced

1–2 cloves garlic, minced

12-oz. can V-8 vegetable juice

1½–2 cups sliced celery

2 tsp. sodium-free beef bouillon powder

2–3 cups vegetables (cauliflower, peas, corn, limas, or your choice of leftovers from your freezer)

1. Combine all ingredients in slow cooker.

2. Cover. Cook on Low 12 hours, or High 4–6 hours.

Exchange List Values: Starch 1.0, Vegetable 2.0, Meat, lean 1.0

Basic Nutritional Values: Calories 179 (Calories from Fat 38), Total Fat 4 gm (Saturated Fat 1.5 gm, Polyunsat Fat 0.4 gm, Monounsat Fat 1.7 gm, Cholesterol 22 mg), Sodium 407 mg, Total Carbohydrate 26 gm, Dietary Fiber 5 gm, Sugars 11 gm, Protein 11 gm

VARIATION: Use 3 cups pre-cooked dried beans or lentils instead of hamburger.

Note: If you are using leftover vegetables that are precooked, add them during last hour if cooking on Low, or during last half hour if cooking on High.

Hamburger Lentil Soup

Juanita Marner • Shipshewana, IN

Makes 8 servings (Ideal slow cooker size: 4-quart)

$\frac{1}{2}$ lb. 85%-lean ground beef

$\frac{1}{2}$ cup chopped onions

4 carrots, diced

3 ribs celery, diced

1 clove garlic, minced, or 1 tsp. garlic powder

1 qt. no-salt-added tomato juice

1$\frac{1}{2}$ tsp. salt

2 cups dry lentils, washed, with stones removed

1 qt. water

$\frac{1}{2}$ tsp. dried marjoram

1 Tbsp. brown sugar

1. Brown ground beef and onions in skillet. Drain.

2. Combine all ingredients in slow cooker.

3. Cover. Cook on Low 8–10 hours, or High 4–6 hours.

Exchange List Values: Starch 2.0, Vegetable 2.0, Meat, lean 1.0

Basic Nutritional Values: Calories 247 (Calories from Fat 32), Total Fat 4 gm (Saturated Fat 1.2 gm, Polyunsat Fat 0.4 gm, Monounsat Fat 1.4 gm, Cholesterol 17 mg), Sodium 508 mg, Total Carbohydrate 38 gm, Dietary Fiber 12 gm, Sugars 10 gm, Protein 18 gm

Have a plan in place in case you get sick—whom to call and when. Don't hesitate to call your doctor if you have questions.

Russian Red Lentil Soup

Naomi E. Fast • Hesston, KS

Makes 8 servings (Ideal slow cooker size: 5-6-quart)

1 Tbsp. canola oil

1 large onion, chopped

3 cloves garlic, minced

$\frac{1}{2}$ cup diced, dried apricots

1$\frac{1}{2}$ cups dried red lentils

$\frac{1}{2}$ tsp. cumin

$\frac{1}{2}$ tsp. dried thyme

3 cups water

2 14$\frac{1}{2}$-oz. cans chicken or vegetable broth

14$\frac{1}{2}$-oz. can diced tomatoes

1 Tbsp. honey

$\frac{1}{2}$ tsp. coarsely ground black pepper

2 Tbsp. chopped fresh mint

1$\frac{1}{2}$ cups plain yogurt

1. Combine all ingredients except mint and yogurt in slow cooker.

2. Cover. Heat on High until soup starts to simmer, then turn to Low and cook 3–4 hours.

3. Add mint and dollop of yogurt to each bowl of soup.

Exchange List Values: Starch 1.5, Fruit 1.0, Vegetable 1.0, Meat, very lean 1.0

Basic Nutritional Values: Calories 244 (Calories from Fat 37), Total Fat 4 gm (Saturated Fat 1.2 gm, Polyunsat Fat 0.8 gm, Monounsat Fat 1.5 gm, Cholesterol 8 mg), Sodium 587 mg, Total Carbohydrate 42 gm, Dietary Fiber 10 gm, Sugars 21 gm, Protein 13 gm

Vegetable Soup with Noodles

Glenda S. Weaver • New Holland, PA

Makes 8 servings (Ideal slow cooker size: 4-quart)

2 tsp. sodium-free beef bouillon powder

1 pint water

1 onion, chopped

$2/3$ lb. 85%-lean ground beef

$1/4$ cup ketchup

$1/8$ tsp. celery salt

$1/2$ cup uncooked noodles

16-oz. pkg. frozen mixed vegetables, or vegetables of your choice

2 cups tomato juice

1. Dissolve bouillon in water.

2. Brown onion and beef in skillet. Drain.

3. Combine all ingredients in slow cooker.

4. Cover. Cook on Low 6 hours, or on High 2–3 hours, until vegetables are tender.

Exchange List Values: Starch 0.5, Vegetable 2.0, Meat, lean 1.0

Basic Nutritional Values: Calories 135 (Calories from Fat 37), Total Fat 4 gm (Saturated Fat 1.5 gm, Polyunsat Fat 0.2 gm, Monounsat Fat 1.7 gm, Cholesterol 25 mg), Sodium 374 mg, Total Carbohydrate 16 gm, Dietary Fiber 2 gm, Sugars 7 gm, Protein 10 gm

Dottie's Creamy Steak Soup

Debbie Zeida • Mashpee, MA

Makes 8 main dish servings (Ideal slow cooker size: 4-quart)

$1/2$ lb. 85%-lean ground beef

half a large onion, chopped

12-oz. can low-sodium V-8 vegetable juice

3 medium potatoes, diced

$10^3/4$-oz. can 98%-fat-free, reduced-sodium cream of mushroom soup

$10^3/4$-oz. can cream of celery soup

16-oz. pkg. frozen mixed vegetables, or your choice of frozen vegetables

$1/2$–$3/4$ tsp. pepper

1. Saute beef and onions in skillet. Drain.

2. Combine all ingredients in slow cooker.

3. Cover. Cook on Low 8–10 hours.

Exchange List Values: Starch 1.0, Vegetable 2.0, Meat, lean 1.0, Fat 0.5

Basic Nutritional Values: Calories 202 (Calories from Fat 54), Total Fat 6 gm (Saturated Fat 2.2 gm, Polyunsat Fat 1.2 gm, Monounsat Fat 1.8 gm, Cholesterol 19 mg), Sodium 506 mg, Total Carbohydrate 28 gm, Dietary Fiber 4 gm, Sugars 7 gm, Protein 10 gm

Sausage Bean Soup

Janie Steele • Moore, OK

Makes 10 servings (Ideal slow cooker size: 5–6-quart)

1-lb. pkg. dried Great Northern beans

28-oz. can whole tomatoes

2 8-oz. cans no-salt-added tomato sauce

2 large onions, chopped

3 cloves garlic, minced

¼–½ tsp. pepper, according to your taste preference

3 ribs celery, sliced

1 bell pepper, sliced

1 large ham bone, all skin and visible fat removed (to yield 6 ozs. ham)

1–2 lbs. low-fat smoked sausage links, sliced

1. Cover beans with water and soak for 8 hours. Rinse and drain.

2. Place beans in 6-qt. cooker and cover with water.

3. Combine all other ingredients, except sausage, in large bowl. Stir into beans in slow cooker.

4. Cover. Cook on High 1–1½ hours. Reduce to Low. Cook 7 hours.

5. Remove ham bone or hock and debone. Stir ham pieces back into soup.

6. Add sausage links.

7. Cover. Cook on Low 1 hour.

Exchange List Values: Starch 2.0, Vegetable 2.0, Meat, lean 1.0

Basic Nutritional Values: Calories 276 (Calories from Fat 34), Total Fat 4 gm (Saturated Fat 1.3 gm, Polyunsat Fat 1.2 gm, Monounsat Fat 1.0 gm, Cholesterol 29 mg), Sodium 760 mg, Total Carbohydrate 41 gm, Dietary Fiber 11 gm, Sugars 12 gm, Protein 21 gm

Note: For enhanced flavor, brown sausage before adding to soup.

If you're angry or tense after a stressful day, you need to get moving to get past it!

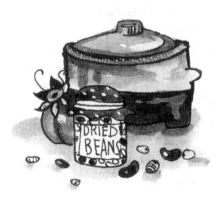

Black Bean Soup

Janie Steele • Moore, OK

Makes 5–6 quarts, or about 18 servings (Ideal slow cooker size: 2 cookers, each 4–5-quart)

4 cups dry black beans

5 qts. water

ham bone, ham pieces, or ham hocks

3 bunches green onions, sliced thin

4 bay leaves

1 tsp. salt

¼–½ tsp. pepper

3 cloves garlic, minced

4 ribs celery, chopped

3 large onions, chopped

10½-oz. can consommé

2½ Tbsp. margarine

2½ Tbsp. flour

1 cup Madeira wine, optional

chopped parsley

1. In each slow cooker, soak half the beans in 2½ qts. water for 8 hours. Rinse. Drain. Pour beans back into slow cookers.

2. Add ham, green onions, bay leaves, salt, pepper, garlic, celery, and onions. Pour in consommé. Add water to cover vegetables and meat.

3. Cover. Cook on High 1½–2 hours. Reduce heat to Low and cook for 6–8 hours.

4. Remove ham bones and bay leaves. Cut ham off bones and set meat aside.

5. Force vegetable mixture through sieve, if you wish.

6. Return cooked ingredients and cut-up ham to cookers.

7. In saucepan, melt margarine. Stir in flour until smooth. Stir into soup to thicken and enrich.

8. Prior to serving, add wine to heated soup mixture. Garnish with chopped parsley.

Exchange List Values: Starch 2.0, Meat, lean 1.0

Basic Nutritional Values: Calories 202 (Calories from Fat 26), Total Fat 3 gm (Saturated Fat 0.6 gm, Polyunsat Fat 0.9 gm, Monounsat Fat 1.0 gm, Cholesterol 6 mg), Sodium 399 mg, Total Carbohydrate 32 gm, Dietary Fiber 11 gm, Sugars 6 gm, Protein 14 gm

You can reduce your risk of eye disease by keeping your blood sugars near normal and getting a regular exam by an eye doctor who specializes in diabetes.

Taco Soup with Black Beans

Alexa Slonin • Harrisonburg, VA

Makes 6–8 servings (Ideal slow cooker size: 4-quart)

¾ lb. 90%-lean ground beef, browned and drained

28-oz. can crushed tomatoes

¼–½ cup water

15¼-oz. can corn, drained and rinsed

15-oz. can no-salt-added black beans, undrained

15½-oz. can no-salt-added red kidney beans, undrained

1 envelope dry Hidden Valley Ranch Dressing mix

2 Tbsp. Low-Sodium Taco Seasoning Mix (see recipe on page 333)

1 small onion, chopped

1. Combine all ingredients in slow cooker.

2. Cover. Cook on Low 4–6 hours.

Exchange List Values: Starch 1.5, Vegetable 2.0, Meat, very lean 2.0

Basic Nutritional Values: Calories 247 (Calories from Fat 41), Total Fat 5 gm (Saturated Fat 1.5 gm, Polyunsat Fat 0.6 gm, Monounsat Fat 1.7 gm, Cholesterol 26 mg), Sodium 652 mg, Total Carbohydrate 35 gm, Dietary Fiber 9 gm, Sugars 9 gm, Protein 17 gm

SUGGESTED GARNISHES:

broken tortilla, or corn, chips

shredded fat-free cheese

fat-free sour cream

Sante Fe Soup

Carla Koslowsky • Hillsboro, KS

Makes 8 servings (Ideal slow cooker size: 4-quart)

8 ozs. fat-free sharp cheddar cheese, cubed

¾ lb. 90%-lean ground beef, browned and drained

15¼-oz. can corn, undrained

15-oz. can no-salt-added kidney beans, undrained

14½-oz. can diced tomatoes with green chilies

14½-oz. can no-salt-added stewed tomatoes

2 Tbsp. Low-Sodium Taco Seasoning Mix (see recipe on page 333)

1. Combine all ingredients in slow cooker.

2. Cover. Cook on High 3 hours.

3. Serve with corn chips as a side, or dip soft tortillas in soup bowls, if your diet allows.

Exchange List Values: Starch 1.0, Vegetable 1.0, Meat, lean 2.0

Basic Nutritional Values: Calories 215 (Calories from Fat 40), Total Fat 4 gm (Saturated Fat 1.5 gm, Polyunsat Fat 0.5 gm, Monounsat Fat 1.7 gm, Cholesterol 29 mg), Sodium 617 mg, Total Carbohydrate 22 gm, Dietary Fiber 5 gm, Sugars 8 gm, Protein 22 gm

Taco Soup with Whole Tomatoes

Marla Folkerts • Holland, OH

Makes 6–8 servings (Ideal slow cooker size: 4-quart)

²/₃ lb. 85%-lean ground beef

½ cup chopped onions

28-oz. can whole tomatoes with juice

14-oz. can kidney beans with juice

1 7-oz. can corn with juice

8-oz. can no-salt-added tomato sauce

2 Tbsp. Low-Sodium Taco Seasoning Mix (see recipe on page 333)

1–2 cups water

salt to taste

pepper to taste

1 cup grated fat-free cheddar cheese

1. Brown beef and onions in skillet. Drain.

2. Combine all ingredients except cheese in slow cooker.

3. Cover. Cook on Low 4–6 hours.

4. Ladle into bowls. Top with cheese and serve with taco/corn chips, if your diet allows.

Exchange List Values: Starch 1.0, Vegetable 1.0, Meat, lean 1.0, Fat 0.5

Basic Nutritional Values: Calories 191 (Calories from Fat 44), Total Fat 5 gm (Saturated Fat 1.6 gm, Polyunsat Fat 0.5 gm, Monounsat Fat 1.9 gm, Cholesterol 24 mg), Sodium 612 mg, Total Carbohydrate 22 gm, Dietary Fiber 5 gm, Sugars 10 gm, Protein 16 gm

Norma's Vegetarian Chili

Kathy Hertzler • Lancaster, PA

Makes 8–10 servings (Ideal slow cooker size: 5–6-quart)

2 Tbsp. canola oil

2 cups minced celery

1½ cups chopped green pepper

1 cup minced onions

4 cloves garlic, minced

5½ cups no-salt-added stewed tomatoes

2 1-lb. cans kidney beans, undrained

1½ cups raisins

¼ cup wine vinegar

1 Tbsp. chopped parsley

1 tsp. salt

1½ tsp. dried oregano

1½ tsp. cumin

¼ tsp. pepper

¼ tsp. Tabasco sauce

1 bay leaf

¾ cup unsalted cashews

1 cup grated cheese, optional

1. Combine all ingredients except cashews and cheese in slow cooker.

2. Cover. Simmer on Low for 8 hours. Add cashews and simmer 30 minutes.

3. Garnish individual servings with grated cheese.

Exchange List Values: Starch 1.0, Fruit 1.0, Vegetable 3.0, Fat 1.5

Basic Nutritional Values: Calories 279 (Calories from Fat 77), Total Fat 9 gm (Saturated Fat 1.4 gm, Polyunsat Fat 2.0 gm, Monounsat Fat 4.7 gm, Cholesterol 0 mg), Sodium 603 mg, Total Carbohydrate 47 gm, Dietary Fiber 7 gm, Sugars 22 gm, Protein 9 gm

Easy Chili

Sheryl Shenk • Harrisonburg, VA

Makes 10–12 servings (Ideal slow cooker size: 5-quart)

1 lb. ground beef

1 onion, chopped

1 medium green pepper, chopped

½ tsp. salt

1 Tbsp. chili powder

2 tsp. Worcestershire sauce

29-oz. can no-salt-added tomato sauce

3 16-oz. cans kidney beans, drained

14½-oz. can crushed, or stewed, tomatoes

6-oz. can tomato paste

4 ozs. grated fat-free cheddar cheese

1. Brown meat in skillet. Add onion and green pepper halfway through browning process. Drain. Pour into slow cooker.

2. Stir in remaining ingredients except cheese.

3. Cover. Cook on High 3 hours, or Low 7–8 hours.

4. Serve in bowls topped with cheddar cheese.

Exchange List Values: Starch 1.0, Vegetable 3.0, Meat, lean 1.0, Fat 0.5

Basic Nutritional Values: Calories 232 (Calories from Fat 41), Total Fat 5 gm (Saturated Fat 1.5 gm, Polyunsat Fat 0.5 gm, Monounsat Fat 1.8 gm, Cholesterol 23 mg), Sodium 456 mg, Total Carbohydrate 30 gm, Dietary Fiber 8 gm, Sugars 9 gm, Protein 18 gm

Note: This chili can be served over cooked rice.

Slow Cooker Chili

Wanda S. Curtin • Bradenton, FL / Ann Sunday McDowell • Newtown, PA

Makes 10 servings (Ideal slow cooker size: 4–5-quart)

2 lbs. ground beef, browned and drained

2 16-oz. cans red kidney beans, drained

2 14½-oz. cans diced tomatoes, drained

2 medium onions, chopped

2 cloves garlic, crushed

2 Tbsp. chili powder

1 tsp. ground cumin

1 tsp. black pepper

1 tsp. salt

1. Combine all ingredients in slow cooker.

2. Cover. Cook on Low 8–10 hours.

Exchange List Values: Starch 1.0, Vegetable 1.0, Meat, lean 3.0

Basic Nutritional Values: Calories 265 (Calories from Fat 89), Total Fat 10 gm (Saturated Fat 3.6 gm, Polyunsat Fat 0.7 gm, Monounsat Fat 4.1 gm, Cholesterol 54 mg), Sodium 568 mg, Total Carbohydrate 21 gm, Dietary Fiber 6 gm, Sugars 6 gm, Protein 23 gm

VARIATIONS:

1. For more flavor, add cayenne pepper or a jalapeno pepper before cooking.

   Dorothy Shank • Sterling, IL

2. Add 1 cup chopped green peppers before cooking.

   Mary V. Warye • West Liberty, OH

Note: Use leftovers over lettuce and other fresh garden vegetables to make a taco salad.

Colleen's Favorite Chili

Colleen Heatwole • Burton, MI

Makes 8 servings (Ideal slow cooker size: 4-quart)

2 medium onions, coarsely chopped

1-1½ lbs. 85%-lean ground beef, browned and drained

2 cloves garlic, minced fine, or ½ tsp. garlic powder

¾ cup finely diced green peppers

2 14½-oz. cans diced tomatoes, or 1 qt. home-canned tomatoes

30-32 ozs. beans—kidney, or pinto, or mixture of the two, drained and rinsed

¼-½ cup water

8-oz. can no-salt-added tomato sauce

1 tsp. ground cumin

½ tsp. pepper

1 tsp. seasoned salt

1 Tbsp., or more, chili powder

1 tsp. dried basil

1. Combine all ingredients in slow cooker.

2. Cover. Cook on Low 8–12 hours, or High 5–6 hours.

Exchange List Values: Starch 1.0, Vegetable 3.0, Meat, lean 2.0, Fat 0.5

Basic Nutritional Values: Calories 296 (Calories from Fat 86), Total Fat 10 gm (Saturated Fat 3.4 gm, Polyunsat Fat 0.7 gm, Monounsat Fat 4.0 gm, Cholesterol 54 mg), Sodium 581 mg, Total Carbohydrate 30 gm, Dietary Fiber 9 gm, Sugars 10 gm, Protein 24 gm

VARIATIONS:

1. Add 1 Tbsp. brown sugar to mixture before cooking.

2. Put in another 1 lb. beans and then decrease ground beef to 1 lb.

Trail Chili

Jeanne Allen • Rye, CO

Makes 10 servings (Ideal slow cooker size: 4-5-quart)

1½ lbs. 90%-lean ground beef

1 large onion, diced

28-oz. can diced tomatoes

2 8-oz. cans tomato puree

16-oz. cans kidney beans, undrained

4-oz. can diced green chilies

1 cup water

2 cloves garlic, minced

2 Tbsp. mild chili powder

½ tsp. salt

2 tsp. ground cumin

1 tsp. pepper

1. Brown beef and onion in skillet. Drain. Place in slow cooker on High.

2. Stir in remaining ingredients. Cook on High 30 minutes.

3. Reduce heat to Low. Cook 4–6 hours.

Exchange List Values: Starch 0.5, Vegetable 2.0, Meat, lean 2.0

Basic Nutritional Values: Calories 195 (Calories from Fat 57), Total Fat 6 gm (Saturated Fat 2.3 gm, Polyunsat Fat 0.5 gm, Monounsat Fat 2.6 gm, Cholesterol 41 mg), Sodium 545 mg, Total Carbohydrate 17 gm, Dietary Fiber 4 gm, Sugars 8 gm, Protein 18 gm

Note: Top individual servings with shredded cheese. Serve with taco chips, if your diet allows.

Quick and Easy Chili

Nan Decker • Albuquerque, NM

Makes 6 servings (Ideal slow cooker size: 3–4-quart)

1 lb. ground beef

1 onion, chopped

16-oz. can stewed tomatoes

11½-oz. can Hot V-8 juice

2 15-oz. cans pinto beans, drained and rinsed

¼–½ cup water

¼ tsp. cayenne pepper

1 Tbsp. chili powder

1. Crumble ground beef in microwave-safe casserole. Add onion. Microwave, covered, on High 15 minutes. Drain. Break meat into pieces.

2. Combine all ingredients in slow cooker.

3. Cook on Low 4–5 hours.

4. Garnish with sour cream, chopped green onions, grated cheese, and sliced ripe olives, if your diet allows.

Exchange List Values: Starch 1.5, Vegetable 2.0, Meat, lean 2.0, Fat 0.5

Basic Nutritional Values: Calories 302 (Calories from Fat 76), Total Fat 8 gm (Saturated Fat 3.0 gm, Polyunsat Fat 0.7 gm, Monounsat Fat 3.5 gm, Cholesterol 45 mg), Sodium 539 mg, Total Carbohydrate 34 gm, Dietary Fiber 10 gm, Sugars 7 gm, Protein 23 gm

Pirate Stew

Nancy Graves • Manhattan, KS

Makes 4–6 servings (Ideal slow cooker size: 4-quart)

¾ cup sliced onion

1 lb. ground beef

¼ cup uncooked long-grain rice

3 cups diced raw potatoes

1 cup diced celery

2 cups canned kidney beans, drained

½ tsp. salt

⅛ tsp. pepper

¼ tsp. chili powder

¼ tsp. Worcestershire sauce

1 cup tomato sauce

½ cup water

1. Brown onions and ground beef in skillet. Drain.

2. Layer ingredients in slow cooker in order given.

3. Cover. Cook on Low 6 hours, or until potatoes and rice are cooked.

Exchange List Values: Starch 2.0, Vegetable 1.0, Meat, lean 2.0, Fat 0.5

Basic Nutritional Values: Calories 310 (Calories from Fat 73), Total Fat 8 gm (Saturated Fat 3.0 gm, Polyunsat Fat 0.5 gm, Monounsat Fat 3.4 gm, Cholesterol 45 mg), Sodium 611 mg, Total Carbohydrate 38 gm, Dietary Fiber 7 gm, Sugars 6 gm, Protein 22 gm

VARIATION: Add a layer of 2 cups sliced carrots between potatoes and celery.

Katrine Rose • Woodbridge, VA

Corn Chili

Gladys Longacre • Susquehanna, PA

Makes 4–6 servings (Ideal slow cooker size: 4-quart)

1 lb. ground beef

1/2 cup chopped onions

1/2 cup chopped green peppers

1/4 tsp. salt

1/8 tsp. pepper

1/4 tsp. dried thyme

14 1/2-oz. can diced tomatoes with Italian herbs

6-oz. can tomato paste, diluted with 1 can water

2 cups frozen whole-kernel corn

16-oz. can kidney beans

1 Tbsp. chili powder

sour cream, optional

shredded cheese, optional

1. Saute ground beef, onions, and green peppers in deep saucepan. Drain and season with salt, pepper, and thyme.

2. Stir in tomatoes, tomato paste, water, and corn. Heat until corn is thawed. Add kidney beans and chili powder. Pour into slow cooker.

3. Cover. Cook on Low 5–6 hours.

4. Top individual servings with dollops of sour cream, or sprinkle with shredded cheese, if your diet allows.

Exchange List Values: Starch 1.5, Vegetable 2.0, Meat, lean 2.0

Basic Nutritional Values: Calories 281 (Calories from Fat 78), Total Fat 9 gm (Saturated Fat 3.1 gm, Polyunsat Fat 0.7 gm, Monounsat Fat 3.5 gm, Cholesterol 45 mg), Sodium 574 mg, Total Carbohydrate 33 gm, Dietary Fiber 7 gm, Sugars 7 gm, Protein 21 gm

White Bean Chili

Tracey Stenger • Gretna, LA

Makes 12 servings (Ideal slow cooker size: 6-quart)

1 lb. ground beef, browned and drained

1 lb. ground turkey, browned and drained

3 bell peppers, chopped

2 onions, chopped

4 cloves garlic, minced

2 14 1/2-oz. cans 98%-fat-free, lower-sodium chicken, or vegetable, broth

15 1/2-oz. can butter beans, rinsed and drained

15-oz. can black-eyed peas, rinsed and drained

15-oz. can garbanzo beans, rinsed and drained

15-oz. can navy beans, rinsed and drained

4-oz. can chopped green chilies

2 Tbsp. chili powder

3 tsp. ground cumin

2 tsp. dried oregano

2 tsp. paprika

1/2 tsp. salt

1/2 tsp. pepper

1. Combine all ingredients in slow cooker.

2. Cover. Cook on Low 8–10 hours.

Exchange List Values: Starch 1.5, Vegetable 1.0, Meat, lean 2.0, Fat 0.5

Basic Nutritional Values: Calories 282 (Calories from Fat 79), Total Fat 9 gm (Saturated Fat 2.5 gm, Polyunsat Fat 1.6 gm, Monounsat Fat 3.3 gm, Cholesterol 50 mg), Sodium 570 mg, Total Carbohydrate 28 gm, Dietary Fiber 8 gm, Sugars 6 gm, Protein 24 gm

Dorothea's Slow Cooker Chili

Dorothea K. Ladd • Ballston Lake, NY

Makes 8 servings (Ideal slow cooker size: 4-quart)

1 lb. ground beef

1/4 lb. bulk pork sausage

1 large onion, chopped

1 large green pepper, chopped

2-3 ribs celery, chopped

2 15 1/2-oz. cans kidney beans, drained and rinsed

1/4-1/2 cup water

29-oz. can no-salt-added tomato puree

6-oz. can tomato paste

2 cloves garlic, minced

2 Tbsp. chili powder

1/2 tsp. salt

1. Brown ground beef and sausage in skillet. Drain.

2. Combine all ingredients in slow cooker.

3. Cover. Cook on Low 8–10 hours.

Exchange List Values: Starch 1.5, Vegetable 3.0, Meat, lean 2.0

Basic Nutritional Values: Calories 298 (Calories from Fat 80), Total Fat 9 gm (Saturated Fat 3.0 gm, Polyunsat Fat 1.0 gm, Monounsat Fat 3.6 gm, Cholesterol 39 mg), Sodium 453 mg, Total Carbohydrate 35 gm, Dietary Fiber 9 gm, Sugars 10 gm, Protein 22 gm

VARIATIONS:

1. For extra flavor, add 1 tsp. cayenne pepper.
2. For more zest, use mild or hot Italian sausage instead of regular pork sausage.
3. Top individual servings with shredded sharp cheddar cheese, if diets permit.

Chili for Twenty

Janie Steele • Moore, OK

Makes 20 servings (Ideal slow cooker size: use 2 slow cookers approx. 4–5-quarts each)

3 lbs. 85%-lean ground beef

3 onions, finely chopped

3 green peppers, finely chopped

2 cloves garlic, minced

4 16-oz. cans Italian-style tomatoes

4 16-oz. cans kidney beans, drained

10-oz. can diced tomatoes and chilies

2 6-oz. cans tomato paste

1 cup water

1 1/4 tsp. salt

1 tsp. pepper

3 whole cloves

2 bay leaves

2 Tbsp. chili powder

1. Brown meat, onions, and peppers in soup pot on top of stove. Drain.

2. Combine all ingredients in large bowl. Divide among several medium-sized slow cookers.

3. Cover. Cook on Low 3–4 hours.

Exchange List Values: Starch 1.0, Vegetable 2.0, Meat, lean 2.0

Basic Nutritional Values: Calories 243 (Calories from Fat 69), Total Fat 8 gm (Saturated Fat 2.7 gm, Polyunsat Fat 0.6 gm, Monounsat Fat 3.1 gm, Cholesterol 40 mg), Sodium 547 mg, Total Carbohydrate 25 gm, Dietary Fiber 7 gm, Sugars 7 gm, Protein 20 gm

Crab Soup

Susan Alexander • Baltimore, MD

Makes 10 servings (Ideal slow cooker size: 5-quart)

1 lb. carrots, sliced

½ bunch celery, sliced

1 large onion, diced

2 10-oz. bags frozen mixed vegetables, or your choice of frozen vegetables

12-oz. can low-sodium tomato juice

8 ozs. extra-lean, lower-sodium ham

1 lb. beef, cubed

6 slices bacon, chopped

¼ tsp. pepper

1 Tbsp. Old Bay seasoning

1 lb. claw crabmeat

1. Combine all ingredients except seasonings and crabmeat in large slow cooker. Pour in water until cooker is half full.

2. Add spices. Stir in thoroughly. Put crab on top.

3. Cover. Cook on Low 8–10 hours.

4. Stir well and serve.

Exchange List Values: Starch 0.5, Vegetable 2.0, Meat, lean 2.0

Basic Nutritional Values: Calories 199 (Calories from Fat 44), Total Fat 5 gm (Saturated Fat 1.5 gm, Polyunsat Fat 0.7 gm, Monounsat Fat 2.0 gm, Cholesterol 74 mg), Sodium 649 mg, Total Carbohydrate 17 gm, Dietary Fiber 4 gm, Sugars 8 gm, Protein 23 gm

Special Seafood Chowder

Dorothea K. Ladd • Ballston Lake, NY

Makes 8–10 servings (Ideal slow cooker size: 4-quart)

½ cup chopped onions

1 Tbsp. canola oil

1 lb. fresh or frozen cod or haddock

4 cups diced potatoes

15-oz. can creamed corn

½ tsp. salt

dash pepper

2 cups water

1 pint fat-free half-and-half

1. Saute onions in oil in skillet until transparent but not brown.

2. Cut fish into ¾" cubes. Combine fish, onions, potatoes, corn, seasonings, and water in slow cooker.

3. Cover. Cook on Low 6 hours, until potatoes are tender.

4. Add half-and-half during last hour.

Exchange List Values: Carbohydrate 1.5, Meat, lean 1.0

Basic Nutritional Values: Calories 172 (Calories from Fat 25), Total Fat 3 gm (Saturated Fat 0.5 gm, Polyunsat Fat 0.6 gm, Monounsat Fat 0.9 gm, Cholesterol 29 mg), Sodium 381 mg, Total Carbohydrate 24 gm, Dietary Fiber 2 gm, Sugars 8 gm, Protein 12 gm

Corn and Shrimp Chowder

Naomi E. Fast • Hesston, KS

Makes 6 servings (Ideal slow cooker size: 4–5-quart)

4 slices bacon, diced

1 cup chopped onions

2 cups diced, unpeeled red potatoes

2 10-oz. pkgs. frozen corn

1 tsp. Worcestershire sauce

½ tsp. paprika

½ tsp. salt

⅛ tsp. pepper

2 6-oz. cans shrimp

2 cups water

2 Tbsp. light, soft tub margarine

12-oz. can fat-free evaporated milk

chopped chives

1. Fry bacon in skillet until lightly crisp. Add onions to drippings and saute until transparent. Using slotted spoon, transfer bacon and onions to slow cooker.

2. Add remaining ingredients except milk and chives to cooker.

3. Cover. Cook on Low 3–4 hours, adding milk and chives 30 minutes before end of cooking time.

4. Serve with broccoli salad for a tasty meal.

Exchange List Values: Starch 3.0, Milk, fat-free 0.5, Meat, very lean 1.0, Fat 0.5

Basic Nutritional Values: Calories 331 (Calories from Fat 50), Total Fat 6 gm (Saturated Fat 0.9 gm, Polyunsat Fat 1.2 gm, Monounsat Fat 2.1 gm, Cholesterol 102 mg), Sodium 488 mg, Total Carbohydrate 49 gm, Dietary Fiber 5 gm, Sugars 11 gm, Protein 24 gm

Note: I learned to make this recipe in a 7th grade home economics class. It made an impression on my father, who liked seafood very much. The recipe calls only for canned shrimp, but I often increase the taste appeal with extra cooked shrimp. I frequently use frozen hash brown potatoes for speedy preparation. There is no difference in the taste.

You might put on weight when you first go on insulin because you're no longer losing calories in your urine, but the benefits of lower blood sugars outweigh the risk of a small weight gain.

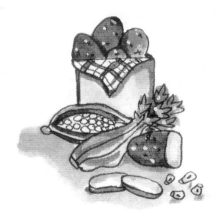

Clam Chowder

Ruth Shank • Gridley, IL

Makes 8-12 servings (Ideal slow cooker size: 5-quart)

2 10¾-oz. cans cream of potato soup

10¾-oz. can cream of celery soup

2 6½-oz. cans minced clams, drained

2 slices bacon, diced and fried

1 soup can water

1 small onion, minced

1 Tbsp. fresh parsley

dash dried marjoram

1 Tbsp. Worcestershire sauce

pepper to taste

1½ cups fat-free milk

1 cup fat-free half-and-half

1. Combine all ingredients, except milk and half-and-half, in slow cooker.

2. Cover. Cook on Low 6–8 hours.

3. Twenty minutes before end of cooking time, stir in milk and half-and-half. Continue cooking until heated through.

Exchange List Values: Carbohydrate 1.0, Meat, very lean 1.0, Fat 0.5

Basic Nutritional Values: Calories 114 (Calories from Fat 34), Total Fat 4 gm (Saturated Fat 1.5 gm, Polyunsat Fat 0.9 gm, Monounsat Fat 0.8 gm, Cholesterol 17 mg), Sodium 634 mg, Total Carbohydrate 13 gm, Dietary Fiber 1 gm, Sugars 5 gm, Protein 7 gm

Manhattan Clam Chowder

Joyce Slaymaker • Strasburg, PA /
Louise Stackhouse • Benton, PA

Makes 8 servings (Ideal slow cooker size: 4-quart)

¼ lb. bacon, diced and fried

1 large onion, chopped

2 carrots, thinly sliced

3 ribs celery, sliced

1 Tbsp. dried parsley flakes

1-lb. 12-oz. can tomatoes

⅛ tsp. salt

2 8-oz. cans clams with liquid

2 whole peppercorns

1 bay leaf

1½ tsp. dried crushed thyme

3 medium potatoes, cubed

1. Combine all ingredients in slow cooker.

2. Cover. Cook on Low 8–10 hours.

Exchange List Values: Starch 0.5, Vegetable 2.0, Meat, lean 1.0

Basic Nutritional Values: Calories 151 (Calories from Fat 25), Total Fat 3 gm (Saturated Fat 0.8 gm, Polyunsat Fat 0.6 gm, Monounsat Fat 0.9 gm, Cholesterol 21 mg), Sodium 427 mg, Total Carbohydrate 22 gm, Dietary Fiber 4 gm, Sugars 8 gm, Protein 11 gm

Chicken Clam Chowder

Irene Klaeger • Inverness, FL

Makes 12 servings (Ideal slow cooker size: 6-quart)

¼ lb. bacon, diced

¼ lb. extra-lean, lower-sodium ham, cubed

2 cups chopped onions

2 cups diced celery

¼ tsp. pepper

2 cups diced potatoes

2 cups cooked, diced chicken

4 tsp. sodium-free chicken bouillon powder mixed with 4 cups water

2 bottles clam juice, or 2 cans clams with juice

1-lb. can whole-kernel corn, drained and rinsed

¼–½ cup water

¾ cup flour

3 cups fat-free milk

1½ cups fat-free half-and-half

4 cups shredded cheddar, or Jack, cheese

½ cup whipping cream (not whipped)

2 Tbsp. fresh parsley

1. Saute bacon, ham, onions, and celery in skillet until bacon is crisp and onions and celery are limp. Add pepper.

2. Combine all ingredients in slow cooker except flour, milk, half-and-half, cheese, cream, and parsley.

3. Cover. Cook on Low 6–8 hours, or on High 3–4 hours.

4. Whisk flour into milk and half-and-half. Stir into soup, along with cheese, whipping cream, and parsley. Cook 1 more hour on High.

Exchange List Values: Carbohydrate 1.5, Meat, lean 2.0

Basic Nutritional Values: Calories 225 (Calories from Fat 37), Total Fat 4 gm (Saturated Fat 1.3 gm, Polyunsat Fat 0.8 gm, Monounsat Fat 1.4 gm, Cholesterol 34 mg), Sodium 517 mg, Total Carbohydrate 26 gm, Dietary Fiber 2 gm, Sugars 9 gm, Protein 21 gm

Get all your prescriptions on the same schedule so that you do not have to go to the pharmacy several times a month.

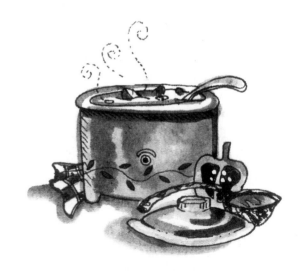

Chicken Broth

Ruth Conrad Liechty • Goshen, IN

Makes about 6 1-cup servings (Ideal slow cooker size: 4-quart)

bony chicken pieces from 2 chickens, skin and visible fat removed

1 onion, quartered

3 whole cloves, optional

3 ribs celery, cut up

1 carrot, quartered

½ tsp. salt

¼ tsp. pepper

4 cups water

1. Place chicken in slow cooker.

2. Stud onion with cloves. Add to slow cooker with other ingredients.

3. Cover. Cook on High 4–5 hours.

4. Remove chicken and vegetables. Discard vegetables. Debone chicken. Cut up meat to equal about 1 cup and add to broth.

5. Place broth in the refrigerator. After broth is cooled, skim fat from the surface. Use as stock for soups.

Exchange List Values: Meat, lean 1.0

Basic Nutritional Values: Calories 42 (Calories from Fat 14), Total Fat 2 gm (Saturated Fat 0.4 gm, Polyunsat Fat 0.4 gm, Monounsat Fat 0.6 gm, Cholesterol 19 mg), Sodium 211 mg, Total Carbohydrate 0 gm, Dietary Fiber 0 gm, Sugars 0 gm, Protein 6 gm

Chicken Noodle Soup

Beth Shank • Wellman, IA

Makes 6–8 servings (Ideal slow cooker size: 4-quart)

2 tsp. sodium-free chicken bouillon powder

5 cups hot water

46-oz. can 100%-fat-free, lower-sodium chicken broth

2 cups cooked chicken

4 cups "homestyle" noodles, uncooked

⅓ cup thinly sliced celery, lightly pre-cooked in microwave

⅓ cup shredded, or chopped, carrots

1. Dissolve bouillon in water. Pour into slow cooker.

2. Add remaining ingredients. Mix well.

3. Cover. Cook on Low 4–6 hours.

Exchange List Values: Starch 1.0, Meat, lean 1.0

Basic Nutritional Values: Calories 155 (Calories from Fat 31), Total Fat 3 gm (Saturated Fat 1.0 gm, Polyunsat Fat 0.8 gm, Monounsat Fat 1.2 gm, Cholesterol 49 mg), Sodium 382 mg, Total Carbohydrate 15 gm, Dietary Fiber 1 gm, Sugars 2 gm, Protein 14 gm

Brown Jug Soup

Dorothy Shank • Sterling, IL

Makes 10–12 servings (Ideal slow cooker size: 6-quart)

10½-oz. can chicken broth

4 tsp. sodium-free chicken bouillon powder

1 qt. water

2 cups (3–4 ribs) diced celery

2 cups (2 medium-sized) diced onions

4 cups diced potatoes

3 cups diced carrots

10-oz. pkg. frozen whole-kernel corn

2 10¾-oz. cans 98%-fat-free, reduced-sodium cream of chicken soup

4 ozs. shredded sharp cheddar cheese

1. Combine all ingredients except cheese in slow cooker.

2. Cover. Cook on Low 10–12 hours, or until vegetables are tender.

3. Just before serving, add cheese. Stir until cheese is melted. Serve.

Exchange List Values: Starch 1.5, Vegetable 1.0

Basic Nutritional Values: Calories 138 (Calories from Fat 13), Total Fat 1 gm (Saturated Fat 0.4 gm, Polyunsat Fat 0.6 gm, Monounsat Fat 0.3 gm, Cholesterol 6 mg), Sodium 464 mg, Total Carbohydrate 25 gm, Dietary Fiber 3 gm, Sugars 6 gm, Protein 7 gm

Chicken Corn Soup

Eleanor Larson • Glen Lyon, PA

Makes 4–6 servings (Ideal slow cooker size: 4-quart)

2 whole boneless, skinless chicken breasts, cubed

1 onion, chopped

1 clove garlic, minced

2 carrots, sliced

2 ribs celery, chopped

2 medium potatoes, cubed

1 tsp. mixed dried herbs

⅓ cup tomato sauce

12-oz. can cream-style corn

14-oz. can whole-kernel corn

3 tsp. sodium-free chicken bouillon powder

3 cups water

¼ cup chopped Italian parsley

¼ tsp. pepper

1. Combine all ingredients except parsley and pepper in slow cooker.

2. Cover. Cook on Low 8–9 hours, or until chicken is tender.

3. Add parsley and seasoning 30 minutes before serving.

Exchange List Values: Starch 2.0, Vegetable 1.0, Meat, very lean 3.0

Basic Nutritional Values: Calories 251 (Calories from Fat 28), Total Fat 3 gm (Saturated Fat 0.6 gm, Polyunsat Fat 0.8 gm, Monounsat Fat 0.9 gm, Cholesterol 49 mg), Sodium 534 mg, Total Carbohydrate 33 gm, Dietary Fiber 5 gm, Sugars 13 gm, Protein 23 gm

Chili, Chicken, Corn Chowder

Jeanne Allen • Rye, CO

Makes 6–8 servings (Ideal slow cooker size: 4-quart)

1 large onion, diced

1 clove garlic, minced

1 rib celery, finely chopped

2 Tbsp. canola oil

2 cups frozen, or canned, corn

2 cups cooked, deboned, diced chicken

4-oz. can diced green chilies

½ tsp. black pepper

2 cups 100%-fat-free, lower-sodium chicken broth

¼ tsp. salt

1 cup fat-free half-and-half

1. In saucepan, saute onion, garlic, and celery in oil until limp.

2. Stir in corn, chicken, and chilies. Saute for 2–3 minutes.

3. Combine all ingredients except half-and-half in slow cooker.

4. Cover. Heat on Low 4 hours.

5. Stir in half-and-half before serving. Do not boil, but be sure cream is heated through.

Exchange List Values: Starch 0.5, Vegetable 1.0, Meat, lean 1.0, Fat 1.0

Basic Nutritional Values: Calories 169 (Calories from Fat 60), Total Fat 7 gm (Saturated Fat 1.2 gm, Polyunsat Fat 1.7 gm, Monounsat Fat 3.0 gm, Cholesterol 33 mg), Sodium 343 mg, Total Carbohydrate 14 gm, Dietary Fiber 2 gm, Sugars 4 gm, Protein 13 gm

White Chili

Esther Martin • Ephrata, PA

Makes 8 servings (Ideal slow cooker size: 5-quart)

3 15-oz. cans Great Northern beans, drained

8 ozs. cooked and shredded chicken breasts

1 cup chopped onions

1½ cups chopped yellow, red, or green bell peppers

2 cloves garlic, minced

2 tsp. ground cumin

½ tsp. salt

½ tsp. dried oregano

3½ cups chicken broth

1. Combine all ingredients in slow cooker.

2. Cover. Cook on Low 8–10 hours, or High 4–5 hours.

3. Ladle into bowls and top individual servings with reduced-fat sour cream, reduced-fat cheddar cheese, and baked tortilla chips, if diets allow.

Exchange List Values: Starch 1.5, Vegetable 1.0, Meat, very lean 1.0

Basic Nutritional Values: Calories 189 (Calories from Fat 15), Total Fat 2 gm (Saturated Fat 0.4 gm, Polyunsat Fat 0.5 gm, Monounsat Fat 0.5 gm, Cholesterol 24 mg), Sodium 561 mg, Total Carbohydrate 25 gm, Dietary Fiber 8 gm, Sugars 5 gm, Protein 19 gm

Try not to think of exercise as a chore, but as play. Get in touch with your inner kid!

White Chili Speciality

Barbara McGinnis • Jupiter, FL

Makes 10 servings (Ideal slow cooker size: 5-quart)

1 lb. large Great Northern beans, soaked overnight

2 lbs. boneless, skinless chicken breasts, cut up

1 medium onion, chopped

2 4½-oz. cans chopped green chilies

2 tsp. cumin

½ tsp. salt

14½-oz. can chicken broth

1 cup water

1. Put soaked beans in medium-sized saucepan and cover with water. Bring to boil and simmer 20 minutes. Discard water.

2. Brown chicken in fat-free cooking spray, in skillet.

3. Combine pre-cooked and drained beans, chicken, and all remaining ingredients in slow cooker.

4. Cover. Cook on Low 10–12 hours, or High 5–6 hours.

Exchange List Values: Starch 2.0, Meat, very lean 3.0

Basic Nutritional Values: Calories 258 (Calories from Fat 28), Total Fat 3 gm (Saturated Fat 0.9 gm, Polyunsat Fat 0.8 gm, Monounsat Fat 1.0 gm, Cholesterol 55 mg), Sodium 571 mg, Total Carbohydrate 26 gm, Dietary Fiber 9 gm, Sugars 4 gm, Protein 30 gm

Mexican Rice and Bean Soup

Esther J. Mast • East Petersburg, PA

Makes 6 servings (Ideal slow cooker size: 4-quart)

½ cup chopped onions

⅓ cup chopped green peppers

1 clove garlic, minced

1 Tbsp. oil

4-oz. pkg. sliced or chipped dried beef

18-oz. can low-sodium tomato juice

15½-oz. can red kidney beans, undrained

1½ cups water

½ cup long-grain rice, uncooked

1 tsp. paprika

½–1 tsp. chili powder

dash pepper

1. Cook onions, green peppers, and garlic in oil in skillet until vegetables are tender but not brown. Transfer to slow cooker.

2. Tear beef into small pieces and add to slow cooker.

3. Add remaining ingredients. Mix well.

4. Cover. Cook on Low 6 hours. Stir before serving.

5. Serve with relish tray and corn bread, home-canned fruit, and cookies.

Exchange List Values: Starch 1.5, Vegetable 2.0, Fat 0.5

Basic Nutritional Values: Calories 190 (Calories from Fat 28), Total Fat 3 gm (Saturated Fat 0.4 gm, Polyunsat Fat 0.9 gm, Monounsat Fat 1.6 gm, Cholesterol 15 mg), Sodium 796 mg, Total Carbohydrate 30 gm, Dietary Fiber 4 gm, Sugars 7 gm, Protein 12 gm

Note: This is a recipe I fixed often when our sons were growing up. We have all enjoyed it in any season of the year.

Chicken Tortilla Soup

Becky Harder • Monument, CO

Makes 6–8 servings (Ideal slow cooker size: 4–5-quart)

4 chicken breast halves

2 15-oz. cans no-salt-added black beans, undrained

2 15-oz. cans Mexican stewed tomatoes, or Rotel tomatoes

1 cup salsa (mild, medium, or hot, whichever you prefer)

4-oz. can chopped green chilies

14½-oz. can no-salt-added tomato sauce

2 ozs. (about 24 chips) tortilla chips

1 cup fat-free cheddar cheese

1. Combine all ingredients except chips and cheese in large slow cooker.

2. Cover. Cook on Low 8 hours.

3. Just before serving, remove chicken breasts and slice into bite-sized pieces. Stir into soup.

4. To serve, put a handful of chips in each individual soup bowl. Ladle soup over chips. Top with cheese.

Exchange List Values: Starch 1.0, Vegetable 2.0, Meat, very lean 3.0, Fat 0.5

Basic Nutritional Values: Calories 263 (Calories from Fat 36), Total Fat 4 gm (Saturated Fat 0.9 gm, Polyunsat Fat 0.8 gm, Monounsat Fat 1.7 gm, Cholesterol 43 mg), Sodium 793 mg, Total Carbohydrate 29 gm, Dietary Fiber 7 gm, Sugars 9 gm, Protein 28 gm

Tortilla Soup

Joy Mintzer • Newark, DE

Makes 6 servings (Ideal slow cooker size: 4-quart)

4 chicken breast halves

1 clove garlic, minced

1½ tsp. canola oil

2 14½-oz. cans 100%-fat-free reduced-sodium chicken broth

2 14½-oz. cans no-salt-added, chopped, stewed tomatoes

1 cup salsa (mild, medium, or hot, whichever you prefer)

½ cup chopped cilantro

1 Tbsp., or more, ground cumin

8 ozs. reduced-fat Monterey Jack cheese, cubed

1. Cook, debone, and shred chicken.

2. Add minced garlic to oil in slow cooker. Saute.

3. Combine all ingredients except cheese.

4. Cover. Cook on Low 8–10 hours.

5. Divide cubed cheese among 6 individual soup bowls. Ladle soup over cheese. Sprinkle with chips and top each bowl with a dollop of sour cream, if diets allow.

Exchange List Values: Vegetable 3.0, Meat, lean 3.0

Basic Nutritional Values: Calories 234 (Calories from Fat 65), Total Fat 7 gm (Saturated Fat 3.4 gm, Polyunsat Fat 1.1 gm, Monounsat Fat 2.6 gm, Cholesterol 69 mg), Sodium 669 mg, Total Carbohydrate 12 gm, Dietary Fiber 2 gm, Sugars 5 gm, Protein 31 gm

Tex-Mex Chicken Chowder

Janie Steele • Moore, OK

Makes 8–10 servings (Ideal slow cooker size: 5-quart or larger)

1 cup chopped onions

1 cup thinly sliced celery

2 cloves garlic, minced

1 Tbsp. canola oil

1½ lbs. boneless, skinless chicken breasts, cubed

4 tsp. sodium-free chicken bouillon powder

4 cups water

1 pkg. country gravy mix

2 cups fat-free milk

16-oz. jar chunky salsa

32-oz. bag frozen hash brown potatoes

4½-oz. can chopped green chilies

4 ozs. fat-free American cheese

1. Combine onions, celery, garlic, oil, chicken, and bouillon mixed with water in 5-quart or larger slow cooker.

2. Cover. Cook on Low 2½ hours, until chicken is no longer pink.

3. In separate bowl, dissolve gravy mix in milk. Stir into chicken mixture. Add salsa, potatoes, chilies, and cheese and combine well. Cook on Low 2–4 hours, or until potatoes are fully cooked.

Exchange List Values: Starch 1.5, Vegetable 1.0, Meat, very lean 2.0, Fat 0.5

Basic Nutritional Values: Calories 247 (Calories from Fat 40), Total Fat 4 gm (Saturated Fat 0.7 gm, Polyunsat Fat 1.3 gm, Monounsat Fat 1.6 gm, Cholesterol 43 mg), Sodium 567 mg, Total Carbohydrate 29 gm, Dietary Fiber 3 gm, Sugars 7 gm, Protein 23 gm

Ham and Potato Chowder

Penny Blosser • Beavercreek, OH

Makes 5 servings (Ideal slow cooker size: 4-quart)

5-oz. pkg. scalloped potatoes

sauce mix from potato package

1 cup extra-lean, reduced-sodium cooked ham, cut into narrow strips

4 tsp. sodium-free bouillon powder

4 cups water

1 cup chopped celery

⅓ cup chopped onions

salt to taste

pepper to taste

2 cups fat-free half-and-half

⅓ cup flour

1. Combine potatoes, sauce mix, ham, bouillon powder, water, celery, onions, salt, and pepper in slow cooker.

2. Cover. Cook on Low 7 hours.

3. Combine half-and-half and flour. Gradually add to slow cooker, blending well.

4. Cover. Cook on Low up to 1 hour, stirring occasionally until thickened.

Exchange List Values: Starch 1.5, Carbohydrate 1.0, Meat, lean 1.0

Basic Nutritional Values: Calories 241 (Calories from Fat 29), Total Fat 3 gm (Saturated Fat 1.2 gm, Polyunsat Fat 0.7 gm, Monounsat Fat 0.2 gm, Cholesterol 21 mg), Sodium 836 mg, Total Carbohydrate 41 gm, Dietary Fiber 3 gm, Sugars 8 gm, Protein 11 gm

Drink plenty of water. You should try to drink eight 8-oz. glasses each day.

Chicken and Ham Gumbo

Barbara Tenney • Delta, PA

Recipe photo appears in color section.

Makes 6 servings (Ideal slow cooker size: 4-quart)

1½ lbs. boneless, skinless chicken thighs

1 Tbsp. oil

10-oz. pkg. frozen okra

½ lb. extra-lean, lower-sodium ham, cut into small chunks

1½ cups coarsely chopped onions

1½ cups coarsely chopped green peppers

2 10-oz. cans no-salt-added cannellini beans, drained

6 cups low-sodium chicken broth

2 10-oz. cans diced tomatoes with green chilies

2 Tbsp. chopped fresh cilantro

1. Cut chicken into bite-sized pieces. Cook in oil in skillet until no longer pink.

2. Run hot water over okra until pieces separate easily.

3. Combine all ingredients except cilantro in slow cooker.

4. Cover. Cook on Low 6–8 hours. Stir in cilantro before serving.

Exchange List Values: Starch 1.0, Vegetable 3.0, Meat, lean 4.0

Basic Nutritional Values: Calories 385 (Calories from Fat 120), Total Fat 13 gm (Saturated Fat 3.1 gm, Polyunsat Fat 3.4 gm, Monounsat Fat 5.2 gm, Cholesterol 96 mg), Sodium 879 mg, Total Carbohydrate 28 gm, Dietary Fiber 7 gm, Sugars 10 gm, Protein 38 gm

VARIATIONS:

1. Stir in ½ cup long-grain, dry rice with rest of ingredients.
2. Add ¼ tsp. pepper with other ingredients.

Easy Southern Brunswick Stew

Barbara Sparks • Glen Burnie, MD

Makes 12 servings (Ideal slow cooker size: 4-quart)

2 lbs. pork butt, visible fat removed

17-oz. can white corn

1¼ cup ketchup

2 cups diced, cooked potatoes

10-oz. pkg. frozen peas

2 10¾-oz. cans reduced-sodium tomato soup

1. Place pork in slow cooker.

2. Cover. Cook on Low 6–8 hours. Remove meat from bone and shred, removing and discarding all visible fat.

3. Combine all ingredients in slow cooker.

4. Cover. Bring to boil on High. Reduce heat to Low and simmer 30 minutes.

Exchange List Values: Starch 1.0, Vegetable 2.0, Meat, lean 1.0, Fat 0.5

Basic Nutritional Values: Calories 213 (Calories from Fat 61), Total Fat 7 gm (Saturated Fat 2.3 gm, Polyunsat Fat 0.9 gm, Monounsat Fat 2.6 gm, Cholesterol 34 mg), Sodium 584 mg, Total Carbohydrate 27 gm, Dietary Fiber 3 gm, Sugars 9 gm, Protein 13 gm

OPTIONAL INGREDIENTS:

hot sauce to taste

salt to taste

pepper to taste

Oriental Pork Soup

Judi Manos • West Islip, NY

Makes 8 servings (Ideal slow cooker size: 5-quart)

½ lb. ground pork

1 clove garlic, minced

2 medium carrots, cut into julienne strips

4 medium green onions, cut into 1" pieces

1 clove garlic, minced

2 Tbsp. light soy sauce

½ tsp. gingerroot, chopped

⅛ tsp. pepper

2 14½-oz. cans chicken broth

2½ tsp. sodium-free chicken bouillon powder

2½ cups water

1 cup sliced mushrooms

1 cup bean sprouts

1. Cook meat with garlic in skillet until brown. Drain.

2. Combine all ingredients except mushrooms and sprouts in slow cooker.

3. Cover. Cook on Low 7–9 hours, or High 3–4 hours.

4. Stir in mushrooms and bean sprouts.

5. Cover. Cook on Low 1 hour.

Exchange List Values: Vegetable 1.0, Meat, medium fat 1.0

Basic Nutritional Values: Calories 97 (Calories from Fat 39), Total Fat 4 gm (Saturated Fat 1.5 gm, Polyunsat Fat 0.4 gm, Monounsat Fat 1.8 gm, Cholesterol 19 mg), Sodium 486 mg, Total Carbohydrate 6 gm, Dietary Fiber 2 gm, Sugars 3 gm, Protein 8 gm

VARIATION: To add flavor to the pork, add ⅛ tsp. five-spice blend to Step 1.

Joy's Brunswick Stew

Joy Sutter • Iowa City, IA

Makes 8 servings (Ideal slow cooker size: 4-quart)

1 lb. boneless, skinless chicken breasts, cut into bite-sized pieces

2 potatoes, thinly sliced

10¾-oz. can tomato soup

16-oz. can stewed tomatoes

10-oz. pkg. frozen corn

10-oz. pkg. frozen lima beans

3 Tbsp. onion flakes

¼ tsp. salt

⅛ tsp. pepper

1. Combine all ingredients in slow cooker.

2. Cover. Cook on High 2 hours. Reduce to Low and cook 2 hours.

Exchange List Values: Starch 2.0, Vegetable 1.0, Meat, very lean 1.0

Basic Nutritional Values: Calories 220 (Calories from Fat 21), Total Fat 2 gm (Saturated Fat 0.6 gm, Polyunsat Fat 0.8 gm, Monounsat Fat 0.6 gm, Cholesterol 34 mg), Sodium 480 mg, Total Carbohydrate 33 gm, Dietary Fiber 5 gm, Sugars 8 gm, Protein 18 gm

VARIATION: For more flavor, add 1 or 2 bay leaves during cooking.

For exercise that lasts longer than an hour and is fairly intense, try sports drinks, which are convenient and easy to digest.

Brunswick Soup Mix

Joyce B. Suiter • Garysburg, NC

Makes 14 servings (Ideal slow cooker size: 5-quart)

1 large onion, chopped

4 cups frozen, cubed hash browns, thawed

4 cups chopped cooked chicken, or 2 20-oz. cans canned chicken

14½-oz. can diced tomatoes

15-oz. can tomato sauce

15¼-oz. can corn

15¼-oz. can lima beans, drained

2 cups 100%-fat-free, lower-sodium chicken broth

¼ tsp. salt

½ tsp. pepper

¼ tsp. Worcestershire sauce

¼ cup sugar

1. Combine all ingredients in large slow cooker.

2. Cover. Cook on High 7 hours.

3. Cool and freeze in 2-cup portions.

4. To use, empty 1 frozen portion into saucepan with small amount of liquid: tomato juice, V-8 juice, or broth. Cook slowly until soup mixture thaws. Stir frequently, adding more liquid until of desired consistency.

Exchange List Values: Starch 1.5, Vegetable 1.0, Meat, lean 1.0

Basic Nutritional Values: Calories 206 (Calories from Fat 34), Total Fat 4 gm (Saturated Fat 1.0 gm, Polyunsat Fat 1.0 gm, Monounsat Fat 1.1 gm, Cholesterol 36 mg), Sodium 578 mg, Total Carbohydrate 28 gm, Dietary Fiber 5 gm, Sugars 10 gm, Protein 16 gm

Oriental Turkey Chili

Kimberly Jensen • Bailey, CO

Makes 6 servings (Ideal slow cooker size: 4-quart)

2 cups yellow onions, diced

1 small red bell pepper, diced

1 lb. ground turkey, browned

2 Tbsp. minced gingerroot

3 cloves garlic, minced

¼ cup dry sherry

¼ cup hoisin sauce

2 Tbsp. chili powder

1 Tbsp. corn oil

2 Tbsp. light soy sauce

1 tsp. sugar

2 cups canned whole tomatoes

16-oz. can no-salt-added dark red kidney beans, undrained

1. Combine all ingredients in slow cooker.

2. Cover. Cook on Low 6 hours.

3. Serve topped with chow mein noodles or over cooked white rice.

Exchange List Values: Starch 1.0, Vegetable 2.0, Meat, lean 2.0, Fat 1.0

Basic Nutritional Values: Calories 279 (Calories from Fat 93), Total Fat 10 gm (Saturated Fat 2.4 gm, Polyunsat Fat 3.5 gm, Monounsat Fat 3.4 gm, Cholesterol 56 mg), Sodium 612 mg, Total Carbohydrate 26 gm, Dietary Fiber 8 gm, Sugars 12 gm, Protein 22 gm

Note: If you serve this chili over rice, this recipe will yield 10–12 servings.

Pumpkin Black-Bean Turkey Chili

Rhoda Atzeff • Harrisburg, PA

Makes 10 servings (Ideal slow cooker size: 4–5-quart)

1 cup chopped onions

1 cup chopped yellow bell pepper

3 cloves garlic, minced

2 Tbsp. canola oil

1½ tsp. dried oregano

1½–2 tsp. ground cumin

2 tsp. chili powder

2 15-oz. cans black beans, rinsed and drained

2½ cups chopped cooked turkey

16-oz. can pumpkin

14½-oz. can diced tomatoes

3 cups 98%-fat-free, lower-sodium chicken broth

1. Saute onions, yellow pepper, and garlic in oil for 8 minutes, or until soft.

2. Stir in oregano, cumin, and chili powder. Cook 1 minute. Transfer to slow cooker.

3. Add remaining ingredients.

4. Cover. Cook on Low 7–8 hours.

Exchange List Values: Starch 1.0, Vegetable 1.0, Meat, lean 1.0, Fat 0.5

Basic Nutritional Values: Calories 189 (Calories from Fat 46), Total Fat 5 gm (Saturated Fat 0.9 gm, Polyunsat Fat 1.5 gm, Monounsat Fat 2.1 gm, Cholesterol 27 mg), Sodium 327 mg, Total Carbohydrate 20 gm, Dietary Fiber 7 gm, Sugars 6 gm, Protein 17 gm

Be sure to tell your doctor right away if you have symptoms such as a change in vision, swelling of the ankles or pain in the feet, or chest pain.

Turkey Chili

Reita F. Yoder • Carlsbad, NM

Makes 6–8 servings (Ideal slow cooker size: 4-quart)

2 lbs. ground turkey, browned and drained

16-oz. can pinto, or kidney, beans

2 cups fresh tomatoes, chopped

2 cups no-salt-added tomato sauce

1 clove garlic, minced

1 small onion, chopped

16-oz. can Rotel tomatoes

1-oz. pkg. Williams chili seasoning

1. Crumble ground turkey in bottom of slow cooker.

2. Add remaining ingredients. Mix well.

3. Cover. Cook on Low 6–8 hours.

Exchange List Values: Starch 0.5, Vegetable 2.0, Meat, lean 3.0, Fat 0.5

Basic Nutritional Values: Calories 294 (Calories from Fat 106), Total Fat 12 gm (Saturated Fat 2.8 gm, Polyunsat Fat 2.9 gm, Monounsat Fat 4.2 gm, Cholesterol 84 mg), Sodium 633 mg, Total Carbohydrate 19 gm, Dietary Fiber 5 gm, Sugars 9 gm, Protein 27 gm

Joyce's Slow-Cooked Chili

Joyce Slaymaker • Strasburg, PA

Makes 10 servings (Ideal slow cooker size: 4-quart)

2 lbs. ground turkey

2 16-oz. cans kidney beans, rinsed and drained

2 14½-oz. cans diced tomatoes, undrained

8-oz. can tomato sauce

2 medium onions, chopped

1 green pepper, chopped

2 cloves garlic, minced

2 Tbsp. chili powder

1 tsp. pepper

1. Brown ground turkey in skillet. Drain. Transfer to slow cooker.

2. Stir in remaining ingredients.

3. Cover. Cook on Low 8–10 hours, or on High 4 hours.

4. Garnish individual servings with cheese.

Exchange List Values: Starch 1.0, Vegetable 2.0, Meat, lean 2.0, Fat 0.5

Basic Nutritional Values: Calories 276 (Calories from Fat 85), Total Fat 9 gm (Saturated Fat 2.2 gm, Polyunsat Fat 2.5 gm, Monounsat Fat 3.3 gm, Cholesterol 67 mg), Sodium 490 mg, Total Carbohydrate 24 gm, Dietary Fiber 6 gm, Sugars 8 gm, Protein 25 gm

Turkey Chili

Dawn Day • Westminster, CA

Makes 8 servings (Ideal slow cooker size: 4-quart)

1 large chopped onion

2 Tbsp. oil

1 lb. ground turkey

3 Tbsp. chili powder

6-oz. can tomato paste

3 1-lb. cans small red beans with liquid

1 cup frozen corn

1. Saute onion in oil in skillet until transparent. Add turkey and brown lightly in skillet.

2. Combine all ingredients in slow cooker. Mix well.

3. Cover. Cook on Low 8–9 hours.

Exchange List Values: Starch 2.0, Vegetable 1.0, Meat, lean 2.0, Fat 0.5

Basic Nutritional Values: Calories 319 (Calories from Fat 91), Total Fat 10 gm (Saturated Fat 1.7 gm, Polyunsat Fat 3.0 gm, Monounsat Fat 4.3 gm, Cholesterol 42 mg), Sodium 678 mg, Total Carbohydrate 37 gm, Dietary Fiber 9 gm, Sugars 7 gm, Protein 22 gm

VARIATION: Serve over rice, topped with shredded fat-free cheddar cheese and fat-free sour cream.

Note: Ground beef can be used in place of turkey.

Chili Sans Cholesterol

Dolores S. Kratz • Souderton, PA

Makes 4 servings (Ideal slow cooker size: 4-quart)

1 lb. ground turkey

½ cup chopped celery

½ cup chopped onions

8-oz. can tomatoes

15-oz. can no-salt-added pinto beans

14½-oz. can diced tomatoes

½ tsp., or more, chili powder

¼ tsp. salt

dash pepper

1. Saute turkey in skillet until browned. Drain.

2. Combine all ingredients in slow cooker.

3. Cover. Cook on Low 6 hours.

Exchange List Values: Starch 1.0, Vegetable 2.0, Meat, lean 3.0, Fat 0.5

Basic Nutritional Values: Calories 317 (Calories from Fat 104), Total Fat 12 gm (Saturated Fat 2.9 gm, Polyunsat Fat 3.0 gm, Monounsat Fat 4.1 gm, Cholesterol 84 mg), Sodium 578 mg, Total Carbohydrate 24 gm, Dietary Fiber 7 gm, Sugars 8 gm, Protein 29 gm

More vegetables = Fewer heart attacks

Italian Vegetable Soup

Patti Boston • Newark, OH

Makes 4–6 servings (Ideal slow cooker size: 4-quart)

3 small carrots, sliced

1 small onion, chopped

2 small potatoes, diced

2 Tbsp. chopped parsley

1 clove garlic, minced

3 tsp. sodium-free beef bouillon powder

1¼ tsp. dried basil

¼ tsp. pepper

16-oz. can red kidney beans, undrained

3 cups water

14½-oz. can stewed tomatoes, with juice

1 cup diced extra-lean, lower-sodium cooked ham

1. Layer carrots, onions, potatoes, parsley, garlic, beef bouillon, basil, pepper, and kidney beans in slow cooker. Do not stir. Add water.

2. Cover. Cook on Low 8–9 hours, or on High 4½–5½ hours, until vegetables are tender.

3. Stir in tomatoes and ham. Cover and cook on High 10–15 minutes.

Exchange List Values: Starch 1.5, Vegetable 2.0

Basic Nutritional Values: Calories 156 (Calories from Fat 7), Total Fat 1 gm (Saturated Fat 0.2 gm, Polyunsat Fat 0.3 gm, Monounsat Fat 0.2 gm, Cholesterol 9 mg), Sodium 614 mg, Total Carbohydrate 29 gm, Dietary Fiber 5 gm, Sugars 8 gm, Protein 9 gm

Chet's Trucker Stew

Janice Muller • Derwood, MD

Makes 12 servings (Ideal slow cooker size: 4–5-quart)

1 lb. bulk pork sausage, cooked and drained

1 lb. ground beef, cooked and drained

31-oz. can pork and beans

2 15-oz. cans no-salt-added kidney beans, drained

14½-oz. can waxed beans, drained

14½-oz. can lima beans, drained

1 cup no-salt-added ketchup

½ cup brown sugar

brown sugar substitute to equal ¼ cup

1 Tbsp. spicy prepared mustard

1. Combine all ingredients in slow cooker.

2. Cover. Simmer on High 2–3 hours.

Exchange List Values: Starch 2.0, Carbohydrate 1.0, Meat, medium fat 2.0

Basic Nutritional Values: Calories 363 (Calories from Fat 100), Total Fat 11 gm (Saturated Fat 3.5 gm, Polyunsat Fat 1.3 gm, Monounsat Fat 4.8 gm, Cholesterol 40 mg), Sodium 708 mg, Total Carbohydrate 46 gm, Dietary Fiber 9 gm, Sugars 21 gm, Protein 20 gm

Spicy Potato Soup

Sharon Kauffman • Harrisonburg, VA

Makes 8 servings (Ideal slow cooker size: 4-quart)

¾ lb. 90%-lean ground beef, browned

4 cups cubed, peeled potatoes

1 small onion, chopped

3 8-oz. cans no-salt-added tomato sauce

1 tsp. salt

1½ tsp. pepper

½–1 tsp. hot pepper sauce

water

1. Combine all ingredients except water in slow cooker. Add enough water to cover ingredients.

2. Cover. Cook on Low 8–10 hours, or High 5 hours, until potatoes are tender.

Exchange List Values: Starch 1.0, Vegetable 1.0, Meat, lean 1.0

Basic Nutritional Values: Calories 152 (Calories from Fat 32), Total Fat 4 gm (Saturated Fat 1.4 gm, Polyunsat Fat 0.2 gm, Monounsat Fat 1.5 gm, Cholesterol 26 mg), Sodium 346 mg, Total Carbohydrate 19 gm, Dietary Fiber 2 gm, Sugars 7 gm, Protein 10 gm

Sauerkraut Soup

Barbara Tenny • Delta, PA

Makes 10 servings (Ideal slow cooker size: 5-quart)

low-fat kielbasa, cut into 1/2" pieces

5 medium potatoes, cubed

2 large onions, chopped

2 large carrots, cut into 1/4" slices

4 tsp. sodium-free chicken bouillon powder

4 cups water

32-oz. can or bag sauerkraut, rinsed and drained

6-oz. can tomato paste

1. Combine all ingredients in large slow cooker. Stir to combine.

2. Cover. Cook on High 2 hours, and then on Low 6–8 hours.

3. Delicious served with rye bread.

Exchange List Values: Starch 1.0, Vegetable 3.0, Meat, lean 1.0

Basic Nutritional Values: Calories 188 (Calories from Fat 22), Total Fat 2 gm (Saturated Fat 0.8 gm, Polyunsat Fat 0.4 gm, Monounsat Fat 1.2 gm, Cholesterol 21 mg), Sodium 772 mg, Total Carbohydrate 33 gm, Dietary Fiber 6 gm, Sugars 9 gm, Protein 10 gm

Hearty Potato Sauerkraut Soup

Kathy Hertzler • Lancaster, PA

Makes 6–8 servings (Ideal slow cooker size: 4-quart)

4 tsp. sodium-free chicken bouillon powder

4 cups water

10 3/4-oz. can 98%-fat-free, reduced-sodium cream of mushroom soup

16-oz. can sauerkraut, rinsed and drained

8 ozs. fresh mushrooms, sliced

1 medium potato, cubed

2 medium carrots, peeled and sliced

2 ribs celery, chopped

8 ozs. low-fat Polish kielbasa (smoked), cubed

2 cups chopped cooked chicken

2 Tbsp. vinegar

2 tsp. dried dill weed

1 1/2 tsp. pepper

1. Mix together bouillon powder and water. Pour into slow cooker.

2. Combine remaining ingredients in large slow cooker.

3. Cover. Cook on Low 10–12 hours.

4. If necessary, skim fat before serving.

Exchange List Values: Carbohydrate 1.0, Vegetable 1.0, Meat, lean 1.0, Fat 0.5

Basic Nutritional Values: Calories 178 (Calories from Fat 44), Total Fat 5 gm (Saturated Fat 1.5 gm, Polyunsat Fat 1.0 gm, Monounsat Fat 1.8 gm, Cholesterol 45 mg), Sodium 664 mg, Total Carbohydrate 17 gm, Dietary Fiber 3 gm, Sugars 5 gm, Protein 16 gm

Kielbasa Soup

Bernice M. Gnidovec • Streator, IL

Makes 8 servings (Ideal slow cooker size: 6-quart)

16-oz. pkg. frozen mixed vegetables, or your choice of vegetables

6-oz. can tomato paste

1 medium onion, chopped

3 medium potatoes, diced

12 ozs. low-fat kielbasa, cut into ¼" pieces

4 qts. water

fresh parsley

1. Combine all ingredients except parsley in large slow cooker.

2. Cover. Cook on Low 12 hours.

3. Garnish individual servings with fresh parsley.

Exchange List Values: Starch 1.5, Vegetable 1.0, Meat, very lean 1.0

Basic Nutritional Values: Calories 167 (Calories from Fat 20), Total Fat 2 gm (Saturated Fat 0.7 gm, Polyunsat Fat 0.3 gm, Monounsat Fat 1.1 gm, Cholesterol 19 mg), Sodium 412 mg, Total Carbohydrate 29 gm, Dietary Fiber 4 gm, Sugars 6 gm, Protein 9 gm

Curried Carrot Soup

Ann Bender • Ft. Defiance, VA

Makes 6–8 servings (Ideal slow cooker size: 4-quart)

1 clove garlic, minced

1 large onion, chopped

2 Tbsp. oil

1 Tbsp. butter

1 tsp. curry powder

1 Tbsp. flour

4 cups 100%-fat-free, lower-sodium chicken broth

6 large carrots, sliced

¼ tsp. salt

¼ tsp. ground red pepper, optional

1½ cups plain yogurt, or light sour cream

1. In skillet cook minced garlic and onion in oil and butter until limp but not brown.

2. Add curry and flour. Cook 30 seconds. Pour into slow cooker.

3. Add chicken broth and carrots.

4. Cover. Cook on High for about 2 hours, or until carrots are soft.

5. Puree mixture in blender. Season with salt and pepper. Return to cooker and keep warm until ready to serve.

6. Add a dollop of yogurt or sour cream to each serving.

Exchange List Values: Vegetable 2.0, Fat 1.0

Basic Nutritional Values: Calories 113 (Calories from Fat 46), Total Fat 5 gm (Saturated Fat 1.2 gm, Polyunsat Fat 1.1 gm, Monounsat Fat 2.5 gm, Cholesterol 5 mg), Sodium 414 mg, Total Carbohydrate 13 gm, Dietary Fiber 2 gm, Sugars 7 gm, Protein 5 gm

Curried Pork and Pea Soup

Kathy Hertzler • Lancaster, PA

Makes 8 servings (Ideal slow cooker size: 4-quart)

1½-lb. boneless pork shoulder roast

1 cup yellow, or green, split peas, rinsed and drained

½ cup finely chopped carrots

½ cup finely chopped celery

½ cup finely chopped onions

49½-oz. can (approximately 6 cups) lower-sodium chicken broth

2 tsp. curry powder

½ tsp. paprika

¼ tsp. ground cumin

¼ tsp. pepper

2 cups torn fresh spinach

1. Trim fat from pork and cut pork into ½" pieces.

2. Combine split peas, carrots, celery, and onions in slow cooker.

3. Stir in broth, curry powder, paprika, cumin, and pepper. Stir in pork.

4. Cover. Cook on Low 10–12 hours, or on High 4 hours.

5. Stir in spinach. Serve immediately.

Exchange List Values: Starch 1.0, Meat, very lean 3.0, Fat 0.5

Basic Nutritional Values: Calories 206 (Calories from Fat 41), Total Fat 5 gm (Saturated Fat 1.5 gm, Polyunsat Fat 0.6 gm, Monounsat Fat 1.9 gm, Cholesterol 43 mg), Sodium 480 mg, Total Carbohydrate 16 gm, Dietary Fiber 6 gm, Sugars 3 gm, Protein 24 gm

Ruth's Split Pea Soup

Ruth Conrad Liechty • Goshen, IN

Makes 8 servings (Ideal slow cooker size: 4-quart)

1 bag (2¼ cups) dry split peas

½ lb. bulk sausage, browned and drained

6 cups water

2 medium potatoes, diced

1 onion, chopped

½ tsp. dried marjoram, or thyme

½ tsp. pepper

1. Wash and sort dried peas, removing any stones. Then combine all ingredients in slow cooker.

2. Cover. Cook on Low 12 hours.

Exchange List Values: Starch 2.5, Meat, medium fat 1.0

Basic Nutritional Values: Calories 257 (Calories from Fat 43), Total Fat 5 gm (Saturated Fat 1.5 gm, Polyunsat Fat 0.8 gm, Monounsat Fat 2.0 gm, Cholesterol 11 mg), Sodium 179 mg, Total Carbohydrate 39 gm, Dietary Fiber 13 gm, Sugars 6 gm, Protein 16 gm

Control the diabetes
so it doesn't control you.

Kelly's Split Pea Soup

Kelly Evenson • Pittsboro, NC

Makes 8 servings (Ideal slow cooker size: 4-quart)

2 cups dry split peas

2 quarts water

2 onions, chopped

2 carrots, peeled and sliced

4 slices Canadian bacon, chopped

2 Tbsp. sodium-free chicken bouillon powder

3/4 tsp. salt

1/4–1/2 tsp. pepper

1. Combine all ingredients in slow cooker.

2. Cover. Cook on Low 8–9 hours.

Exchange List Values: Starch 2.0, Meat, very lean 1.0

Basic Nutritional Values: Calories 195 (Calories from Fat 14), Total Fat 2 gm (Saturated Fat 0.4 gm, Polyunsat Fat 0.3 gm, Monounsat Fat 0.6 gm, Cholesterol 7 mg), Sodium 411 mg, Total Carbohydrate 32 gm, Dietary Fiber 11 gm, Sugars 7 gm, Protein 14 gm

VARIATION: For a creamier soup, remove half of soup when done and puree. Stir back into rest of soup.

Karen's Split Pea Soup

Karen Stoltzfus • Alto, MI

Makes 6 servings (Ideal slow cooker size: 4–5-quart)

2 carrots

2 ribs celery

1 onion

1 parsnip

1 leek (do not use top 3" of green)

1 ripe tomato

6 ozs. extra-lean lower-sodium ham, cubed

1 3/4 cups (1 lb.) dried split peas, washed, with stones removed

2 Tbsp. olive oil

1 bay leaf

1 tsp. dried thyme

4 cups chicken broth

4 cups water

1 tsp. salt

1/4 tsp. pepper

2 tsp. chopped fresh parsley

1. Cut all vegetables into 1/4" pieces and place in slow cooker. Add remaining ingredients except salt, pepper, and parsley.

2. Cover. Cook on High 7 hours.

3. Season soup with salt and pepper. Stir in parsley. Serve immediately.

Exchange List Values: Starch 2.0, Vegetable 2.0, Meat, lean 1.0

Basic Nutritional Values: Calories 275 (Calories from Fat 41), Total Fat 5 gm (Saturated Fat 0.7 gm, Polyunsat Fat 0.7 gm, Monounsat Fat 2.8 gm, Cholesterol 10 mg), Sodium 453 mg, Total Carbohydrate 41 gm, Dietary Fiber 14 gm, Sugars 7 gm, Protein 20 gm

Dorothy's Split Pea Soup

Dorothy M. Van Deest • Memphis, TN

Makes 8 servings (Ideal slow cooker size: 5-quart)

2 Tbsp. canola oil

1 cup minced onions

8 cups water

2 cups (1 lb.) green split peas, washed and stones removed

4 whole cloves

1 bay leaf

$\frac{1}{4}$ tsp. pepper

6 ozs. extra-lean, lower-sodium ham, cubed

1 cup finely minced celery

1 cup diced carrots

$\frac{1}{8}$ tsp. dried marjoram

$\frac{3}{4}$ tsp. salt

$\frac{1}{8}$ tsp. dried savory

1. Combine all ingredients in slow cooker.

2. Cover. Cook on Low 8–10 hours.

Exchange List Values: Starch 2.0, Vegetable 1.0, Meat, lean 1.0

Basic Nutritional Values: Calories 239 (Calories from Fat 40), Total Fat 4 gm (Saturated Fat 0.5 gm, Polyunsat Fat 1.4 gm, Monounsat Fat 2.3 gm, Cholesterol 10 mg), Sodium 419 mg, Total Carbohydrate 35 gm, Dietary Fiber 13 gm, Sugars 7 gm, Protein 16 gm

VARIATION: For a thick soup, uncover soup after 8-10 hours and turn heat to High. Simmer, stirring occasionally, until the desired consistency is reached.

Skipping meals only makes you hungrier and can cause you to overeat at the next meal.

Rosemarie's Pea Soup

Rosemarie Fitzgerald • Gibsonia, PA /
Shirley Sears • Tiskilwa, IL

Makes 6 servings (Ideal slow cooker size: 4-quart)

2 cups dried split peas

4 cups water

1 rib celery, chopped

1 cup chopped potatoes

1 large carrot, chopped

1 medium onion, chopped

$\frac{1}{4}$ tsp. dried thyme, or marjoram

1 bay leaf

$\frac{1}{2}$ tsp. salt

1 clove garlic

$\frac{1}{2}$ tsp. dried basil

1. Combine all ingredients in slow cooker.

2. Cover. Cook on Low 8–12 hours, or on High 6 hours, until peas are tender.

Exchange List Values: Starch 2.5, Vegetable 1.0

Basic Nutritional Values: Calories 230 (Calories from Fat 7), Total Fat 1 gm (Saturated Fat 0.1 gm, Polyunsat Fat 0.3 gm, Monounsat Fat 0.1 gm, Cholesterol 0 mg), Sodium 216 mg, Total Carbohydrate 43 gm, Dietary Fiber 15 gm, Sugars 7 gm, Protein 15 gm

VARIATION: For increased flavor, use chicken broth instead of water. Stir in curry powder, coriander, or red pepper flakes to taste.

French Market Soup

Ethel Mumaw • Berlin, OH

Makes about 2½ quarts total (Ideal slow cooker size: 4-quart)

2 cups dry bean mix, washed, with stones removed

2 quarts water

1 ham hock, all visible fat removed

1 tsp. salt

¼ tsp. pepper

16-oz. can tomatoes

1 large onion, chopped

1 clove garlic, minced

1 chili pepper, chopped, or 1 tsp. chili powder

¼ cup lemon juice

1. Combine all ingredients in slow cooker.

2. Cover. Cook on Low 8 hours. Turn to High and cook an additional 2 hours, or until beans are tender.

3. Debone ham, cut meat into bite-sized pieces, and stir back into soup.

Exchange List Values: Starch 1.5, Vegetable 1.0, Meat, lean 1.0

Basic Nutritional Values: Calories 191 (Calories from Fat 34), Total Fat 4 gm (Saturated Fat 1.3 gm, Polyunsat Fat 0.6 gm, Monounsat Fat 1.5 gm, Cholesterol 9 mg), Sodium 488 mg, Total Carbohydrate 29 gm, Dietary Fiber 7 gm, Sugars 5 gm, Protein 12 gm

Nine-Bean Soup with Tomatoes

Violette Harris Denney • Carrollton, GA

Makes 8 servings (Ideal slow cooker size: 5-quart)

2 cups dry nine-bean soup mix

12 ozs. extra-lean, lower-sodium ham, diced

1 large onion, chopped

1 clove garlic, minced

2 qts. water

16-oz. can no-salt-added tomatoes, undrained and chopped

10-oz. can tomatoes with green chilies, undrained

1. Sort and wash bean mix. Place in slow cooker. Cover with water to 2" above beans. Let soak overnight. Drain.

2. Add ham, onion, garlic, and 2 quarts fresh water.

3. Cover. Cook on Low 7 hours.

4. Add remaining ingredients and continue cooking on Low another hour. Stir occasionally.

Exchange List Values: Starch 2.0, Vegetable 1.0, Meat, very lean 1.0

Basic Nutritional Values: Calories 231 (Calories from Fat 14), Total Fat 2 gm (Saturated Fat 0.4 gm, Polyunsat Fat 0.5 gm, Monounsat Fat 0.4 gm, Cholesterol 20 mg), Sodium 518 mg, Total Carbohydrate 37 gm, Dietary Fiber 9 gm, Sugars 9 gm, Protein 19 gm

Note: Nine-Bean Soup mix is a mix of barley pearls, black beans, red beans, pinto beans, navy beans, Great Northern beans, lentils, split peas, and black-eyed peas.

Lentil Soup with Ham Bone

Rhoda Atzeff • Harrisburg, PA

Makes 6-8 servings (Ideal slow cooker size: 5-quart)

1 lb. lentils, washed and drained

1 rib celery, chopped

1 large carrot, grated

½ cup chopped onions

1 bay leaf

¼ tsp. dried thyme

7-8 cups water

1 ham bone, skin and visible fat removed

¼–½ tsp. crushed red hot pepper flakes

pepper to taste

salt to taste

1. Combine all ingredients except pepper and salt in slow cooker.

2. Cover. Cook on Low 8–9 hours. Remove bay leaf and ham bone. Dice meat from bone and return to cooker.

3. Season to taste with pepper and salt.

4. Serve alone, or over rice with grated cheese on top.

Exchange List Values: Starch 2.0, Meat, lean 1.0

Basic Nutritional Values: Calories 220 (Calories from Fat 17), Total Fat 2 gm (Saturated Fat 0.5 gm, Polyunsat Fat 0.4 gm, Monounsat Fat 0.6 gm, Cholesterol 12 mg), Sodium 298 mg, Total Carbohydrate 33 gm, Dietary Fiber 13 gm, Sugars 4 gm, Protein 19 gm

Calico Ham and Bean Soup

Esther Martin • Ephrata, PA

Makes 8 servings (Ideal slow cooker size: 5-6-quart)

1 lb. dry bean mix, rinsed and drained, with stones removed

6 cups water

2 cups extra-lean, lower-sodium, cubed, cooked ham

1 cup chopped onions

1 cup chopped carrots

1 tsp. dried basil

1 tsp. dried oregano

¾ tsp. salt

¼ tsp. pepper

2 bay leaves

6 cups water

1 tsp. liquid smoke, optional

1. Combine beans and 6 cups water in large saucepan. Bring to boil, reduce heat, and simmer uncovered for 10 minutes. Drain, discarding cooking water, and rinse beans.

2. Combine all ingredients in slow cooker.

3. Cover. Cook on Low 8–10 hours, or High 4–5 hours. Discard bay leaves before serving.

Exchange List Values: Starch 2.0, Vegetable 1.0, Meat, very lean 1.0

Basic Nutritional Values: Calories 228 (Calories from Fat 12), Total Fat 1 gm (Saturated Fat 0.4 gm, Polyunsat Fat 0.5 gm, Monounsat Fat 0.3 gm, Cholesterol 13 mg), Sodium 462 mg, Total Carbohydrate 38 gm, Dietary Fiber 10 gm, Sugars 6 gm, Protein 17 gm

Bean and Herb Soup

LaVerne A. Olson • Willow Street, PA

Makes 6 servings (Ideal slow cooker size: 5–6-quart)

1½ cups dry mixed beans

5 cups water

6 ozs. extra-lean, lower-sodium ham

1 cup chopped onions

1 cup chopped celery

1 cup chopped carrots

2–3 cups water

½ tsp. salt

¼–½ tsp. pepper

1–2 tsp. fresh basil, or ½ tsp. dried basil

1–2 tsp. fresh oregano, or ½ tsp. dried oregano

1–2 tsp. fresh thyme, or ½ tsp. dried thyme

2 cups fresh tomatoes, crushed

1. Combine beans, water, and ham in saucepan. Bring to boil. Turn off heat and let stand 1 hour.

2. Combine onions, celery, and carrots in 2–3 cups water in another saucepan. Cook until soft. Mash slightly.

3. Combine all ingredients in slow cooker.

4. Cover. Cook on High 2 hours, and then on Low 2 hours.

Exchange List Values: Starch 2.0, Vegetable 1.0, Meat, very lean 1.0

Basic Nutritional Values: Calories 222 (Calories from Fat 13), Total Fat 1 gm (Saturated Fat 0.3 gm, Polyunsat Fat 0.5 gm, Monounsat Fat 0.3 gm, Cholesterol 13 mg), Sodium 465 mg, Total Carbohydrate 38 gm, Dietary Fiber 10 gm, Sugars 8 gm, Protein 16 gm

If you plan to drink alcohol, be sure you will be eating, too.

Northern Bean Soup

Patricia Howard • Albuquerque, NM

Makes 6–8 servings (Ideal slow cooker size: 4-quart)

1 lb. dry Great Northern beans

1 lb. extra-lean, lower-sodium ham

2 medium onions, chopped

half a green pepper, chopped

1 cup chopped celery

16-oz. can diced tomatoes

4 carrots, peeled and chopped

4-oz. can green chili peppers

1 tsp. garlic powder

1–2 qts. water

1. Wash beans. Cover with water and soak overnight. Drain. Pour into slow cooker.

2. Dice ham into 1" pieces. Add to beans.

3. Stir in remaining ingredients.

4. Cover. Cook on High 2 hours, then on Low 10–12 hours, or until beans are tender.

Exchange List Values: Starch 2.0, Vegetable 2.0, Meat, very lean 2.0

Basic Nutritional Values: Calories 272 (Calories from Fat 17), Total Fat 2 gm (Saturated Fat 0.6 gm, Polyunsat Fat 0.6 gm, Monounsat Fat 0.4 gm, Cholesterol 26 mg), Sodium 674 mg, Total Carbohydrate 42 gm, Dietary Fiber 13 gm, Sugars 11 gm, Protein 23 gm

Easy Lima Bean Soup

Barbara Tenney • Delta, PA

Makes 8–10 servings (Ideal slow cooker size: 5–6-quart)

1-lb. bag large dry lima beans

1 large onion, chopped

6 ribs celery, chopped

3 large potatoes, cut in $\frac{1}{2}$" cubes

2 large carrots, cut in $\frac{1}{4}$" rounds

2 cups extra-lean, lower-sodium ham

1 tsp. salt

1 tsp. pepper

2 bay leaves

3 quarts water, or combination water and beef broth

1. Sort beans. Soak overnight. Drain.

2. Combine all ingredients in slow cooker.

3. Cover. Cook on Low 8–10 hours.

Exchange List Values: Starch 2.5, Vegetable 1.0, Meat, very lean 1.0

Basic Nutritional Values: Calories 258 (Calories from Fat 12), Total Fat 1 gm (Saturated Fat 0.4 gm, Polyunsat Fat 0.5 gm, Monounsat Fat 0.4 gm, Cholesterol 21 mg), Sodium 648 mg, Total Carbohydrate 43 gm, Dietary Fiber 11 gm, Sugars 9 gm, Protein 19 gm

VARIATION: For extra flavor, add 1 tsp. dried oregano before cooking.

Navy Bean and Bacon Chowder

Ruth A. Feister • Narvon, PA

Makes 6 servings (Ideal slow cooker size: 4-quart)

$1\frac{1}{2}$ cups dried navy beans

2 cups cold water

5 slices bacon, cooked and crumbled

2 medium carrots, sliced

1 rib celery, sliced

1 medium onion, chopped

1 tsp. dried Italian seasoning

$\frac{1}{8}$ tsp. pepper

46-oz. can 100%-fat-free, 30–50%-less-sodium chicken broth

1 cup milk

1. Soak beans in water for 8 hours.

2. After beans have soaked, drain, if necessary, and place in slow cooker.

3. Add all remaining ingredients, except milk, to slow cooker.

4. Cover. Cook on Low 7–9 hours, or until beans are crisp-tender.

5. Place 2 cups cooked bean mixture into blender. Process until smooth. Return to slow cooker.

6. Add milk. Cover and heat on High 10 minutes.

7. Serve with crusty French bread and additional herbs and seasonings for diners to add as they wish.

Exchange List Values: Starch 2.5, Vegetable 1.0, Meat, very lean 1.0, Fat 0.5

Basic Nutritional Values: Calories 263 (Calories from Fat 37), Total Fat 4 gm (Saturated Fat 1.4 gm, Polyunsat Fat 0.6 gm, Monounsat Fat 1.6 gm, Cholesterol 7 mg), Sodium 623 mg, Total Carbohydrate 41 gm, Dietary Fiber 9 gm, Sugars 8 gm, Protein 17 gm

Slow-Cooked Navy Beans with Ham

Julia Lapp • New Holland, PA

Makes 10 servings (Ideal slow cooker size: 4-quart)

1 lb. dry navy beans (2½ cups)

5 cups water

1 clove garlic, minced

1 ham hock, skin and all visible fat removed

1 tsp. salt

1. Soak beans in water at least 4 hours in slow cooker.

2. Add garlic and ham hock.

3. Cover. Cook on Low 7–8 hours, or High 4 hours. Add salt during last hour of cooking time.

4. Remove ham hock from cooker. Allow to cool. Cut ham from hock and stir back into bean mixture. Correct seasonings and serve in soup bowls with hot corn bread.

Exchange List Values: Starch 2.0, Meat, very lean 1.0, Fat 0.5

Basic Nutritional Values: Calories 199 (Calories from Fat 34), Total Fat 4 gm (Saturated Fat 1.3 gm, Polyunsat Fat 0.6 gm, Monounsat Fat 1.4 gm, Cholesterol 9 mg), Sodium 418 mg, Total Carbohydrate 30 gm, Dietary Fiber 7 gm, Sugars 3 gm, Protein 12 gm

VARIATION: For added flavor, stir 1 chopped onion, 2-3 chopped celery stalks, 2-3 sliced carrots, and 3-4 cups canned tomatoes into cooker with garlic and ham hock.

Navy Bean Soup

Joyce Bowman • Lady Lake, FL

Makes 8 servings (Ideal slow cooker size: 4-quart)

1 lb. dry navy beans

8 cups water

1 onion, finely chopped

2 bay leaves

½ tsp. ground thyme

½ tsp. nutmeg

½ tsp. salt

½ tsp. lemon pepper

3 cloves garlic, minced

1 lb. extra-lean, lower-sodium ham pieces

1. Soak beans in water overnight. Strain out stones but reserve liquid.

2. Combine all ingredients in slow cooker.

3. Cover. Cook on Low 8–10 hours. Debone meat and cut into bite-sized pieces. Set ham aside.

4. Puree three-fourths of soup in blender in small batches. When finished blending, stir in meat.

Exchange List Values: Starch 2.5, Meat, very lean 2.0

Basic Nutritional Values: Calories 264 (Calories from Fat 17), Total Fat 2 gm (Saturated Fat 0.6 gm, Polyunsat Fat 0.5 gm, Monounsat Fat 0.5 gm, Cholesterol 26 mg), Sodium 631 mg, Total Carbohydrate 40 gm, Dietary Fiber 9 gm, Sugars 7 gm, Protein 22 gm

VARIATION: Add small chunks of cooked potatoes when stirring in ham pieces after blending.

Old-Fashioned Bean Soup

Gladys M. High • Ephrata, PA

Makes 7 servings (Ideal slow cooker size: 4-quart)

1 lb. dry navy beans, or dry green split peas

1 lb. extra-lean, lower-sodium ham pieces

1/8 tsp. salt

1/4 tsp. ground pepper

1/2 cup chopped celery leaves

2 qts. water

1 medium onion, chopped

1 bay leaf, optional

1. Soak beans or peas overnight. Drain, discarding soaking water.

2. Combine all ingredients in slow cooker.

3. Cover. Cook on High 8–9 hours.

Exchange List Values: Starch 3.0, Meat, very lean 2.0

Basic Nutritional Values: Calories 300 (Calories from Fat 19), Total Fat 2 gm (Saturated Fat 0.7 gm, Polyunsat Fat 0.6 gm, Monounsat Fat 0.5 gm, Cholesterol 30 mg), Sodium 576 mg, Total Carbohydrate 46 gm, Dietary Fiber 11 gm, Sugars 7 gm, Protein 25 gm

Don't be afraid to use insulin if the doctor says you need it.

Black Bean Chili con Carne

Janie Steele • Moore, OK

Makes 18 1-cup servings (Ideal slow cooker size: 2 cookers, each 4–5-quarts)

1 lb. dried black beans

3 lbs. ground beef

2 large onions, chopped

1 green pepper, chopped

3 cloves garlic, minced

2 tsp. salt

1 tsp. pepper

6-oz. can tomato paste

3 cups tomato juice, or more

1 tsp. celery salt

1 Tbsp. Worcestershire sauce

1 tsp. dry mustard

cayenne pepper to taste

cumin to taste

3 Tbsp. chili powder

1. Cover beans with water and soak 8 hours or overnight. Rinse and drain.

2. Brown ground beef in batches in large skillet. Drain.

3. Combine all ingredients and then divide between 2 cookers.

4. Cover. Cook on Low 8 hours.

5. Serve over salad greens or wrapped in tortillas, topped with lettuce and grated cheese.

Exchange List Values: Starch 1.0, Vegetable 1.0, Meat, lean 2.0, Fat 0.5

Basic Nutritional Values: Calories 237 (Calories from Fat 76), Total Fat 8 gm (Saturated Fat 3.1 gm, Polyunsat Fat 0.5 gm, Monounsat Fat 3.4 gm, Cholesterol 45 mg), Sodium 510 mg, Total Carbohydrate 21 gm, Dietary Fiber 7 gm, Sugars 5 gm, Protein 20 gm

Caribbean-Style Black Bean Soup

Sheryl Shenk • Harrisonburg, VA

Makes 8–10 servings (Ideal slow cooker size: 4-quart)

1 lb. dried black beans, washed and stones removed

4 qts. water

3 medium onions, chopped

1 medium green pepper, chopped

4 cloves garlic, minced

¾ cup cubed ham

1 Tbsp. canola oil

1 Tbsp. ground cumin

2 tsp. dried oregano

1 tsp. dried thyme

2 tsp. salt

½ tsp. pepper

3 cups water

2 Tbsp. vinegar

fresh chopped cilantro

1. Soak beans overnight in 4 quarts water. Drain.

2. Combine beans, onions, green pepper, garlic, ham, oil, cumin, oregano, thyme, salt, pepper, and 3 cups fresh water. Stir well.

3. Cover. Cook on Low 8–10 hours, or on High 4–5 hours.

4. For a thick soup, remove half of cooked bean mixture and puree until smooth in blender or mash with potato masher. Return to cooker. If you like a soupier soup, leave as is.

5. Add vinegar and stir well.

6. Serve in soup bowls topped with fresh cilantro.

Exchange List Values: Starch 1.5, Vegetable 1.0, Meat, very lean 1.0

Basic Nutritional Values: Calories 188 (Calories from Fat 24), Total Fat 3 gm (Saturated Fat 0.4 gm, Polyunsat Fat 0.8 gm, Monounsat Fat 1.2 gm, Cholesterol 5 mg), Sodium 582 mg, Total Carbohydrate 30 gm, Dietary Fiber 10 gm, Sugars 6 gm, Protein 12 gm

A registered dietitian can help you create the right meal plan for you, and your health insurance company may even cover the sessions!

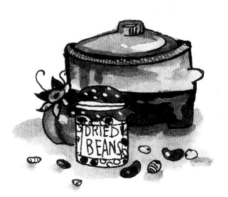

Katelyn's Black Bean Soup

Katelyn Bailey • Mechanicsburg, PA

Makes 4–6 servings (Ideal slow cooker size: 4-quart)

1/3 cup chopped onions

1 clove garlic, minced

1–2 Tbsp. oil

2 15½-oz. cans black beans, undrained

1 cup water

1 tsp. sodium-free chicken bouillon powder

1/2 cup diced, cooked smoked ham

1/2 cup diced carrots

1 dash, or more, cayenne pepper

1–2 drops, or more, Tabasco sauce

sour cream

1. Saute onion and garlic in oil in saucepan.

2. Puree or mash contents of one can of black beans. Add to sauteed ingredients.

3. Combine all ingredients except sour cream in slow cooker.

4. Cover. Cook on Low 6–8 hours.

5. Add dollop of sour cream to each individual bowl before serving.

Exchange List Values: Starch 1.5, Meat, very lean 1.0

Basic Nutritional Values: Calories 161 (Calories from Fat 29), Total Fat 3 gm (Saturated Fat 0.4 gm, Polyunsat Fat 0.9 gm, Monounsat Fat 1.6 gm, Cholesterol 5 mg), Sodium 540 mg, Total Carbohydrate 22 gm, Dietary Fiber 6 gm, Sugars 3 gm, Protein 11 gm

Vegetable Bean Soup

Kathi Rogge • Alexandria, IN

Makes 8 servings (Ideal slow cooker size: 4-quart)

6 cups cooked beans: navy, pinto, Great Northern

1 meaty ham bone (about 6 ozs. ham), visible fat and skin removed

1 cup cooked ham, diced

1/4 tsp. garlic powder

1 small bay leaf

1 cup cubed potatoes

1 cup chopped onions

1 cup chopped celery

1 cup chopped carrots

water

1. Combine all ingredients except water in 4-quart slow cooker. Add water to about 1" from top.

2. Cover. Cook on Low 5–8 hours.

3. Remove bay leaf before serving.

Exchange List Values: Starch 2.0, Vegetable 1.0, Meat, very lean 2.0

Basic Nutritional Values: Calories 261 (Calories from Fat 25), Total Fat 3 gm (Saturated Fat 0.8 gm, Polyunsat Fat 0.6 gm, Monounsat Fat 1.0 gm, Cholesterol 20 mg), Sodium 499 mg, Total Carbohydrate 39 gm, Dietary Fiber 11 gm, Sugars 5 gm, Protein 21 gm

Slow Cooker Black Bean Chili

Mary Seielstad • Sparks, NV

Makes 8 servings (Ideal slow cooker size: 4-quart)

1-lb. pork tenderloin, cut into 1" chunks

16-oz. jar thick chunky salsa

3 15-oz. cans black beans, rinsed and drained

1/2 cup chicken broth

1 medium red bell pepper, chopped

1 medium onion, chopped

1 tsp. ground cumin

2 tsp. chili powder

1-1/2 tsp. dried oregano

1/4 cup sour cream

1. Combine all ingredients except sour cream in slow cooker.

2. Cover. Cook on Low 6–8 hours, or until pork is tender.

3. Garnish individual servings with sour cream.

Exchange List Values: Starch 1.5, Vegetable 1.0, Meat, very lean 2.0, Fat 0.5

Basic Nutritional Values: Calories 231 (Calories from Fat 38), Total Fat 4 gm (Saturated Fat 1.6 gm, Polyunsat Fat 0.6 gm, Monounsat Fat 1.4 gm, Cholesterol 36 mg), Sodium 389 mg, Total Carbohydrate 28 gm, Dietary Fiber 9 gm, Sugars 6 gm, Protein 21 gm

Ask your doctor if you should take an aspirin every day—it may prevent a heart attack.

Mjeddrah or Esau's Lentil Soup

Dianna Milhizer • Springfield, VA

Makes 12 servings (Ideal slow cooker size: 4-quart)

1 cup chopped carrots

1 cup diced celery

2 cups chopped onions

1 Tbsp. olive oil, or butter

2 cups brown rice

1 Tbsp. olive oil, or butter

6 cups water

1 lb. lentils, washed and drained

garden salad

vinaigrette

1. Saute carrots, celery, and onions in 1 Tbsp. oil in skillet. When soft and translucent, place in slow cooker.

2. Brown rice in 1 Tbsp. oil until dry. Add to slow cooker.

3. Stir in water and lentils.

4. Cover. Cook on High 6–8 hours.

5. When thoroughly cooked, serve in individual soup bowls. Cover each with a serving of fresh garden salad (lettuce, spinach leaves, chopped tomatoes, minced onions, chopped bell peppers, sliced olives, sliced radishes). Pour favorite vinaigrette over all.

Exchange List Values: Starch 3.0, Meat, very lean 1.0

Basic Nutritional Values: Calories 269 (Calories from Fat 33), Total Fat 4 gm (Saturated Fat 0.5 gm, Polyunsat Fat 0.7 gm, Monounsat Fat 2.1 gm, Cholesterol 0 mg), Sodium 21 mg, Total Carbohydrate 48 gm, Dietary Fiber 10 gm, Sugars 4 gm, Protein 12 gm

French Onion Soup

Jenny R. Unternahrer • Wayland, IA /
Janice Yoskovich • Carmichaels, PA

Makes 10 servings (Ideal slow cooker size: 4-quart)

8-10 large onions, sliced

1/2 cup light, soft tub margarine

3 14-oz. cans 98%-fat-free, lower-sodium beef broth

2 1/2 cups water

3 tsp. sodium-free chicken bouillon powder

1 1/2 tsp. Worcestershire sauce

3 bay leaves

10 1-oz. slices French bread, toasted

1. Saute onions in margarine until crisp-tender. Transfer to slow cooker.

2. Add beef broth, water, and bouillon powder. Mix well. Add Worcestershire sauce and bay leaves.

3. Cover. Cook on Low 5–7 hours, or until onions are tender. Discard bay leaves.

4. Ladle into bowls. Top each with a slice of bread.

Exchange List Values: Starch 1.0, Vegetable 3.0, Fat 0.5

Basic Nutritional Values: Calories 178 (Calories from Fat 35), Total Fat 4 gm (Saturated Fat 0.3 gm, Polyunsat Fat 0.9 gm, Monounsat Fat 2.0 gm, Cholesterol 0 mg), Sodium 476 mg, Total Carbohydrate 31 gm, Dietary Fiber 4 gm, Sugars 12 gm, Protein 6 gm

Note: For a more intense beef flavor, add one beef bouillon cube, or use home-cooked beef broth instead of canned broth.

Potato Soup

Jeanne Hertzog • Bethlehem, PA /
Marcia S. Myer • Manheim, PA /
Rhonda Lee Schmidt • Scranton, PA / Mitzi
McGlynchey • Downingtown, PA /
Vera Schmucker • Goshen, IN / Kaye Schnell •
Falmouth, MA / Elizabeth Yoder • Millersburg, OH

Makes 10 servings (Ideal slow cooker size: 4-quart)

6 potatoes, peeled and cubed

2 leeks, chopped

2 onions, chopped

1 rib celery, sliced

4 chicken bouillon cubes

1 Tbsp. dried parsley flakes

5 cups water

pepper to taste

3 Tbsp. light, soft tub margarine

12-oz. can fat-free evaporated milk

chopped chives

1. Combine all ingredients except milk and chives in slow cooker.

2. Cover. Cook on Low 10–12 hours, or High 3–4 hours. Stir in milk during last hour.

3. If desired, mash potatoes before serving.

4. Garnish with chives.

Exchange List Values: Carbohydrate 1.5

Basic Nutritional Values: Calories 123 (Calories from Fat 14), Total Fat 2 gm (Saturated Fat 0.1 gm, Polyunsat Fat 0.4 gm, Monounsat Fat 0.8 gm, Cholesterol 0 mg), Sodium 447 mg, Total Carbohydrate 23 gm, Dietary Fiber 2 gm, Sugars 7 gm, Protein 5 gm

VARIATIONS:

1. Add one carrot, sliced, to vegetables before cooking.

2. Instead of water and bouillon cubes, use 4–5 cups chicken stock.

No-Fuss Potato Soup

Lucille Amos • Greensboro, NC /
Lavina Hochstedler • Grand Blanc, MI /
Betty Moore • Plano, IL

Makes 8–10 servings (Ideal slow cooker size: 5–6-quart)

6 cups diced, peeled potatoes

5 cups water

2 cups diced onions

1/2 cup diced celery

1/2 cup chopped carrots

1/4 cup light, soft tub margarine

4 tsp. sodium-free chicken bouillon powder

1 tsp. salt

1/4 tsp. pepper

12-oz. can fat-free evaporated milk

3 Tbsp. chopped fresh parsley

8 ozs. fat-free cheddar, shredded

1. Combine all ingredients except milk, parsley, and cheese in slow cooker.

2. Cover. Cook on High 7–8 hours, or until vegetables are tender.

3. Stir in milk and parsley. Stir in cheese until it melts. Heat thoroughly.

Exchange List Values: Starch 1.5, Vegetable 1.0, Meat, very lean 1.0

Basic Nutritional Values: Calories 173 (Calories from Fat 19), Total Fat 2 gm (Saturated Fat 0.2 gm, Polyunsat Fat 0.5 gm, Monounsat Fat 1.0 gm, Cholesterol 2 mg), Sodium 493 mg, Total Carbohydrate 27 gm, Dietary Fiber 2 gm, Sugars 8 gm, Protein 12 gm

VARIATIONS:

1. For added flavor, stir in 3 slices bacon, browned until crisp, and crumbled.

2. Top individual servings with chopped chives.

Baked Potato Soup

Kristina Shuil • Timberville, VA

Makes 6–8 servings (Ideal slow cooker size: 4-quart)

4 large baked potatoes

3 Tbsp. light, soft tub margarine

2/3 cup flour

3 cups fat-free milk

3 cups fat-free half-and-half

1/4 tsp. salt

1/2 tsp. pepper

4 green onions, chopped

4 slices bacon, fried, patted dry, and crumbled

1 1/2 cups shredded fat-free cheddar cheese

3/4 cup fat-free sour cream

1. Cut potatoes in half. Scoop out pulp and put in small bowl.

2. Melt margarine in large kettle. Add flour. Gradually stir in milk and half-and-half. Continue to stir until smooth, thickened, and bubbly.

3. Stir in potato pulp, salt, pepper, and three-quarters of the onions, bacon, and cheese. Cook until heated. Stir in sour cream.

4. Transfer to slow cooker set on Low. Top with remaining onions, bacon, and cheese. Take to a potluck, or serve on a buffet table, straight from the cooker.

Exchange List Values: Carbohydrate 3.0, Meat, very lean 1.0, Fat 1.0

Basic Nutritional Values: Calories 307 (Calories from Fat 57), Total Fat 6 gm (Saturated Fat 1.5 gm, Polyunsat Fat 1.0 gm, Monounsat Fat 2.6 gm, Cholesterol 14 mg), Sodium 541 mg, Total Carbohydrate 45 gm, Dietary Fiber 2 gm, Sugars 14 gm, Protein 17 gm

VARIATION: Add several slices of Velveeta cheese to make soup extra cheesy and creamy.

German Potato Soup

Lee Ann Hazlett • Freeport, IL

Makes 8 servings (Ideal slow cooker size: 4-quart)

1 onion, chopped

1 leek, trimmed and diced

2 carrots, diced

1 cup chopped cabbage

¼ cup chopped fresh parsley

4 cups 99%-fat-free, lower-sodium beef broth

1 lb. potatoes, diced

1 bay leaf

1–2 tsp. black pepper

1 tsp. salt, optional

½ tsp. caraway seeds, optional

¼ tsp. nutmeg

½ cup fat-free sour cream

½ lb. bacon, cooked and crumbled

1. Combine all ingredients except sour cream and bacon.

2. Cover. Cook on Low 8–10 hours, or High 4–5 hours.

3. Remove bay leaf. Use a slotted spoon to remove potatoes. Mash potatoes and mix with sour cream. Return to slow cooker. Stir in. Add bacon and mix together thoroughly.

Exchange List Values: Starch 1.0, Vegetable 1.0, Fat 0.5

Basic Nutritional Values: Calories 130 (Calories from Fat 37), Total Fat 4 gm (Saturated Fat 1.3 gm, Polyunsat Fat 0.5 gm, Monounsat Fat 1.9 gm, Cholesterol 8 mg), Sodium 384 mg, Total Carbohydrate 17 gm, Dietary Fiber 2 gm, Sugars 4 gm, Protein 6 gm

Veggie Chili

Wanda Roth • Napoleon, OH

Makes 6 servings (Ideal slow cooker size: 4-quart)

2 qts. no-salt-added whole or diced tomatoes, undrained

6-oz. can tomato paste

½ cup chopped onions

½ cup chopped celery

½ cup chopped green peppers

2 cloves garlic, minced

½ tsp. salt

1½ tsp. ground cumin

1 tsp. dried oregano

¼ tsp. cayenne pepper

3 Tbsp. brown sugar

15-oz. can garbanzo beans

1. Combine all ingredients except beans in slow cooker.

2. Cook on Low 6–8 hours, or High 3–4 hours. Add beans 1 hour before serving.

Exchange List Values: Starch 1.0, Carbohydrate 0.5, Vegetable 4.0

Basic Nutritional Values: Calories 214 (Calories from Fat 16), Total Fat 2 gm (Saturated Fat 0.1 gm, Polyunsat Fat 0.8 gm, Monounsat Fat 0.4 gm, Cholesterol 0 mg), Sodium 571 mg, Total Carbohydrate 47 gm, Dietary Fiber 11 gm, Sugars 22 gm, Protein 8 gm

VARIATION: If you prefer a less-tomatoey taste, substitute 2 vegetable bouillon cubes and 1 cup water for tomato paste.

Black-Eye and Vegetable Chili

Julie Weaver • Reinholds, PA

Makes 4–6 servings (Ideal slow cooker size: 4-quart)

1 cup finely chopped onions

1 cup finely chopped carrots

1 cup finely chopped red or green pepper, or mixture of two

1 clove garlic, minced

4 tsp. chili powder

1 tsp. ground cumin

2 Tbsp. chopped cilantro

14½-oz. can diced tomatoes

3 cups cooked black-eyed beans, or 2 15-oz. cans black-eyed beans, drained

4-oz. can chopped green chilies

¾ cup orange juice

¾ cup water, or broth

1 Tbsp. cornstarch

2 Tbsp. water

½ cup shredded cheddar cheese

2 Tbsp. chopped cilantro

1. Combine all ingredients except cornstarch, 2 Tbsp. water, cheese, and cilantro.

2. Cover. Cook on Low 6–8 hours, or High 4 hours.

3. Dissolve cornstarch in water. Stir into soup mixture 30 minutes before serving.

4. Garnish individual servings with cheese and cilantro.

Exchange List Values: Starch 1.5, Vegetable 2.0, Fat 0.5

Basic Nutritional Values: Calories 205 (Calories from Fat 38), Total Fat 4 gm (Saturated Fat 2.1 gm, Polyunsat Fat 0.6 gm, Monounsat Fat 1.1 gm, Cholesterol 10 mg), Sodium 317 mg, Total Carbohydrate 33 gm, Dietary Fiber 9 gm, Sugars 12 gm, Protein 11 gm

Note: Black-eyed beans are also known as black-eyed peas or crowder peas.

Walking keeps you younger in mind and body.

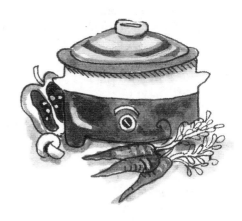

Vegetarian Chili

Connie Johnson • Loudon, NH

Makes 6 servings (Ideal slow cooker size: 4-quart)

3 cloves garlic, minced

2 onions, chopped

1 cup textured vegetable protein (T.V.P.)

1-lb. can beans of your choice, drained

1 green bell pepper, chopped

1 jalapeno pepper, seeds removed, chopped

28-oz. can diced Italian tomatoes

1 bay leaf

1 Tbsp. dried oregano

$\frac{1}{2}$ tsp. salt

$\frac{1}{4}$ tsp. pepper

1. Combine all ingredients in slow cooker.

2. Cover. Cook on Low 6–8 hours.

Exchange List Values: Starch 1.0, Vegetable 2.0, Meat, very lean 1.0

Basic Nutritional Values: Calories 157 (Calories from Fat 6), Total Fat 1 gm (Saturated Fat 0.1 gm, Polyunsat Fat 0.3 gm, Monounsat Fat 0.1 gm, Cholesterol 0 mg), Sodium 518 mg, Total Carbohydrate 28 gm, Dietary Fiber 9 gm, Sugars 11 gm, Protein 14 gm

Hearty Black Bean Soup

Della Yoder • Kalona, IA

Makes 6–8 servings (Ideal slow cooker size: 4-quart)

3 medium carrots, halved and thinly sliced

2 ribs celery, thinly sliced

1 medium onion, chopped

4 cloves garlic, minced

20-oz. can black beans, drained and rinsed

2 14$\frac{1}{2}$-oz. cans 98%-fat-free, lower-sodium chicken broth

15-oz. can crushed tomatoes

1$\frac{1}{2}$ tsp. dried basil

$\frac{1}{2}$ tsp. dried oregano

$\frac{1}{2}$ tsp. ground cumin

$\frac{1}{2}$ tsp. chili powder

$\frac{1}{2}$ tsp. hot pepper sauce

1. Combine all ingredients in slow cooker.

2. Cover. Cook on Low 9–10 hours.

Exchange List Values: Starch 0.5, Vegetable 2.0

Basic Nutritional Values: Calories 104 (Calories from Fat 4), Total Fat 0 gm (Saturated Fat 0.1 gm, Polyunsat Fat 0.2 gm, Monounsat Fat 0.1 gm, Cholesterol 0 mg), Sodium 481 mg, Total Carbohydrate 19 gm, Dietary Fiber 6 gm, Sugars 7 gm, Protein 6 gm

VARIATION: If you prefer a thicker soup, use only 1 can chicken broth.

Note: May be served over cooked rice.

Black Bean and Corn Soup

Joy Sutter • Iowa City, IA

Makes 6–8 servings (Ideal slow cooker size: 4-quart)

2 15-oz. cans black beans, drained and rinsed

14½-oz. can Mexican stewed tomatoes, undrained

14½-oz. can diced tomatoes, undrained

11-oz. can whole-kernel corn, drained

4 green onions, sliced

2 Tbsp. chili powder

1 tsp. ground cumin

½ tsp. dried minced garlic

1. Combine all ingredients in slow cooker.

2. Cover. Cook on High 5–6 hours.

Exchange List Values: Starch 1.5, Vegetable 1.0

Basic Nutritional Values: Calories 134 (Calories from Fat 10), Total Fat 1 gm (Saturated Fat 0.1 gm, Polyunsat Fat 0.5 gm, Monounsat Fat 0.2 gm, Cholesterol 0 mg), Sodium 366 mg, Total Carbohydrate 26 gm, Dietary Fiber 8 gm, Sugars 7 gm, Protein 7 gm

VARIATIONS:

1. Use 2 cloves fresh garlic, minced, instead of dried garlic.
2. Add 1 large rib celery, sliced thinly, and 1 small green pepper, chopped.

Tuscan Garlicky Bean Soup

Sara Harter Fredette • Williamsburg, MA

Makes 8–10 servings (Ideal slow cooker size: 4-quart)

1 lb. dry Great Northern, or other dry white, beans

1 qt. water

1 qt. 99%-fat-free, lower-sodium beef broth

2 cloves garlic, minced

4 Tbsp. chopped parsley

3 Tbsp. olive oil

1¼ tsp. salt

½ tsp. pepper

1. Place beans in large soup pot. Cover with water and bring to boil. Cook 2 minutes. Remove from heat. Cover pot and allow to stand for 1 hour. Drain, discarding water.

2. Combine beans, 1 quart fresh water, and beef broth in slow cooker.

3. Saute garlic and parsley in olive oil in skillet. Stir into slow cooker. Add salt and pepper.

4. Cover. Cook on Low 8–10 hours, or until beans are tender.

Exchange List Values: Starch 1.5, Meat, very lean 1.0, Fat 0.5

Basic Nutritional Values: Calories 174 (Calories from Fat 41), Total Fat 5 gm (Saturated Fat 0.7 gm, Polyunsat Fat 0.5 gm, Monounsat Fat 3.0 gm, Cholesterol 0 mg), Sodium 470 mg, Total Carbohydrate 24 gm, Dietary Fiber 8 gm, Sugars 3 gm, Protein 10 gm

Green Bean Soup

Loretta Krahn • Mountain Lake, MN

Makes 6 servings (Ideal slow cooker size: 4-quart)

2 cups cubed, extra-lean, lower-sodium ham

1½ qts. water

1 large onion, chopped

2-3 cups cut-up green beans

3 large carrots, sliced

2 large potatoes, peeled and cubed

1 Tbsp. parsley

1 Tbsp. summer savory

¼ tsp. pepper

1 cup fat-free half-and-half

1. Combine all ingredients except half-and-half in slow cooker.

2. Cover. Cook on High 4–6 hours.

3. Turn to Low. Stir in half-and-half. Heat through and serve.

Exchange List Values: Starch 1.0, Vegetable 2.0, Meat, lean 1.0

Basic Nutritional Values: Calories 170 (Calories from Fat 15), Total Fat 2 gm (Saturated Fat 0.6 gm, Polyunsat Fat 0.3 gm, Monounsat Fat 0.4 gm, Cholesterol 24 mg), Sodium 468 mg, Total Carbohydrate 27 gm, Dietary Fiber 4 gm, Sugars 10 gm, Protein 12 gm

Invite a friend or family member to do any 10 of the tips in this book with you. It's easier when you have company!

Bean Soup

Joyce Cox • Port Angeles, WA

Makes 10-12 servings (Ideal slow cooker size: 4-quart)

1 cup dry Great Northern beans

1 cup dry red beans, or pinto beans

4 cups water

28-oz. can diced tomatoes

1 medium onion, chopped

2 Tbsp. vegetable bouillon granules, or 4 bouillon cubes

2 cloves garlic, minced

2 tsp. Italian seasoning, crushed

9-oz. pkg. frozen green beans, thawed

1. Soak and rinse dried beans. Drain.

2. Combine all ingredients except green beans in slow cooker.

3. Cover. Cook on High 5½–6½ hours, or on Low 11–13 hours.

4. Stir green beans into soup during last 2 hours.

Exchange List Values: Starch 1.0, Vegetable 1.0

Basic Nutritional Values: Calories 114 (Calories from Fat 5), Total Fat 1 gm (Saturated Fat 0.1 gm, Polyunsat Fat 0.2 gm, Monounsat Fat 0 gm, Cholesterol 0 mg), Sodium 435 mg, Total Carbohydrate 22 gm, Dietary Fiber 7 gm, Sugars 5 gm, Protein 7 gm

Vegetarian Minestrone Soup

Connie Johnson • Loudon, NH

Makes 8 servings (Ideal slow cooker size: 4-quart)

6 cups fat-free, 60%-lower-sodium vegetable broth

2 carrots, chopped

2 large onions, chopped

3 ribs celery, chopped

2 cloves garlic, minced

1 small zucchini, cubed

1 handful fresh kale, chopped

$\frac{1}{2}$ cup dry barley

1 can chickpeas, or white kidney beans, drained

1 Tbsp. parsley

$\frac{1}{2}$ tsp. dried thyme

1 tsp. dried oregano

28-oz. can crushed Italian tomatoes

$\frac{1}{4}$ tsp. pepper

1. Combine all ingredients in slow cooker.

2. Cover. Cook on Low 6–8 hours, or until vegetables are tender.

Exchange List Values: Starch 1.5, Vegetable 4.0

Basic Nutritional Values: Calories 200 (Calories from Fat 13), Total Fat 1 gm (Saturated Fat 0.1 gm, Polyunsat Fat 0.6 gm, Monounsat Fat 0.3 gm, Cholesterol 0 mg), Sodium 641 mg, Total Carbohydrate 41 gm, Dietary Fiber 9 gm, Sugars 12 gm, Protein 7 gm

Joyce's Minestrone

Joyce Shackelford • Green Bay, Wisconsin

Makes 6 servings (Ideal slow cooker size: 4–5-quart)

$3\frac{1}{2}$ cups 99%-fat-free, lower-sodium beef broth

28-oz. can crushed tomatoes

2 medium carrots, thinly sliced

$\frac{1}{2}$ cup chopped onion

$\frac{1}{2}$ cup chopped celery

2 medium potatoes, thinly sliced

1-2 cloves garlic, minced

15-oz. can no-salt-added red kidney beans, drained

2 ozs. thin spaghetti, broken into 2" pieces

2 Tbsp. parsley flakes

2-3 tsp. dried basil

1-2 tsp. dried oregano

1 bay leaf

1. Combine all ingredients in slow cooker.

2. Cover. Cook on Low 10–16 hours, or on High 4–6 hours.

3. Remove bay leaf. Serve.

Exchange List Values: Starch 2.0, Vegetable 2.0

Basic Nutritional Values: Calories 213 (Calories from Fat 7), Total Fat 1 gm (Saturated Fat 0 gm, Polyunsat Fat 0.4 gm, Monounsat Fat 0.1 gm, Cholesterol 0 mg), Sodium 655 mg, Total Carbohydrate 42 gm, Dietary Fiber 9 gm, Sugars 11 gm, Protein 10 gm

Grace's Minestrone Soup

Grace Ketcham • Marietta, GA

Makes 8 servings (Ideal slow cooker size: 4–5-quart)

¾ cup dry elbow macaroni

2 qts. 98%-fat-free, lower-sodium chicken stock

2 large onions, diced

2 carrots, sliced

half a head of cabbage, shredded

½ cup celery, diced

1-lb. can no-salt-added tomatoes

½ tsp. dried oregano

1 Tbsp. minced parsley

¼ cup each frozen corn, peas, and lima beans

¼ tsp. pepper

1. Cook macaroni according to package directions. Set aside.

2. Combine all ingredients except macaroni in large slow cooker.

3. Cover. Cook on Low 8 hours. Add macaroni during last 30 minutes of cooking time.

Exchange List Values: Starch 1.0, Vegetable 2.0

Basic Nutritional Values: Calories 112 (Calories from Fat 5), Total Fat 1 gm (Saturated Fat 0 gm, Polyunsat Fat 0.3 gm, Monounsat Fat 0.1 gm, Cholesterol 0 mg), Sodium 559 mg, Total Carbohydrate 22 gm, Dietary Fiber 4 gm, Sugars 8 gm, Protein 6 gm

Winter Squash and White Bean Stew

Mary E. Herr • Three Rivers, MI

Makes 6 servings (Ideal slow cooker size: 4-quart)

1 cup chopped onions

1 Tbsp. olive oil

½ tsp. ground cumin

¼ tsp. cinnamon

1 clove garlic, minced

3 cups peeled butternut squash, cut into ¾" cubes

1½ cups chicken broth

19-oz. can cannellini beans, drained

14½-oz. can diced tomatoes, undrained

1 Tbsp. chopped fresh cilantro

1. Combine all ingredients in slow cooker.

2. Cover. Cook on High 1 hour. Reduce heat to Low and cook 2–3 hours.

Exchange List Values: Starch 1.5, Vegetable 1.0, Fat 0.5

Basic Nutritional Values: Calories 164 (Calories from Fat 30), Total Fat 3 gm (Saturated Fat 0.5 gm, Polyunsat Fat 0.6 gm, Monounsat Fat 1.9 gm, Cholesterol 1 mg), Sodium 586 mg, Total Carbohydrate 28 gm, Dietary Fiber 7 gm, Sugars 6 gm, Protein 8 gm

VARIATIONS:

1. Beans can be pureed in blender and added during the last hour.
2. Eight ounces dried beans can be soaked overnight, cooked until soft, and used in place of canned beans.

Cabbage Soup

Margaret Jarrett • Anderson, IN

Makes 8 servings (Ideal slow cooker size: 4-quart)

half a head of cabbage, sliced thin

2 ribs celery, sliced thin

2–3 carrots, sliced thin

1 onion, chopped

2 tsp. sodium-free chicken bouillon powder

2 cloves garlic, minced

1 qt. tomato juice

1/4 tsp. pepper

water

1. Combine all ingredients except water in slow cooker. Add water to within 3" of top of slow cooker.

2. Cover. Cook on High 3½–4 hours, or until vegetables are tender.

Exchange List Values: Vegetable 2.0

Basic Nutritional Values: Calories 55 (Calories from Fat 3), Total Fat 0 gm (Saturated Fat 0 gm, Polyunsat Fat 0.1 gm, Monounsat Fat 0 gm, Cholesterol 0 mg), Sodium 474 mg, Total Carbohydrate 13 gm, Dietary Fiber 3 gm, Sugars 8 gm, Protein 2 gm

Cheese and Corn Chowder

Loretta Krahn • Mt. Lake, MN

Makes 8 servings (Ideal slow cooker size: 4-quart)

3/4 cup water

1/2 cup chopped onions

1½ cups sliced carrots

1½ cups chopped celery

1/4 tsp. salt

1/2 tsp. pepper

15¼-oz. can whole-kernel corn, drained

15-oz. can no-salt-added cream-style corn

1½ cups fat-free milk

1½ cups fat-free half-and-half

1 cup grated fat-free cheddar cheese

1. Combine water, onions, carrots, celery, salt, and pepper in slow cooker.

2. Cover. Cook on High 4–6 hours.

3. Add corn, milk, half-and-half, and cheese. Heat on High 1 hour, and then turn to Low until you are ready to eat.

Exchange List Values: Starch 1.0, Milk, fat-free 1.0

Basic Nutritional Values: Calories 168 (Calories from Fat 29), Total Fat 3 gm (Saturated Fat 1.3 gm, Polyunsat Fat 0.4 gm, Monounsat Fat 0.9 gm, Cholesterol 12 mg), Sodium 391 mg, Total Carbohydrate 26 gm, Dietary Fiber 3 gm, Sugars 13 gm, Protein 11 gm

Broccoli-Cheese Soup

Darla Sathre • Baxter, MN

Makes 8 servings (Ideal slow cooker size: 4-quart)

2 16-oz. pkgs. frozen chopped broccoli

10¾-oz. can cheddar cheese soup

12-oz. can fat-free evaporated milk

2½ cups fat-free half-and-half

¼ cup finely chopped onions

1 Tbsp. Italian Seasoning Mix (see recipe on page 333)

¼ tsp. pepper

2 oz. fat-free cheddar cheese

sunflower seeds, optional

crumbled bacon, optional

1. Combine all ingredients except sunflower seeds and bacon in slow cooker.

2. Cover. Cook on Low 8–10 hours.

3. Garnish with sunflower seeds and bacon.

Exchange List Values: Milk, fat-free 1.0, Vegetable 2.0, Fat 0.5

Basic Nutritional Values: Calories 171 (Calories from Fat 36), Total Fat 4 gm (Saturated Fat 1.6 gm, Polyunsat Fat 0.9 gm, Monounsat Fat 0.9 gm, Cholesterol 12 mg), Sodium 581 mg, Total Carbohydrate 22 gm, Dietary Fiber 4 gm, Sugars 12 gm, Protein 12 gm

Make your goals realistic and specific. Instead of thinking, "I'll walk more often," you might say, "I'm going to walk for 30 minutes, 5 days a week."

Corn Chowder

Mary Rogers • Waseca, MN

Makes 12 servings (Ideal slow cooker size: 6-quart)

6 ozs. bacon

4 cups diced potatoes

2 cups chopped onions

2 cups fat-free sour cream

1½ cups reduced-fat (2%) milk

1 cup fat-free half-and-half

2 10¾-oz. cans 98%-fat-free, lower-sodium cream of chicken soup

2 15¼-oz. cans corn, undrained

1. Cut bacon into 1" pieces. Cook for 5 minutes in large skillet.

2. Add potatoes and onions and a bit of water. Cook 15–20 minutes, until tender, stirring occasionally. Drain. Transfer to slow cooker.

3. Combine sour cream, milk, half-and-half, chicken soup, and corn. Place in slow cooker.

4. Cover. Cook on Low for 2 hours.

5. Serve with homemade biscuits or a pan of steaming corn bread fresh from the oven.

Exchange List Values: Starch 1.0, Carbohydrate 1.0, Fat 1.0

Basic Nutritional Values: Calories 202 (Calories from Fat 41), Total Fat 5 gm (Saturated Fat 1.5 gm, Polyunsat Fat 0.9 gm, Monounsat Fat 1.5 gm, Cholesterol 14 mg), Sodium 568 mg, Total Carbohydrate 32 gm, Dietary Fiber 3 gm, Sugars 13 gm, Protein 8 gm

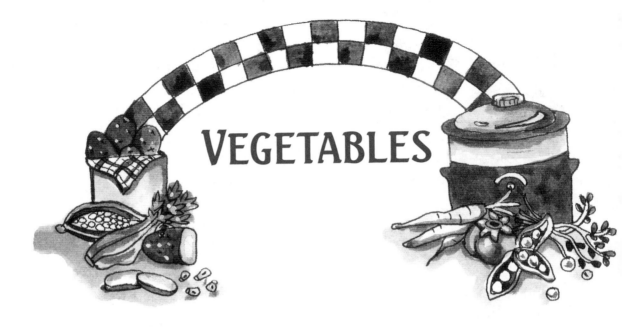

VEGETABLES

Very Special Spinach

Jeanette Oberholtzer • Manheim, PA

Makes 8 servings (Ideal slow cooker size: 4-quart)

3 10-oz. boxes frozen spinach, thawed and drained

2 cups low-fat (1%) cottage cheese

1½ cups grated fat-free cheddar cheese

3 eggs

¼ cup flour

4 Tbsp. (¼ cup) light, soft tub margarine, melted

1. Mix together all ingredients.

2. Pour into slow cooker.

3. Cook on High 1 hour. Reduce heat to Low and cook 4 more hours.

Exchange List Values: Starch 0.5, Vegetable 1.0, Meat, lean 2.0

Basic Nutritional Values: Calories 160 (Calories from Fat 44), Total Fat 5 gm (Saturated Fat 1.3 gm, Polyunsat Fat 0.9 gm, Monounsat Fat 2.1 gm, Cholesterol 84 mg), Sodium 520 mg, Total Carbohydrate 11 gm, Dietary Fiber 3 gm, Sugars 3 gm, Protein 19 gm

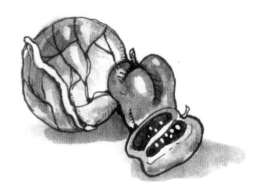

Caramelized Onions

Mrs. J. E. Barthold • Bethlehem, PA

Makes 8 servings (Ideal slow cooker size: 4-quart)

6 large Vidalia or other sweet onions

4 Tbsp. margarine

10-oz. can chicken, or vegetable, broth

1. Peel onions. Remove stems and root ends. Place in slow cooker.

2. Pour margarine and broth over.

3. Cook on Low 12 hours.

Exchange List Values: Vegetable 3.0, Fat 1.0

Basic Nutritional Values: Calories 123 (Calories from Fat 57), Total Fat 6 gm (Saturated Fat 1.1 gm, Polyunsat Fat 2.0 gm, Monounsat Fat 2.7 gm, Cholesterol 1 mg), Sodium 325 mg, Total Carbohydrate 15 gm, Dietary Fiber 3 gm, Sugars 11 gm, Protein 2 gm

Note: Serve as a side dish, or use onions and liquid to flavor soups or stews, or as topping for pizza.

Barbecued Green Beans

Arlene Wengerd • Millersburg, OH

Makes 6 servings (Ideal slow cooker size: 3-4-quart)

4 slices bacon

1/4 cup chopped onions

1/2 cup ketchup

2 Tbsp. brown sugar

brown sugar substitute to equal 2 Tbsp.

3 tsp. Worcestershire sauce

1/8 tsp. salt

4 cups green beans

1. Brown bacon in skillet until crisp and then break into pieces.

2. Saute onions in non-fat cooking spray in skillet.

3. Combine ketchup, brown sugar, sugar substitute, Worcestershire sauce, and salt. Stir into bacon and onions.

4. Pour mixture over green beans and mix lightly.

5. Pour into slow cooker and cook on High 3-4 hours, or on Low 6-8 hours.

Exchange List Values: Carbohydrate 0.5, Vegetable 2.0, Fat 0.5

Basic Nutritional Values: Calories 98 (Calories from Fat 22), Total Fat 2 gm (Saturated Fat 0.7 gm, Polyunsat Fat 0.3 gm, Monounsat Fat 0.9 gm, Cholesterol 3 mg), Sodium 386 mg, Total Carbohydrate 18 gm, Dietary Fiber 3 gm, Sugars 9 gm, Protein 3 gm

Dutch Green Beans

Edwina Stoltzfus • Narvon, PA

Makes 12 servings (Ideal slow cooker size: 4–5-quart)

6 slices bacon

4 medium onions, sliced

2 Tbsp. canola oil

2 qts. fresh, frozen, or canned green beans

4 cups diced, fresh tomatoes

$\frac{1}{2}$ tsp. salt

$\frac{1}{4}$ tsp. pepper

1. Brown bacon until crisp in skillet. Drain. Crumble bacon into small pieces.

2. Saute onions in canola oil.

3. Combine all ingredients in slow cooker.

4. Cover. Cook on Low $4\frac{1}{2}$ hours.

Exchange List Values: Vegetable 3.0, Fat 0.5

Basic Nutritional Values: Calories 99 (Calories from Fat 39), Total Fat 4 gm (Saturated Fat 0.7 gm, Polyunsat Fat 1.1 gm, Monounsat Fat 2.1 gm, Cholesterol 3 mg), Sodium 154 mg, Total Carbohydrate 14 gm, Dietary Fiber 4 gm, Sugars 6 gm, Protein 4 gm

Select a mix of colorful vegetables each day. Different colored vegetables provide different nutrients.

Easy Flavor-Filled Green Beans

Paula Showalter • Weyers Cave, VA

Makes 10 servings (Ideal slow cooker size: 4–5-quart)

2 qts. green beans, drained

$\frac{1}{3}$ cup chopped onions

4-oz. can mushrooms, drained

1 Tbsp. brown sugar

brown sugar substitute to equal $1\frac{1}{2}$ tsp.

3 Tbsp. light, soft tub margarine

pepper to taste

1. Combine beans, onions, and mushrooms in slow cooker.

2. Sprinkle with brown sugar and sugar substitute.

3. Dot with margarine.

4. Sprinkle with pepper.

5. Cover. Cook on High 3–4 hours. Stir just before serving.

Exchange List Values: Vegetable 2.0

Basic Nutritional Values: Calories 47 (Calories from Fat 14), Total Fat 2 gm (Saturated Fat 0 gm, Polyunsat Fat 0.4 gm, Monounsat Fat 0.8 gm, Cholesterol 0 mg), Sodium 339 mg, Total Carbohydrate 7 gm, Dietary Fiber 3 gm, Sugars 4 gm, Protein 2 gm

Green Bean Casserole

Vicki Dinkel • Sharon Springs, KS

Makes 9–11 servings (Ideal slow cooker size: 3–4-quart)

3 10-oz. pkgs. frozen, cut green beans

1½ 10½-oz. cans cheddar cheese soup

½ cup water

¼ cup chopped green onions

4-oz. can sliced mushrooms, drained

8-oz. can water chestnuts, drained and sliced, optional

½ cup slivered almonds

¼ tsp. pepper

1. Combine all ingredients in lightly greased slow cooker. Mix well.

2. Cover. Cook on Low 8–10 hours, or on High 3–4 hours.

Exchange List Values: Carbohydrate 0.5, Vegetable 1.0, Fat 1.0

Basic Nutritional Values: Calories 102 (Calories from Fat 51), Total Fat 6 gm (Saturated Fat 1.4 gm, Polyunsat Fat 1.6 gm, Monounsat Fat 2.6 gm, Cholesterol 7 mg), Sodium 407 mg, Total Carbohydrate 10 gm, Dietary Fiber 3 gm, Sugars 3 gm, Protein 4 gm

Creamy Cheesy Bean Casserole

Martha Hershey • Ronks, PA

Makes 5 servings (Ideal slow cooker size: 3–4-quart)

16-oz. bag frozen green beans, cooked

¾ cup fat-free milk

1 cup grated fat-free American cheese

2 slices bread, crumbled

1. Place beans in slow cooker.

2. Combine milk and cheese in saucepan. Heat, stirring continually, until cheese melts. Fold in bread cubes and pour mixture over beans.

3. Cover. Heat on High 2 hours.

Exchange List Values: Carbohydrate 0.5, Vegetable 1.0, Meat, very lean 1.0

Basic Nutritional Values: Calories 94 (Calories from Fat 5), Total Fat 1 gm (Saturated Fat 0.1 gm, Polyunsat Fat 0.3 gm, Monounsat Fat 0.1 gm, Cholesterol 4 mg), Sodium 366 mg, Total Carbohydrate 14 gm, Dietary Fiber 3 gm, Sugars 5 gm, Protein 9 gm

VARIATION: Use 15-oz. container of Cheez Whiz instead of making cheese sauce. Mix crumbled bread into Cheez Whiz and pour over beans. Proceed with Step 3.

Stewed Tomatoes

Michelle Showalter • Bridgewater, VA

Makes 10-12 servings (Ideal slow cooker size: 4-quart)

2 qts. canned tomatoes

2½ Tbsp. sugar

sugar substitute to equal 1½ Tbsp.

½ tsp. salt

dash pepper

2 cups bread cubes

1½ Tbsp. light, soft tub margarine

1. Place tomatoes in slow cooker.

2. Sprinkle with sugar, sugar substitute, salt, and pepper.

3. Lightly toast bread cubes in melted margarine. Spread over tomatoes.

4. Cover. Cook on High 3-4 hours.

Exchange List Values: Vegetable 2.0

Basic Nutritional Values: Calories 62 (Calories from Fat 9), Total Fat 1 gm (Saturated Fat 0 gm, Polyunsat Fat 0.4 gm, Monounsat Fat 0.4 gm, Cholesterol 0 mg), Sodium 377 mg, Total Carbohydrate 13 gm, Dietary Fiber 2 gm, Sugars 7 gm, Protein 2 gm

VARIATION: If you prefer bread that is less moist and soft, add bread cubes 15 minutes before serving and continue cooking without lid.

Orange Glazed Carrots

Cyndie Marrara • Port Matilda, PA

Makes 8 servings (Ideal slow cooker size: 4-quart)

32-oz. (2 lbs.) pkg. baby carrots

3 Tbsp. brown sugar

brown sugar substitute to equal 2 Tbsp.

½ cup orange juice

2 Tbsp. margarine

¾ tsp. cinnamon

¼ tsp. nutmeg

2 Tbsp. cornstarch

¼ cup water

1. Combine all ingredients except cornstarch and water in slow cooker.

2. Cover. Cook on Low 3-4 hours, until carrots are tender-crisp.

3. Put carrots in serving dish and keep warm, reserving cooking juices. Put reserved juices in small saucepan. Bring to boil.

4. Mix cornstarch and water in small bowl until blended. Add to juices. Boil 1 minute, or until thickened, stirring constantly.

5. Pour over carrots and serve.

Exchange List Values: Carbohydrate 0.5, Vegetable 2.0, Fat 0.5

Basic Nutritional Values: Calories 108 (Calories from Fat 29), Total Fat 3 gm (Saturated Fat 0.6 gm, Polyunsat Fat 1.0 gm, Monounsat Fat 1.3 gm, Cholesterol 0 mg), Sodium 115 mg, Total Carbohydrate 20 gm, Dietary Fiber 4 gm, Sugars 12 gm, Protein 1 gm

Glazed Tzimmes

Elaine Vigoda • Rochester, NY

Makes 6-8 servings (Ideal slow cooker size: 2 4-5-qt. cookers)

1 sweet potato

6 carrots, sliced

1 potato, peeled and diced

1 onion, chopped

2 apples, peeled and sliced

1 medium (about 1½ lbs.) butternut squash, peeled and sliced

¼ cup dry white wine or apple juice

½ lb. dried apricots

1 Tbsp. ground cinnamon

1 Tbsp. apple pie spice

1 Tbsp. maple syrup or honey

1 tsp. salt

1 tsp. ground ginger

1. Combine all ingredients in large slow cooker, or mix all ingredients in large bowl and then divide between 2 4- or 5-qt. cookers.

2. Cover. Cook on Low 10 hours.

Exchange List Values: Starch 1.0, Fruit 1.5, Vegetable 1.0

Basic Nutritional Values: Calories 179 (Calories from Fat 5), Total Fat 1 gm (Saturated Fat 0.1 gm, Polyunsat Fat 0.2 gm, Monounsat Fat 0.1 gm, Cholesterol 0 mg), Sodium 332 mg, Total Carbohydrate 45 gm, Dietary Fiber 6 gm, Sugars 27 gm, Protein 3 gm

Note: This is a special dish served primarily on Jewish holidays, such as Rosh Hashanah and Passover. The sweetness of the vegetables and fruit signifies wishes for a sweet year.

Vegetable Medley

Teena Wagner • Waterloo, ON

Makes 8 servings (Ideal slow cooker size: 4-quart)

2 medium parsnips

4 medium carrots

1 turnip, about 4½" around

1 tsp. salt

½ cup water

3 Tbsp. sugar

2 Tbsp. canola or olive oil

½ tsp. salt

1. Clean and peel vegetables. Cut in 1" pieces.

2. Dissolve 1 tsp. salt in water in saucepan. Add vegetables and boil for 10 minutes. Drain, reserving ½ cup liquid.

3. Place vegetables in slow cooker. Add liquid.

4. Stir in sugar, oil, and ½ tsp. salt.

5. Cover. Cook on Low 2–3 hours.

6. Remove vegetables from juice in pot to serve.

Exchange List Values: Starch 1.0

Basic Nutritional Values: Calories 63 (Calories from Fat 17), Total Fat 2 gm (Saturated Fat 0.1 gm, Polyunsat Fat 0.6 gm, Monounsat Fat 1.0 gm, Cholesterol 0 mg), Sodium 327 mg, Total Carbohydrate 12 gm, Dietary Fiber 2 gm, Sugars 6 gm, Protein 1 gm

Start liking yourself.
If you're going to lose weight or
make other changes, you need to
be your own cheerleader.

Easy Olive Bake

Jean Robinson • Cinnaminson, NJ

Makes 8 servings (Ideal slow cooker size: 4-quart)

1 cup uncooked rice

2 medium onions, chopped

2 Tbsp. light, soft tub margarine, melted

2 cups stewed tomatoes

2 cups water

1 cup black olives, quartered

$\frac{1}{2}$ tsp. chili powder

1 Tbsp. Worcestershire sauce

4-oz. can mushrooms with juice

$\frac{1}{2}$ cup grated fat-free cheese

1. Wash and drain rice. Place in slow cooker.

2. Add remaining ingredients except cheese. Mix well.

3. Cover. Cook on High 1 hour, then on Low 2 hours, or until rice is tender but not mushy.

4. Add cheese before serving.

5. This is a good accompaniment to baked ham.

Exchange List Values: Starch 1.0, Vegetable 2.0, Fat 0.5

Basic Nutritional Values: Calories 163 (Calories from Fat 28), Total Fat 3 gm (Saturated Fat 0.2 gm, Polyunsat Fat 0.5 gm, Monounsat Fat 1.9 gm, Cholesterol 1 mg), Sodium 492 mg, Total Carbohydrate 29 gm, Dietary Fiber 2 gm, Sugars 5 gm, Protein 6 gm

Zucchini Special

Louise Stackhouse • Benten, PA

Makes 8 servings (Ideal slow cooker size: 4-quart)

1 medium to large zucchini, peeled and sliced

1 medium onion, sliced

1 qt. stewed, no-salt-added tomatoes with juice, or 2 14$\frac{1}{2}$-oz. cans stewed, no-salt-added tomatoes with juice

$\frac{1}{2}$ tsp. salt

1 tsp. dried basil

4 ozs. (1 cup) reduced-fat mozzarella cheese, shredded

1. Layer zucchini, onion, and tomatoes in slow cooker.

2. Sprinkle with salt, basil, and cheese.

3. Cover. Cook on Low 6–8 hours.

Exchange List Values: Vegetable 2.0, Fat 0.5

Basic Nutritional Values: Calories 79 (Calories from Fat 21), Total Fat 2 gm (Saturated Fat 1.3 gm, Polyunsat Fat 0.3 gm, Monounsat Fat 0.4 gm, Cholesterol 8 mg), Sodium 273 mg, Total Carbohydrate 11 gm, Dietary Fiber 2 gm, Sugars 5 gm, Protein 6 gm

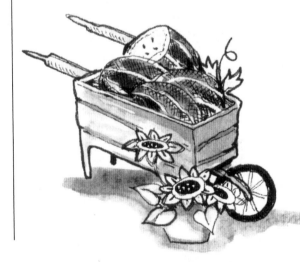

Squash Casserole

Sharon Anders • Alburtis, PA

Makes 9 servings (Ideal slow cooker size: 4-quart)

2 lbs. yellow summer squash or zucchini, thinly sliced (about 6 cups)

half a medium onion, chopped

1 cup peeled, shredded carrot

10¾-oz. can 98%-fat-free, reduced-sodium condensed cream of chicken soup

½ cup fat-free sour cream

2 Tbsp. flour

4 ozs. (½ of 8-oz. pkg.) seasoned stuffing crumbs

2 Tbsp. canola oil

1. Combine squash, onion, carrots, and soup.

2. Mix together sour cream and flour. Stir into vegetables.

3. Toss stuffing mix with oil. Spread half in bottom of slow cooker. Add vegetable mixture. Top with remaining crumbs.

4. Cover. Cook on Low 7–9 hours.

Exchange List Values: Starch 1.0, Vegetable 1.0, Fat 1.0

Basic Nutritional Values: Calories 140 (Calories from Fat 38), Total Fat 4 gm (Saturated Fat 0.5 gm, Polyunsat Fat 1.4 gm, Monounsat Fat 2.1 gm, Cholesterol 4 mg), Sodium 486 mg, Total Carbohydrate 21 gm, Dietary Fiber 3 gm, Sugars 5 gm, Protein 4 gm

Squash Medley

Evelyn Page • Riverton, WY

Makes 8 servings (Ideal slow cooker size: 4-quart)

8 (up to 8 ozs. total) summer squash, each about 4" long, thinly sliced

½ tsp. salt

2 tomatoes, peeled and chopped

¼ cup sliced green onions

half a small sweet green pepper, chopped

1 chicken bouillon cube

¼ cup hot water

4 slices bacon, fried and crumbled

¼ cup fine dry bread crumbs

1. Sprinkle squash with salt.

2. In slow cooker, layer half the squash, tomatoes, onions, and pepper. Repeat layers.

3. Dissolve bouillon in hot water. Pour into slow cooker.

4. Top with bacon. Sprinkle bread crumbs over top.

5. Cover. Cook on Low 4–6 hours.

Exchange List Values: Vegetable 1.0, Fat 0.5

Basic Nutritional Values: Calories 47 (Calories from Fat 17), Total Fat 2 gm (Saturated Fat 0.5 gm, Polyunsat Fat 0.3 gm, Monounsat Fat 0.8 gm, Cholesterol 3 mg), Sodium 339 mg, Total Carbohydrate 6 gm, Dietary Fiber 1 gm, Sugars 2 gm, Protein 2 gm

VARIATION: For a sweeter touch, sprinkle 1 Tbsp. brown sugar over half the layered vegetables. Repeat over second half of layered vegetables.

Baked Acorn Squash

Dale Peterson • Rapid City, SD

Makes 4 servings (Ideal slow cooker size: 3–4-quart)

2 small (1¼ lbs. each) acorn squash

½ cup cracker crumbs

¼ cup coarsely chopped pecans

2 Tbsp. light, soft tub margarine, melted

2 Tbsp. brown sugar

brown sugar substitute to equal 1 Tbsp.

¼ tsp. salt

¼ tsp. ground nutmeg

2 Tbsp. orange juice

1. Cut squash in half. Remove seeds.

2. Combine remaining ingredients. Spoon into squash halves. Place squash in slow cooker.

3. Cover. Cook on Low 5–6 hours, or until squash is tender.

Exchange List Values: Starch 2.0, Carbohydrate 0.5, Fat 1.0

Basic Nutritional Values: Calories 229 (Calories from Fat 82), Total Fat 9 gm (Saturated Fat 0.8 gm, Polyunsat Fat 2.3 gm, Monounsat Fat 5.1 gm, Cholesterol 0 mg), Sodium 314 mg, Total Carbohydrate 38 gm, Dietary Fiber 8 gm, Sugars 15 gm, Protein 3 gm

Apple Walnut Squash

Michele Ruvola • Selden, NY

Makes 4 servings (Ideal slow cooker size: 3–4-quart)

¼ cup water

2 small (1¼ lbs. each) acorn squash

2 Tbsp. brown sugar

brown sugar substitute to equal 1 Tbsp.

2 Tbsp. light, soft tub margarine

3 Tbsp. apple juice

1½ tsp. ground cinnamon

¼ tsp. salt

1 cup toasted walnut halves

1 medium apple, unpeeled, chopped

1. Pour water into slow cooker.

2. Cut squash crosswise in half. Remove seeds. Place in slow cooker, cut sides up.

3. Combine brown sugar, sugar substitute, margarine, apple juice, cinnamon, and salt. Spoon into squash.

4. Cover. Cook on High 3–4 hours, or until squash is tender.

5. Combine walnuts and chopped apple. Add to center of squash and mix with sauce to serve.

6. Serve with a pork dish.

Exchange List Values: Starch 1.5, Fruit 1.0, Fat 1.5

Basic Nutritional Values: Calories 244 (Calories from Fat 96), Total Fat 11 gm (Saturated Fat 0.8 gm, Polyunsat Fat 6.5 gm, Monounsat Fat 2.4 gm, Cholesterol 0 mg), Sodium 202 mg, Total Carbohydrate 39 gm, Dietary Fiber 9 gm, Sugars 19 gm, Protein 4 gm

Stuffed Acorn Squash

Jean Butzer • Batavia, NY

Makes 6 servings (Ideal slow cooker size: 4-quart)

3 small (1¼ lbs. each) acorn squash

5 Tbsp. dry instant brown rice

3 Tbsp. dried cranberries

3 Tbsp. diced celery

3 Tbsp. minced onion

pinch ground or dried sage

1 tsp. butter, divided

3 Tbsp. orange juice

½ cup water

1. Slice off points on the bottoms of squash so they will stand in slow cooker. Slice off tops and discard. Scoop out seeds. Place squash in slow cooker.

2. Combine rice, cranberries, celery, onion, and sage. Stuff into squash.

3. Dot with butter.

4. Pour 1 Tbsp. orange juice into each squash.

5. Pour water into bottom of slow cooker.

6. Cover. Cook on Low 2½ hours.

7. Serve with cooked turkey breast.

Exchange List Values: Starch 2.0

Basic Nutritional Values: Calories 131 (Calories from Fat 10), Total Fat 1 gm (Saturated Fat 0.4 gm, Polyunsat Fat 0.2 gm, Monounsat Fat 0.3 gm, Cholesterol 2 mg), Sodium 18 mg, Total Carbohydrate 31 gm, Dietary Fiber 7 gm, Sugars 11 gm, Protein 2 gm

Note: To make squash easier to slice, microwave whole squash on High 5 minutes to soften skin.

Caponata

Katrine Rose • Woodbridge, VA

Makes 10 servings (Ideal slow cooker size: 4-quart)

1 medium (1 lb.) eggplant, peeled and cut into ½" cubes

14-oz. can diced tomatoes

1 medium onion, chopped

1 red bell pepper, cut into ½" pieces

¾ cup salsa

¼ cup olive oil

2 Tbsp. capers, drained

3 Tbsp. balsamic vinegar

3 cloves garlic, minced

1¼ tsp. dried oregano

⅓ cup chopped fresh basil, packed in measuring cup

1. Combine all ingredients except basil in slow cooker.

2. Cover. Cook on Low 7–8 hours, or until vegetables are tender.

3. Stir in basil. Serve spread on toasted French bread.

Exchange List Values: Vegetable 2.0, Fat 1.0

Basic Nutritional Values: Calories 84 (Calories from Fat 51), Total Fat 6 gm (Saturated Fat 0.7 gm, Polyunsat Fat 0.6 gm, Monounsat Fat 4.0 gm, Cholesterol 0 mg), Sodium 182 mg, Total Carbohydrate 9 gm, Dietary Fiber 2 gm, Sugars 5 gm, Protein 1 gm

Julia's Broccoli and Cauliflower with Cheese

Julia Lapp • New Holland, PA

Makes 6 servings (Ideal slow cooker size: 4-quart)

5 cups raw broccoli and cauliflower

¼ cup water

2 Tbsp. margarine

2 Tbsp. flour

½ tsp. salt

1 cup fat-free milk

1 cup shredded fat-free cheddar cheese

1. Cook broccoli and cauliflower in saucepan in water, until just crisp-tender. Set aside.

2. Make white sauce by melting margarine in another pan over Low heat. Blend in flour and salt. Add milk all at once. Cook quickly, stirring constantly, until mixture thickens and bubbles. Add cheese. Stir until melted and smooth.

3. Combine vegetables and sauce in slow cooker. Mix well.

4. Cook on Low 1½ hours.

Exchange List Values: Carbohydrate 0.5, Vegetable 1.0, Meat, lean 1.0

Basic Nutritional Values: Calories 108 (Calories from Fat 37), Total Fat 4 gm (Saturated Fat 0.8 gm, Polyunsat Fat 1.3 gm, Monounsat Fat 1.7 gm, Cholesterol 3 mg), Sodium 412 mg, Total Carbohydrate 9 gm, Dietary Fiber 2 gm, Sugars 5 gm, Protein 10 gm

VARIATION: Substitute green beans and carrots or other vegetables for broccoli and cauliflower.

Golden Cauliflower

Carol Peachey • Lancaster, PA

Makes 4–6 servings (Ideal slow cooker size: 4-quart)

2 10-oz. pkgs. frozen cauliflower, thawed

2 Tbsp. light, soft tub margarine, melted

1 Tbsp. flour

1 cup evaporated fat-free milk

1 oz. (¼ cup) fat-free cheddar cheese

2 Tbsp. low-fat (1%) cottage cheese

2 tsp. Parmesan cheese

4 slices bacon, crisply browned and crumbled

1. Place cauliflower in slow cooker.

2. Melt margarine on stove. Add flour and evaporated milk. Heat till thickened. Add cheeses.

3. Pour sauce over cauliflower. Top with bacon.

4. Cover. Cook on High 1½ hours, and then reduce to Low for an additional 2 hours. Or cook only on Low 4–5 hours.

Exchange List Values: Carbohydrate 0.5, Meat, lean 1.0

Basic Nutritional Values: Calories 106 (Calories from Fat 37), Total Fat 4 gm (Saturated Fat 0.8 gm, Polyunsat Fat 0.6 gm, Monounsat Fat 1.9 gm, Cholesterol 5 mg), Sodium 228 mg, Total Carbohydrate 10 gm, Dietary Fiber 2 gm, Sugars 6 gm, Protein 8 gm

Quick Broccoli Fix

Willard E. Roth • Elkhart, IN

Makes 6 servings (Ideal slow cooker size: 4-quart)

1 lb. fresh or frozen broccoli, cut up

10¾-oz. can 98%-fat-free, reduced-sodium cream of mushroom soup

¼ cup fat-free mayonnaise

½ cup fat-free plain yogurt

½ lb. sliced fresh mushrooms

1 cup shredded fat-free cheddar cheese, divided

1 cup crushed saltine crackers with unsalted tops

sliced almonds, optional

1. Microwave broccoli for 3 minutes. Place in greased slow cooker.

2. Combine soup, mayonnaise, yogurt, mushrooms, and ½ cup cheese. Pour over broccoli.

3. Cover. Cook on Low 5–6 hours.

4. Top with remaining cheese and crackers for last half hour of cooking time.

5. Top with sliced almonds, for a special touch, before serving.

Exchange List Values: Carbohydrate 1.0, Vegetable 1.0, Meat, lean 1.0

Basic Nutritional Values: Calories 158 (Calories from Fat 28), Total Fat 3 gm (Saturated Fat 0.4 gm, Polyunsat Fat 0.8 gm, Monounsat Fat 1.0 gm, Cholesterol 3 mg), Sodium 523 mg, Total Carbohydrate 22 gm, Dietary Fiber 3 gm, Sugars 5 gm, Protein 12 gm

Eat breakfast every day. People who eat breakfast are less likely to overeat later in the day.

Broccoli and Rice Casserole

Deborah Swartz • Grottoes, VA

Makes 4–6 servings (Ideal slow cooker size: 4-quart)

1 lb. chopped broccoli, fresh or frozen, thawed

1 medium onion, chopped

1 Tbsp. canola oil

1 cup minute rice, or 1½ cups cooked rice

10¾-oz. can 99%-fat-free, reduced-sodium cream of chicken, or mushroom, soup

¼ cup fat-free milk

1⅓ cups shredded fat-free cheddar cheese

1. Cook broccoli for 5 minutes in saucepan in boiling water. Drain and set aside.

2. Saute onion in oil in saucepan until tender. Add to broccoli.

3. Combine remaining ingredients. Add to broccoli mixture. Pour into greased slow cooker.

4. Cover. Cook on Low 3–4 hours.

Exchange List Values: Starch 1.5, Vegetable 1.0, Meat, lean 1.0

Basic Nutritional Values: Calories 188 (Calories from Fat 33), Total Fat 4 gm (Saturated Fat 0.5 gm, Polyunsat Fat 1.2 gm, Monounsat Fat 1.6 gm, Cholesterol 7 mg), Sodium 404 mg, Total Carbohydrate 26 gm, Dietary Fiber 3 gm, Sugars 5 gm, Protein 13 gm

Sweet-Sour Cabbage

Irma H. Schoen • Windsor, CT

Recipe photo appears in color section.

Makes 6 servings (Ideal slow cooker size: 4-quart)

1 medium-sized head red or green cabbage, shredded

2 medium onions, chopped

4 medium tart apples, pared, quartered

$1/2$ cup raisins

$1/4$ cup lemon juice

$1/4$ cup cider, or apple juice

1 Tbsp. honey

1 Tbsp. caraway seeds

$1/8$ tsp. allspice

$1/2$ tsp. salt

1. Combine all ingredients in slow cooker.

2. Cook on High 3–5 hours, depending upon how crunchy or soft you want the cabbage and onions.

Exchange List Values: Fruit 1.0, Vegetable 2.0

Basic Nutritional Values: Calories 112 (Calories from Fat 6), Total Fat 1 gm (Saturated Fat 0 gm, Polyunsat Fat 0.3 gm, Monounsat Fat 0.1 gm, Cholesterol 0 mg), Sodium 154 mg, Total Carbohydrate 27 gm, Dietary Fiber 5 gm, Sugars 21 gm, Protein 3 gm

Bavarian Cabbage

Joyce Shackelford • Green Bay, WI

Makes 4–8 servings, depending upon the size of the cabbage head (Ideal slow cooker size: 4-quart)

1 small ($1\frac{1}{2}$ lbs.) head red cabbage, sliced

1 medium onion, chopped

3 medium tart apples, unpeeled, cored and quartered

1 tsp. salt

1 cup hot water

1 Tbsp. sugar

sugar substitute to equal $1/2$ Tbsp.

$1/3$ cup vinegar

$1\frac{1}{2}$ Tbsp. bacon drippings

1. Place all ingredients in slow cooker in order listed.

2. Cover. Cook on Low 8 hours, or on High 3 hours. Stir well before serving.

Exchange List Values: Fruit 0.5, Vegetable 1.0, Fat 0.5

Basic Nutritional Values: Calories 85 (Calories from Fat 24), Total Fat 3 gm (Saturated Fat 1.1 gm, Polyunsat Fat 0.3 gm, Monounsat Fat 1.0 gm, Cholesterol 2 mg), Sodium 313 mg, Total Carbohydrate 16 gm, Dietary Fiber 3 gm, Sugars 12 gm, Protein 1 gm

VARIATION: Add 6 slices bacon, browned until crisp and crumbled.

Jean M. Butzer • Batavia, NY

Cabbage Casserole

Edwina Stoltzfus • Narvon, PA

Makes 6 servings (Ideal slow cooker size: 4-quart)

1 large head cabbage, chopped

2 cups water

3 Tbsp. margarine

¼ cup flour

¼ tsp. salt

¼ tsp. pepper

1⅓ cups fat-free milk

1⅓ cups shredded fat-free cheddar

1. Cook cabbage in saucepan in boiling water for 5 minutes. Drain. Place in slow cooker.

2. In saucepan, melt margarine. Stir in flour, salt, and pepper. Add milk, stirring constantly on Low heat for 5 minutes. Remove from heat. Stir in cheese. Pour over cabbage.

3. Cover. Cook on Low 4–5 hours.

Exchange List Values: Carbohydrate 0.5, Vegetable 2.0, Meat, lean 1.0, Fat 0.5

Basic Nutritional Values: Calories 179 (Calories from Fat 57), Total Fat 6 gm (Saturated Fat 1.1 gm, Polyunsat Fat 2.1 gm, Monounsat Fat 2.6 gm, Cholesterol 4 mg), Sodium 400 mg, Total Carbohydrate 19 gm, Dietary Fiber 5 gm, Sugars 10 gm, Protein 13 gm

VARIATION: Replace cabbage with cauliflower.

Vegetable Curry

Sheryl Shenk • Harrisonburg, VA

Makes 8–10 servings (Ideal slow cooker size: 4–5-quart)

16-oz. pkg. baby carrots

3 medium potatoes, unpeeled, cubed

1 lb. fresh, or frozen, green beans, cut in 2" pieces

1 medium green pepper, chopped

1 medium onion, chopped

1–2 cloves garlic, minced

15-oz. can garbanzo beans, drained

28-oz. can crushed tomatoes

3 Tbsp. minute tapioca

3 tsp. curry powder

1½ tsp. chicken bouillon granules

1¾ cups boiling water

1. Combine carrots, potatoes, green beans, green pepper, onion, garlic, garbanzo beans, and crushed tomatoes in large bowl.

2. Stir in tapioca and curry powder.

3. Dissolve bouillon in boiling water. Pour over vegetables. Mix well. Spoon into large cooker, or two medium-sized ones.

4. Cover. Cook on Low 8–10 hours, or High 3–4 hours. Serve with cooked rice.

Exchange List Values: Starch 1.0, Vegetable 3.0

Basic Nutritional Values: Calories 166 (Calories from Fat 10), Total Fat 1 gm (Saturated Fat 0.1 gm, Polyunsat Fat 0.5 gm, Monounsat Fat 0.2 gm, Cholesterol 0 mg), Sodium 436 mg, Total Carbohydrate 35 gm, Dietary Fiber 8 gm, Sugars 10 gm, Protein 6 gm

VARIATION: Substitute canned green beans for fresh beans, but add toward the end of the cooking time.

Wild Mushrooms Italian

Connie Johnson • Loudon, NH

Makes 10 servings (Ideal slow cooker size: 4-quart)

2 large onions, chopped

3 large red bell peppers, chopped

3 large green bell peppers, chopped

2 Tbsp. canola oil

12-oz. pkg. oyster mushrooms, cleaned and chopped

4 cloves garlic, minced

3 fresh bay leaves

10 fresh basil leaves, chopped

1 tsp. salt

1½ tsp. pepper

28-oz. can Italian plum tomatoes, crushed or chopped

1. Saute onions and peppers in oil in skillet until soft. Stir in mushrooms and garlic. Saute just until mushrooms begin to turn brown. Pour into slow cooker.

2. Add remaining ingredients. Stir well.

3. Cover. Cook on Low 6–8 hours.

Exchange List Values: Vegetable 3.0, Fat 0.5

Basic Nutritional Values: Calories 82 (Calories from Fat 29), Total Fat 3 gm (Saturated Fat 0.2 gm, Polyunsat Fat 1.0 gm, Monounsat Fat 1.7 gm, Cholesterol 0 mg), Sodium 356 mg, Total Carbohydrate 13 gm, Dietary Fiber 4 gm, Sugars 8 gm, Protein 3 gm

Note: Good as an appetizer or on pita bread, or serve over rice or pasta for a main dish.

Stuffed Mushrooms

Melanie L. Thrower • McPherson, KS

Makes 6 servings (Ideal slow cooker size: 3–4-quart)

12 large mushrooms

1 Tbsp. canola oil

¼ tsp. minced garlic

dash salt

dash pepper

dash cayenne pepper

¼ cup grated reduced-fat Monterey Jack cheese

1. Remove stems from mushrooms and dice.

2. Heat oil in skillet. Saute diced stems with garlic until softened. Remove skillet from heat.

3. Stir in seasonings and cheese. Stuff into mushroom shells. Place in slow cooker.

4. Cover. Heat on Low 2–4 hours.

Exchange List Values: Vegetable 1.0, Fat 0.5

Basic Nutritional Values: Calories 46 (Calories from Fat 30), Total Fat 3 gm (Saturated Fat 0.8 gm, Polyunsat Fat 0.8 gm, Monounsat Fat 1.6 gm, Cholesterol 3 mg), Sodium 39 mg, Total Carbohydrate 2 gm, Dietary Fiber 1 gm, Sugars 1 gm, Protein 3 gm

VARIATIONS:

1. Add 1 Tbsp. minced onion to Step 2.

2. Use Monterey Jack cheese with jalapenos.

Corn Pudding

Barbara A. Yoder • Goshen, IN

Makes 15-plus servings (Ideal slow cooker size: 4–5-quart)

2 10-oz. cans whole-kernel corn with juice

2 1-lb. cans no-salt-added creamed corn

2 6½-oz. boxes corn muffin mix, requiring only water

2 Tbsp. margarine

8-oz. fat-free sour cream

1. Combine all ingredients in slow cooker.

2. Cover. Heat on Low 2–3 hours, until thickened and set.

Exchange List Values: Starch 2.0, Fat 0.5

Basic Nutritional Values: Calories 166 (Calories from Fat 39), Total Fat 4 gm (Saturated Fat 0.7 gm, Polyunsat Fat 0.9 gm, Monounsat Fat 1.6 gm, Cholesterol 1 mg), Sodium 456 mg, Total Carbohydrate 30 gm, Dietary Fiber 2 gm, Sugars 8 gm, Protein 4 gm

Corn on the Cob

Donna Conto • Saylorsburg, PA

Makes 6 servings (Ideal slow cooker size: 5–6-quart)

6 small (5½"–6½" long) ears of corn (in husk)

½ cup water

1. Remove silk from corn, as much as possible, but leave husks on.

2. Cut off ends of corn so ears can stand in the cooker.

3. Add water.

4. Cover. Cook on Low 2–3 hours.

Exchange List Values: Starch 1.0

Basic Nutritional Values: Calories 68 (Calories from Fat 5), Total Fat 1 gm (Saturated Fat 0.1 gm, Polyunsat Fat 0.3 gm, Monounsat Fat 0.2 gm, Cholesterol 0 mg), Sodium 3 mg, Total Carbohydrate 16 gm, Dietary Fiber 2 gm, Sugars 2 gm, Protein 2 gm

Eat one more serving of vegetables today than you usually would.

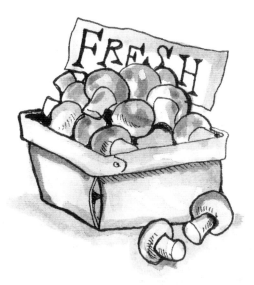

Cheesy Corn

Tina Snyder • Manheim, PA / Jeannine Janzen • Elbing, KS / Nadine Martinitz • Salina, KS

Makes 10 servings (Ideal slow cooker size: 4-quart)

3 16-oz. pkgs. frozen corn

8-oz. pkg. fat-free cream cheese, cubed

2 Tbsp. light, soft tub margarine

3 Tbsp. water

3 Tbsp. fat-free milk

2 Tbsp. sugar

6 slices reduced-fat American cheese, cut into squares

1. Combine all ingredients in slow cooker. Mix well.

2. Cover. Cook on Low 4 hours, or until heated through and cheese is melted.

Exchange List Values: Starch 2.0, Fat 0.5

Basic Nutritional Values: Calories 176 (Calories from Fat 29), Total Fat 3 gm (Saturated Fat 1.3 gm, Polyunsat Fat 0.5 gm, Monounsat Fat 1.2 gm, Cholesterol 8 mg), Sodium 220 mg, Total Carbohydrate 33 gm, Dietary Fiber 3 gm, Sugars 7 gm, Protein 7 gm

Super Creamed Corn

Ruth Ann Penner • Hillsboro, KS / Alix Nancy Botsford • Seminole, OK

Makes 8-12 servings (Ideal slow cooker size: 4-quart)

2 lbs. frozen corn

8-oz. pkg. fat-free cream cheese, cubed

2 Tbsp. margarine, melted

1 Tbsp. sugar

sugar substitute to equal ½ Tbsp.

2–3 Tbsp. water, optional

1. Combine ingredients in slow cooker.

2. Cover. Cook on Low 4 hours.

3. Serve with meat loaf, turkey, or hamburgers.

Exchange List Values: Starch 1.0, Fat 0.5

Basic Nutritional Values: Calories 99 (Calories from Fat 20), Total Fat 2 gm (Saturated Fat 0.4 gm, Polyunsat Fat 0.8 gm, Monounsat Fat 0.9 gm, Cholesterol 2 mg), Sodium 129 mg, Total Carbohydrate 17 gm, Dietary Fiber 2 gm, Sugars 3 gm, Protein 5 gm

A great addition to a holiday that is easy and requires no last-minute preparation. It also frees the stove and oven for other food preparation.

Baked Corn

Velma Stauffer • Akron, PA

Makes 8 servings (Ideal slow cooker size: 3-quart)

1 qt. corn, frozen or fresh

2 eggs, beaten

1 tsp. salt

1 cup fat-free milk

⅛ tsp. pepper

2 tsp. oil

1½ Tbsp. sugar

sugar substitute to equal 2 tsp.

3 Tbsp. flour

1. Combine all ingredients well. Pour into greased slow cooker.

2. Cover. Cook on High 3 hours, and then on Low 45 minutes.

Exchange List Values: Starch 1.5, Fat 0.5

Basic Nutritional Values: Calories 125 (Calories from Fat 25), Total Fat 3 gm (Saturated Fat 0.7 gm, Polyunsat Fat 0.7 gm, Monounsat Fat 1.3 gm, Cholesterol 54 mg), Sodium 324 mg, Total Carbohydrate 22 gm, Dietary Fiber 2 gm, Sugars 6 gm, Protein 5 gm

Note: If you use home-grown sweet corn, you could reduce the amount of sugar.

Scalloped Corn

Rebecca Plank Leichty • Harrisonburg, VA

Makes 8 servings (Ideal slow cooker size: 4-quart)

2 eggs

10¾-oz. can cream of celery soup

⅔ cup unseasoned bread crumbs

2 cups whole-kernel corn, drained, or cream-style corn

1 tsp. minced onion

⅛ tsp. pepper

1 Tbsp. sugar

1 Tbsp. light, soft tub margarine, melted

1. Beat eggs with fork. Add soup and bread crumbs. Mix well.

2. Add remaining ingredients and mix thoroughly. Pour into greased slow cooker.

3. Cover. Cook on High 3 hours, or on Low 6 hours.

Exchange List Values: Starch 1.0, Fat 1.0

Basic Nutritional Values: Calories 132 (Calories from Fat 44), Total Fat 5 gm (Saturated Fat 1.4 gm, Polyunsat Fat 1.5 gm, Monounsat Fat 1.5 gm, Cholesterol 55 mg), Sodium 473 mg, Total Carbohydrate 19 gm, Dietary Fiber 1 gm, Sugars 3 gm, Protein 4 gm

Baked Corn and Noodles

Ruth Hershey • Paradise, PA

Makes 6 servings (Ideal slow cooker size: 4-quart)

3 cups noodles, cooked al dente

2 cups fresh or frozen corn, thawed

¾ cup grated fat-free cheddar cheese or cubed Velveeta cheese

1 egg, beaten

2 Tbsp. light, soft tub margarine, melted

½ tsp. salt

1. Combine all ingredients in slow cooker.

2. Cover. Cook on Low 6–8 hours, or on High 3–4 hours.

Exchange List Values: Starch 2.0, Fat 0.5

Basic Nutritional Values: Calories 198 (Calories from Fat 34), Total Fat 4 gm (Saturated Fat 0.6 gm, Polyunsat Fat 0.9 gm, Monounsat Fat 1.6 gm, Cholesterol 63 mg), Sodium 343 mg, Total Carbohydrate 32 gm, Dietary Fiber 2 gm, Sugars 3 gm, Protein 11 gm

Mexican Corn

Betty K. Drescher • Quakertown, PA

Makes 8 servings (Ideal slow cooker size: 3–4-quart)

2 10-oz. pkgs. frozen corn, partially thawed

4-oz. jar chopped pimentos

⅓ cup chopped green peppers

⅓ cup water

1 tsp. salt

¼ tsp. pepper

½ tsp. paprika

½ tsp. chili powder

1. Combine all ingredients in slow cooker.

2. Cover. Cook on High 45 minutes, then on Low 2–4 hours. Stir occasionally.

Exchange List Values: Starch 1.0

Basic Nutritional Values: Calories 63 (Calories from Fat 3), Total Fat 0 gm (Saturated Fat 0.1 gm, Polyunsat Fat 0.2 gm, Monounsat Fat 0.1 gm, Cholesterol 0 mg), Sodium 298 mg, Total Carbohydrate 15 gm, Dietary Fiber 2 gm, Sugars 2 gm, Protein 2 gm

VARIATIONS: For more fire, add ⅓ cup salsa to the ingredients, and increase the amounts of pepper, paprika, and chili powder to match your taste.

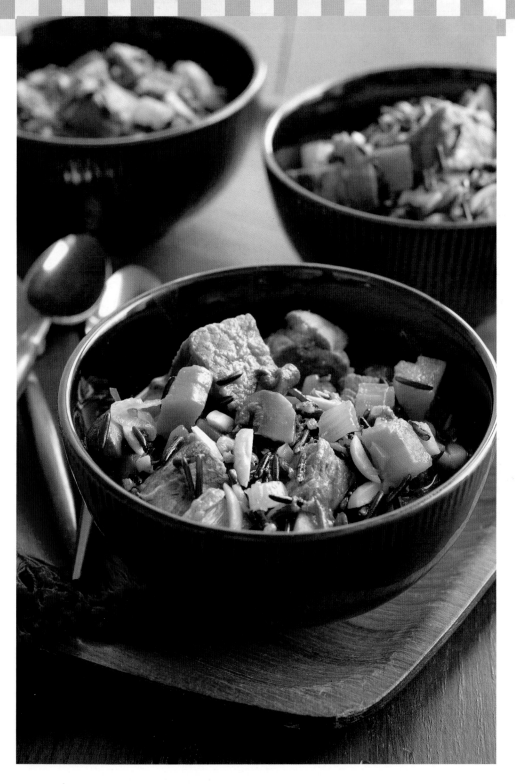

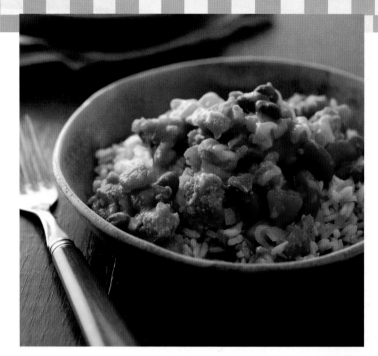

Chili and Cheese on
Rice ■ 39

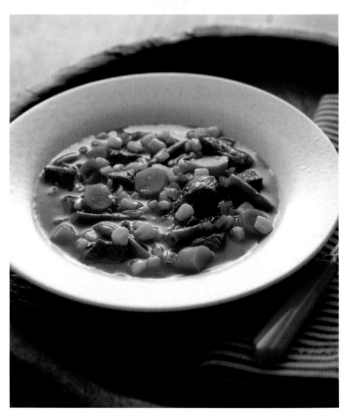

Sante Fe Stew ■ 18

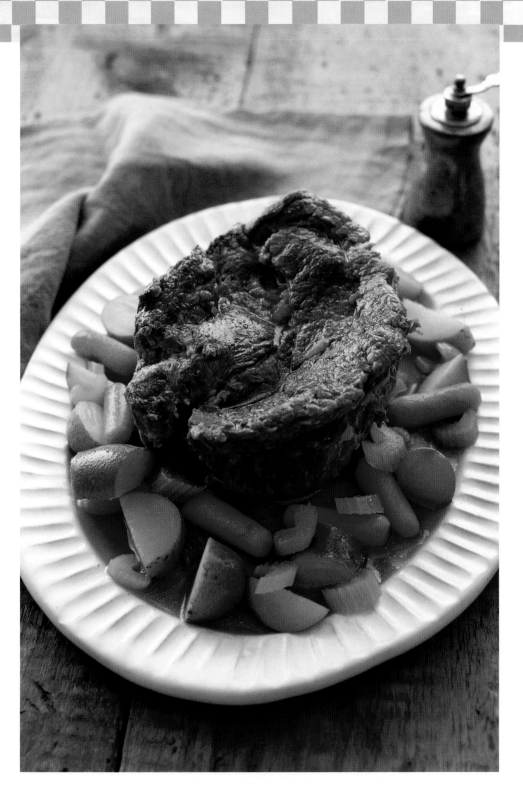

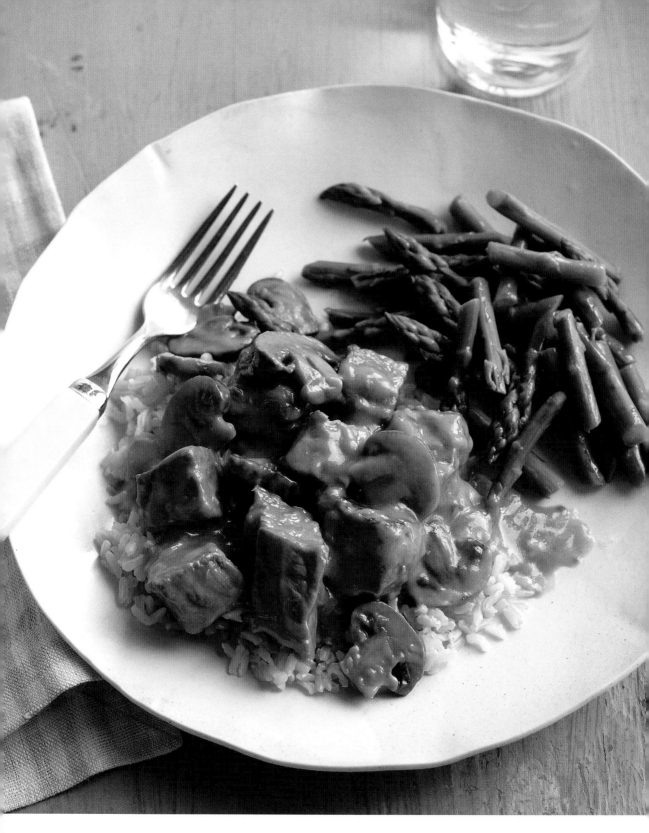

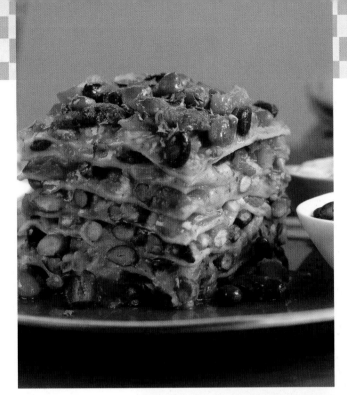

Three-Bean Burrito
Bake ■ 26

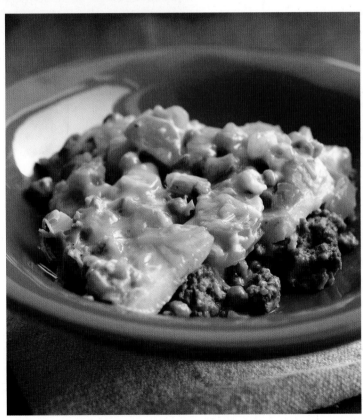

Supper-in-a-Dish
■ 43

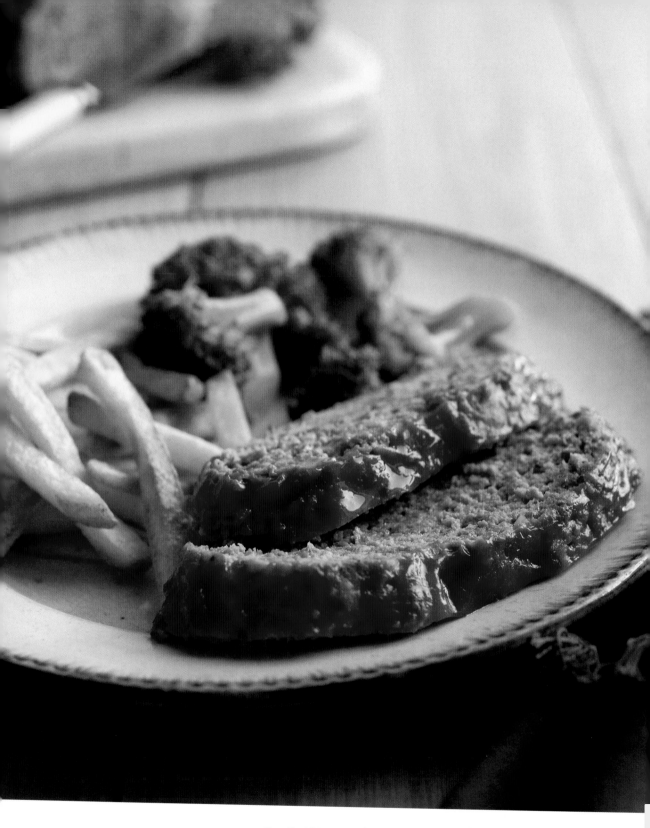

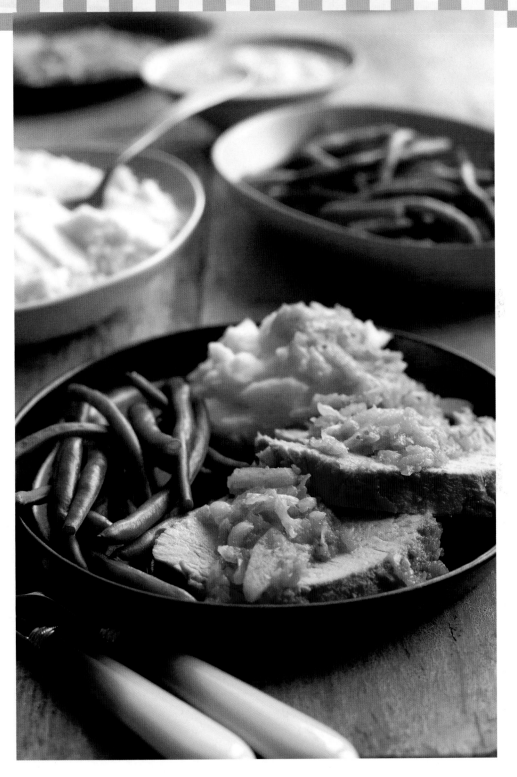

Pork Roast with Sauerkraut

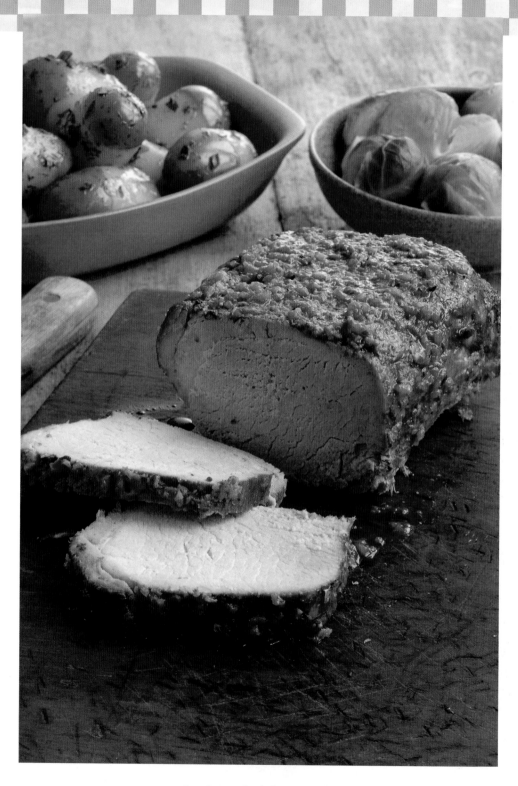

Cranberry Pork Roast ■ 57

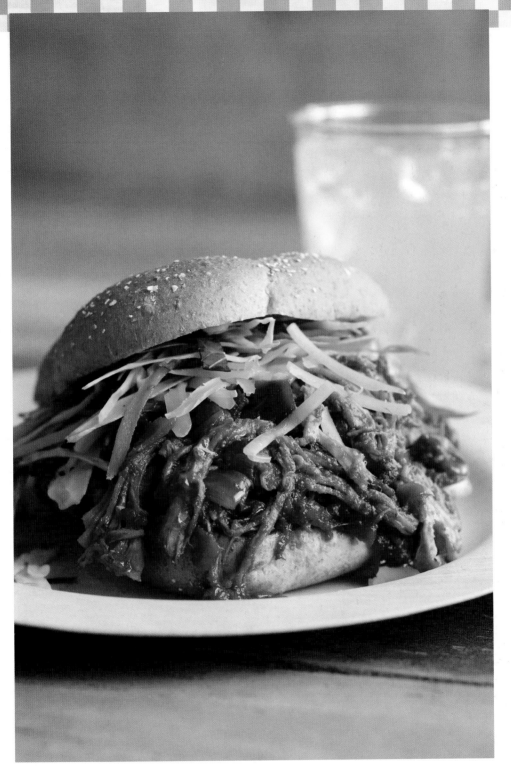

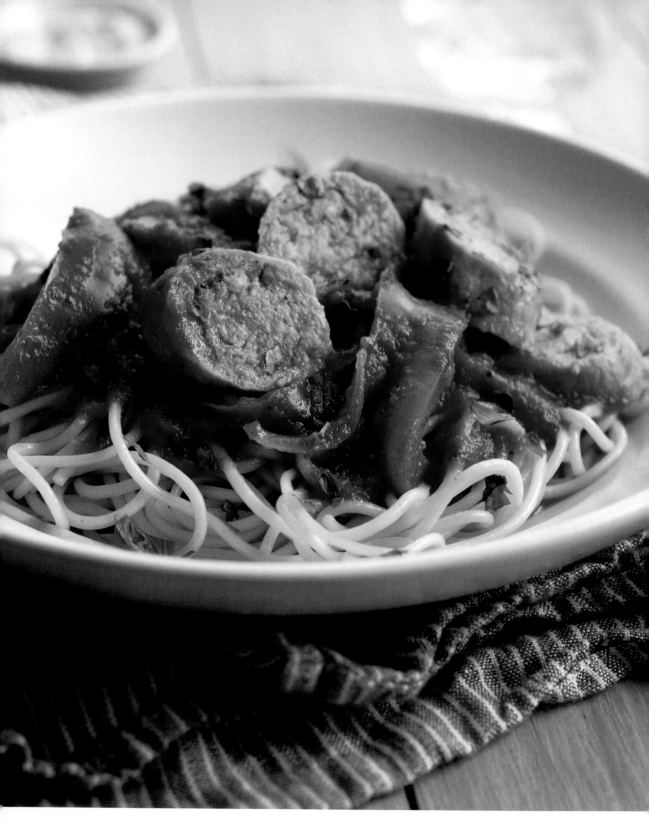

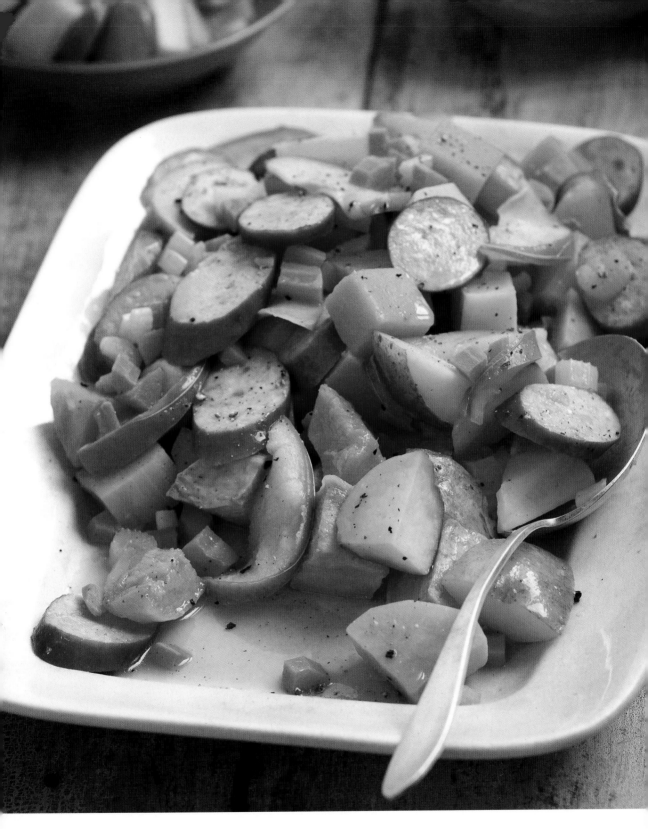

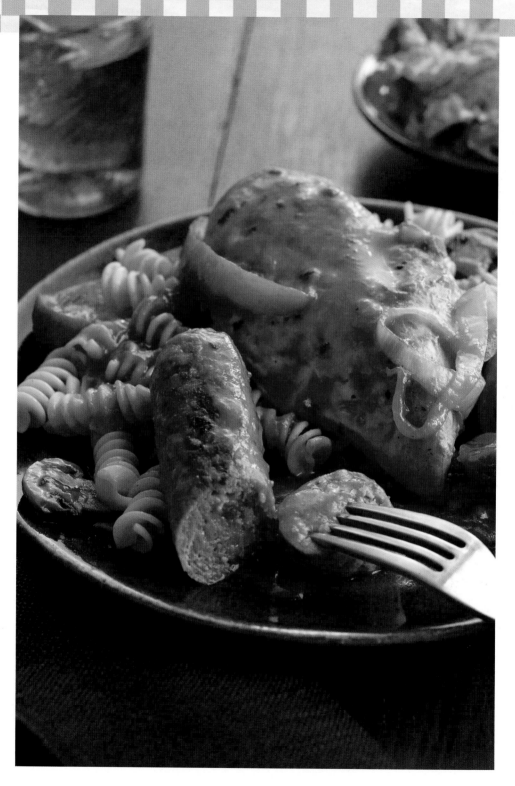

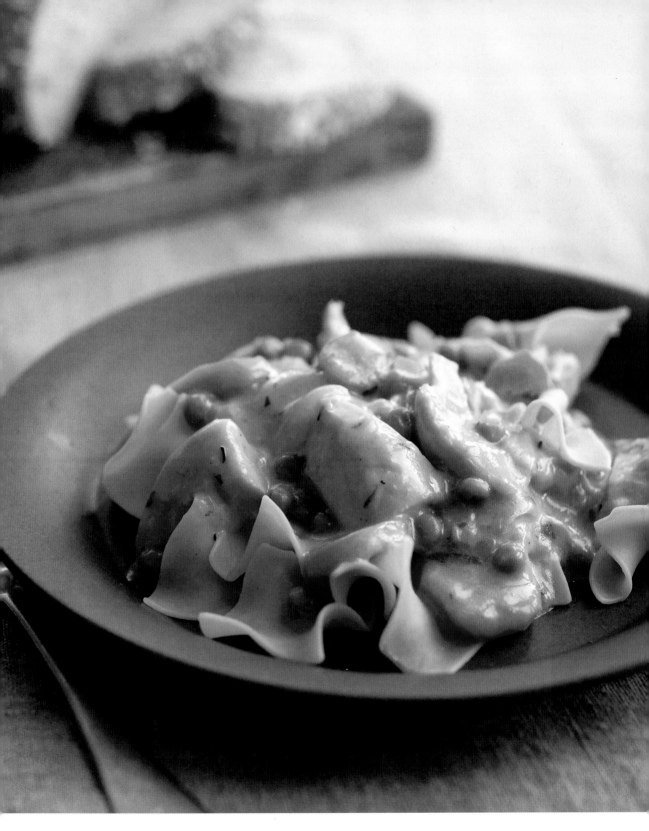

Creamy Chicken and Noodles

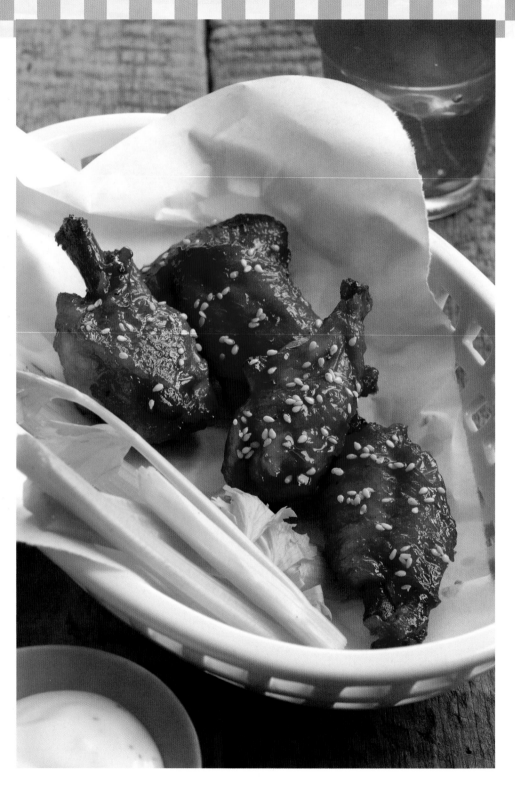

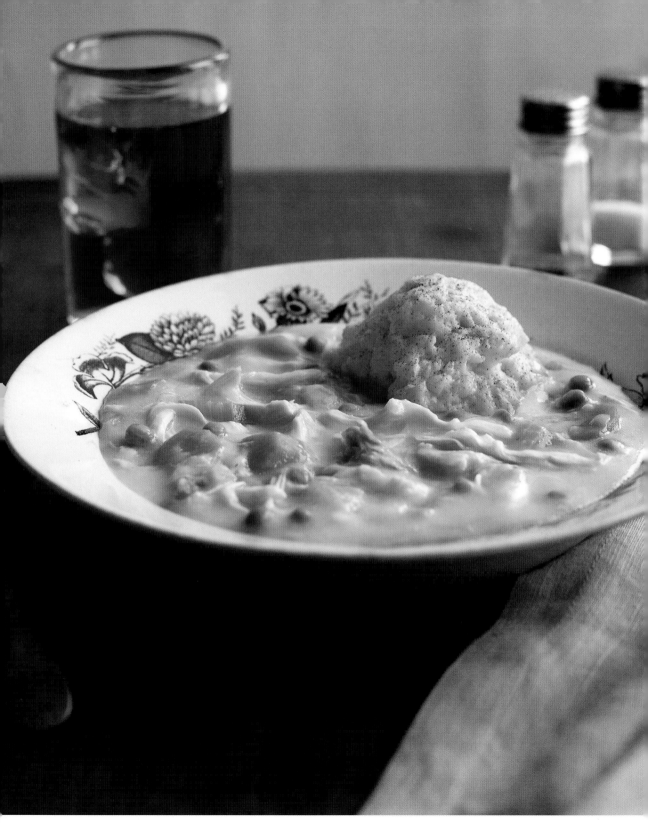

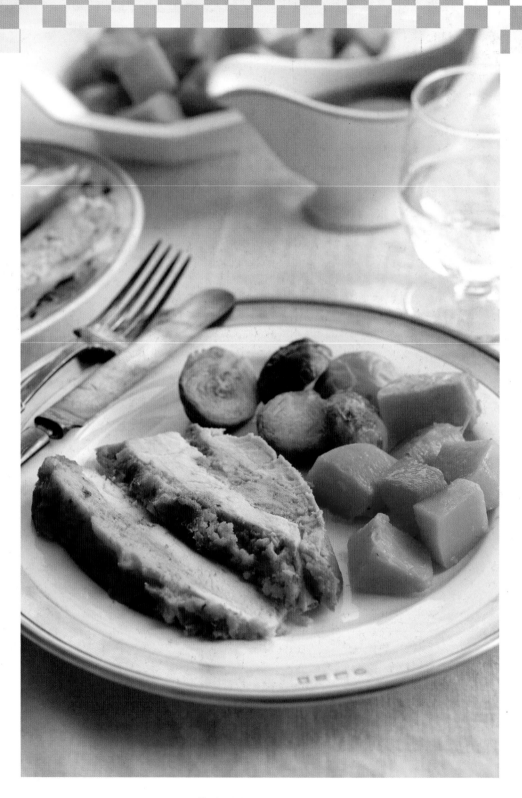

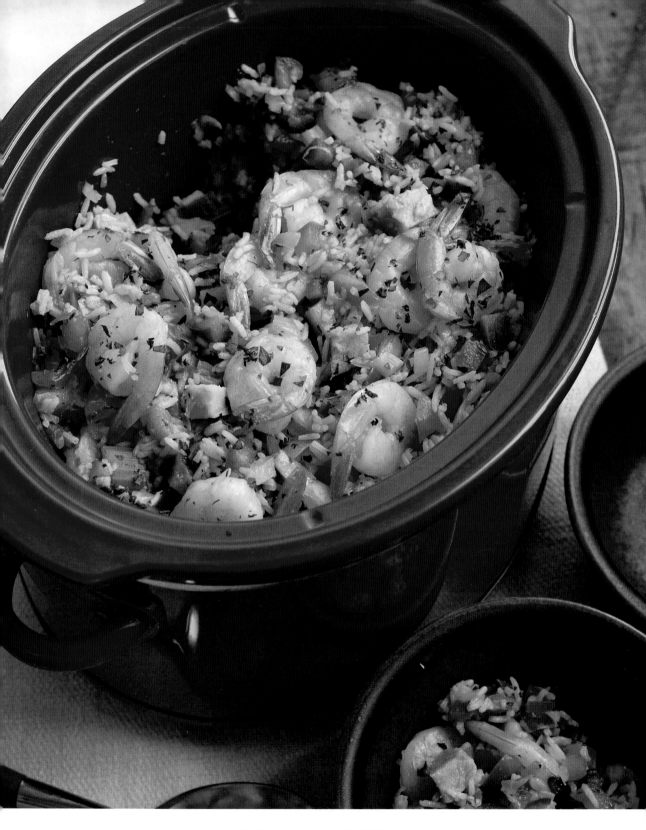

Shrimp Jambalaya ■ 140

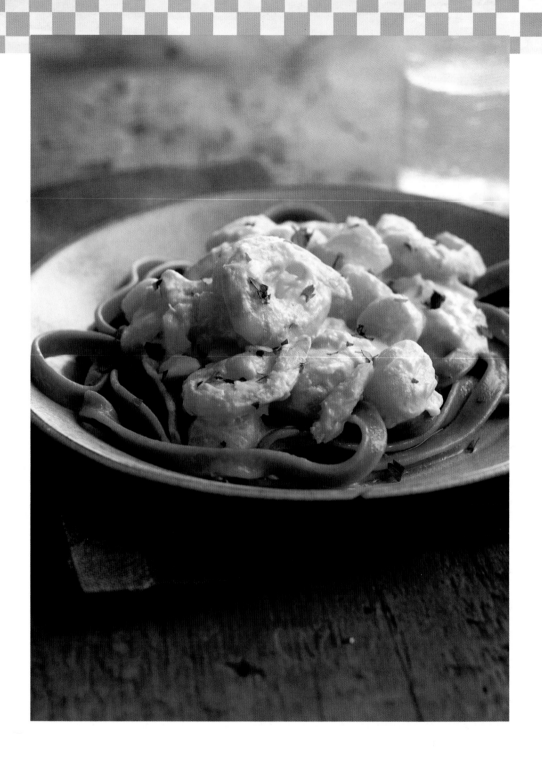

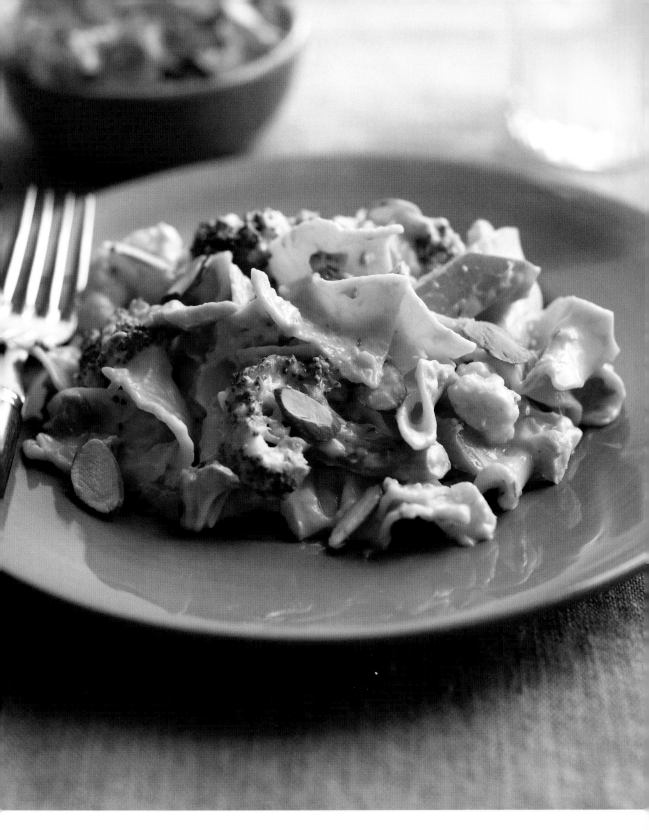

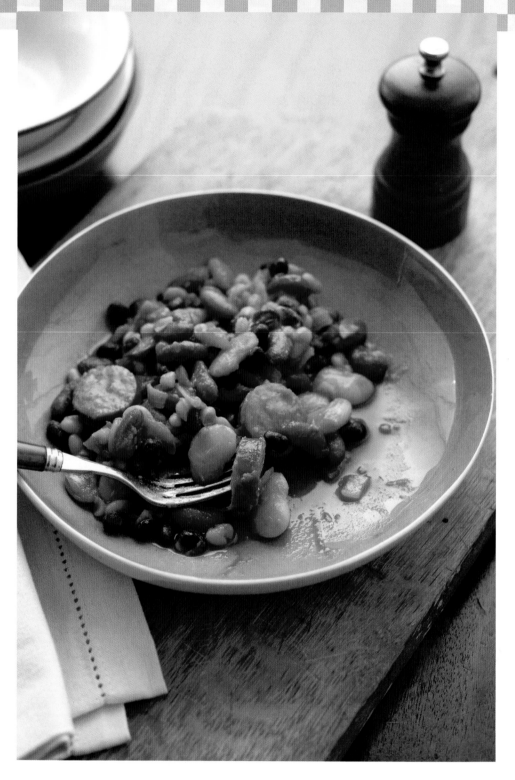

Four Beans and Sausage

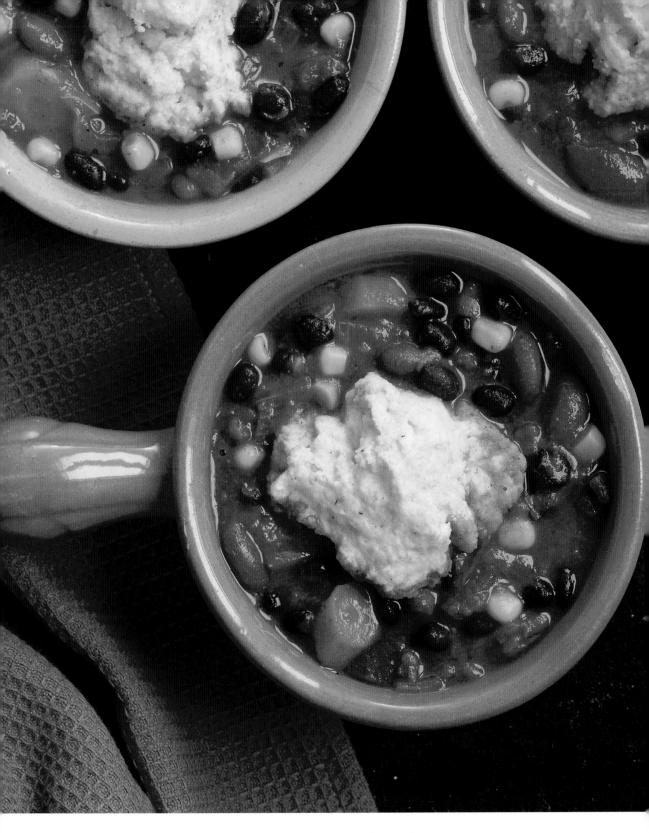

Southwestern Bean Soup with Cornmeal Dumplings

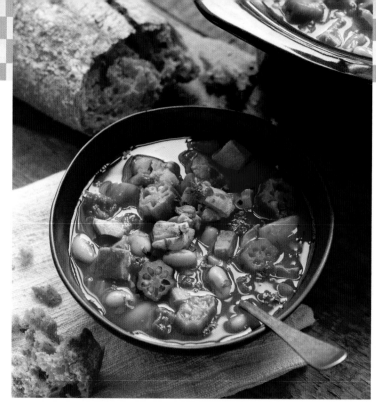

 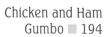

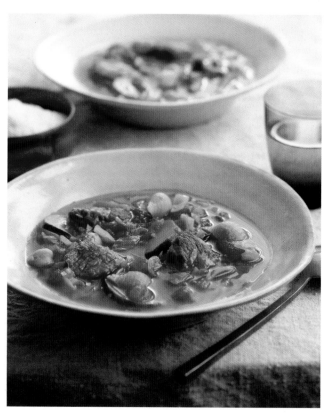

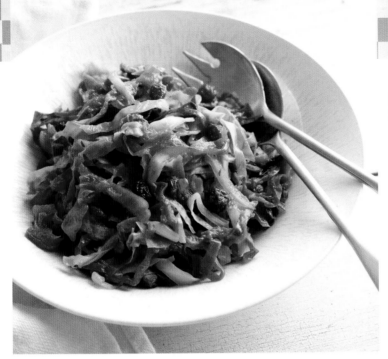

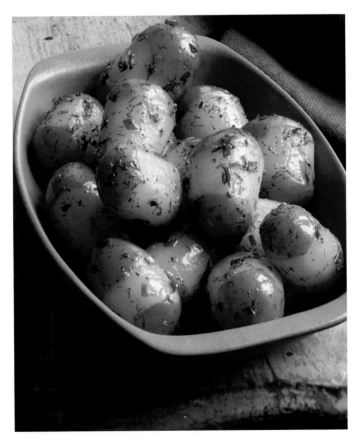

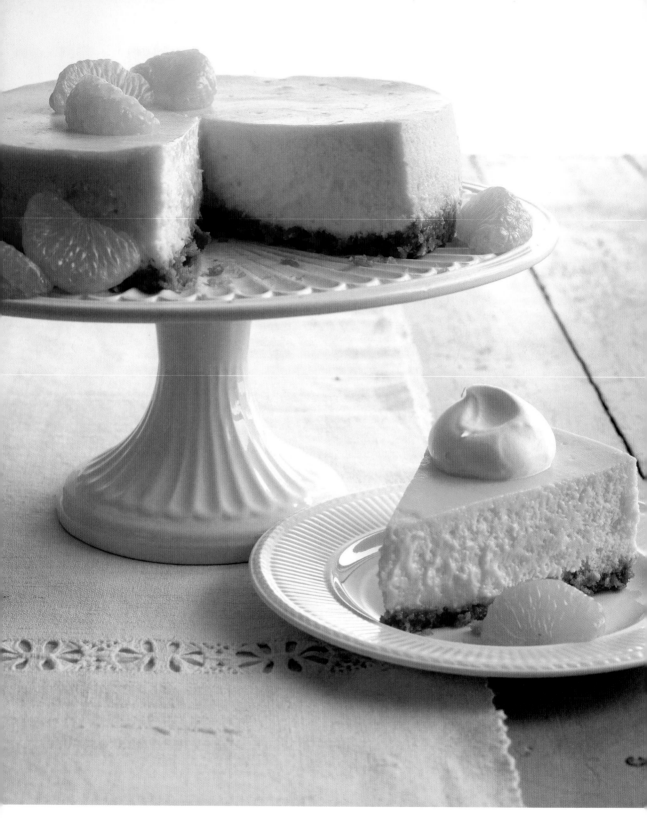

Creamy Orange Cheesecake ■ 282

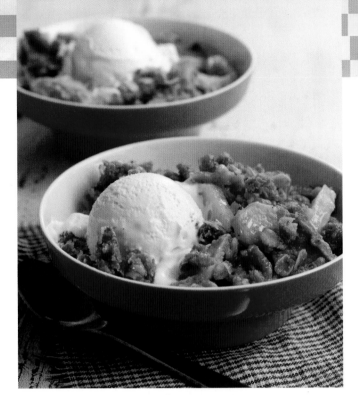

Apple Peanut Crumble ▦ 286

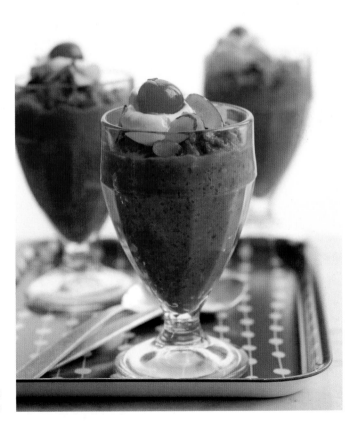

Chocolate Rice
Pudding ▦ 289

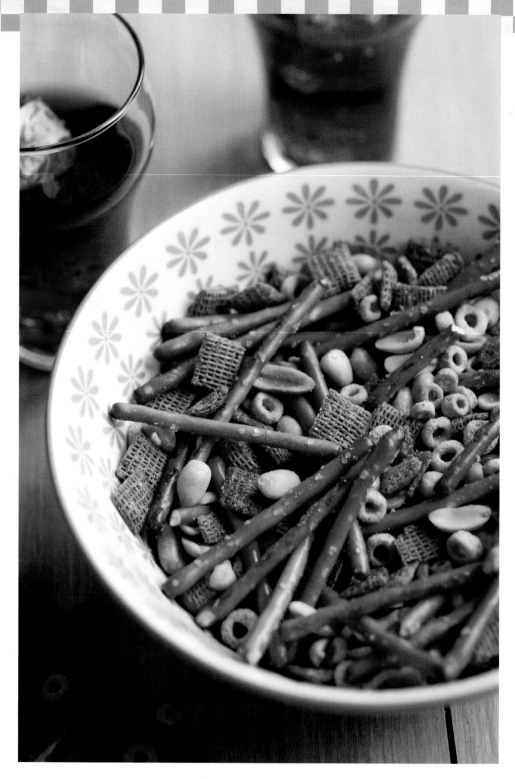

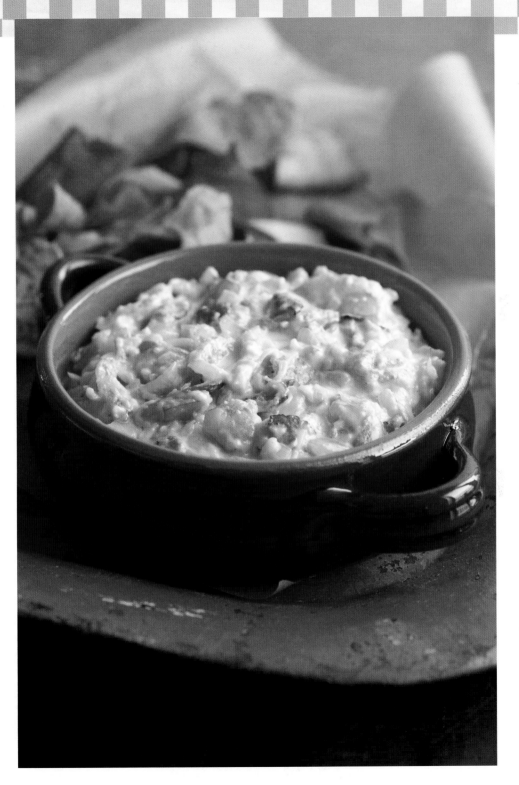

Cheesy New Orleans Shrimp Dip ▪ 298

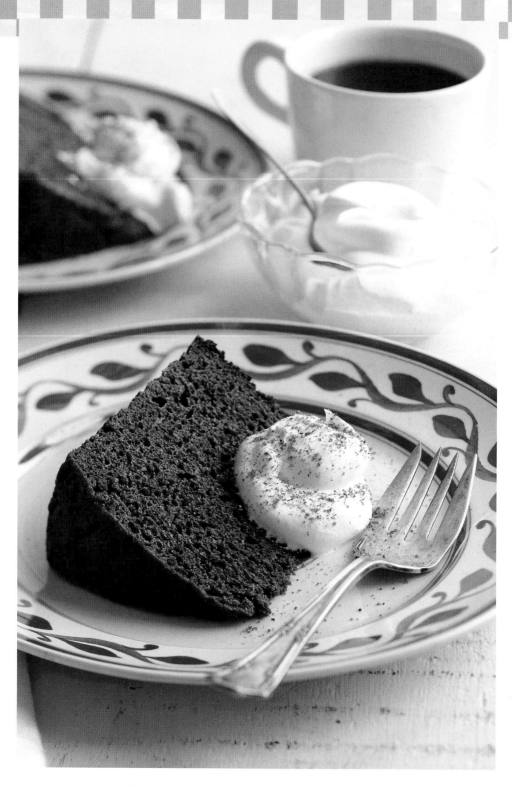

Old-Fashioned Gingerbread ■ 332

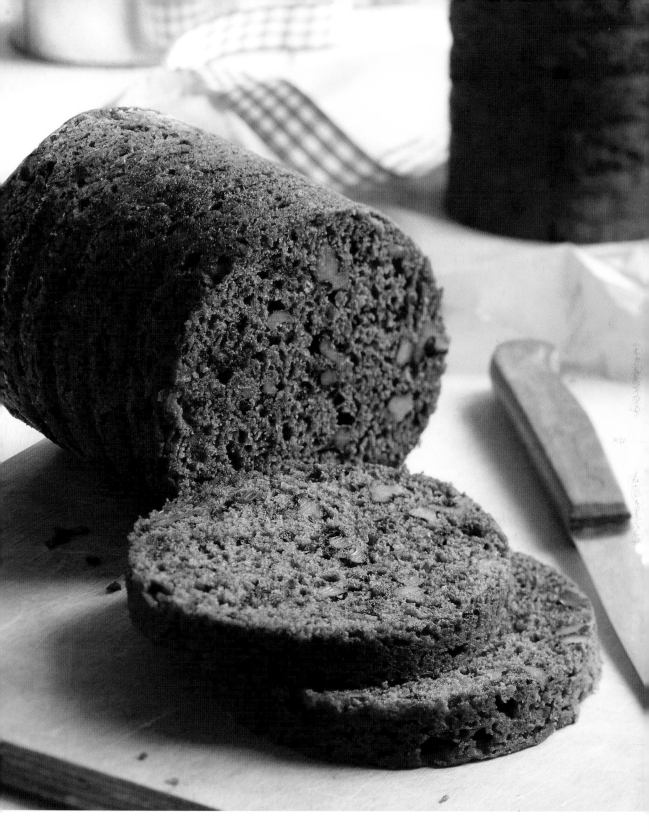

Date and Nut Loaf ■ 328

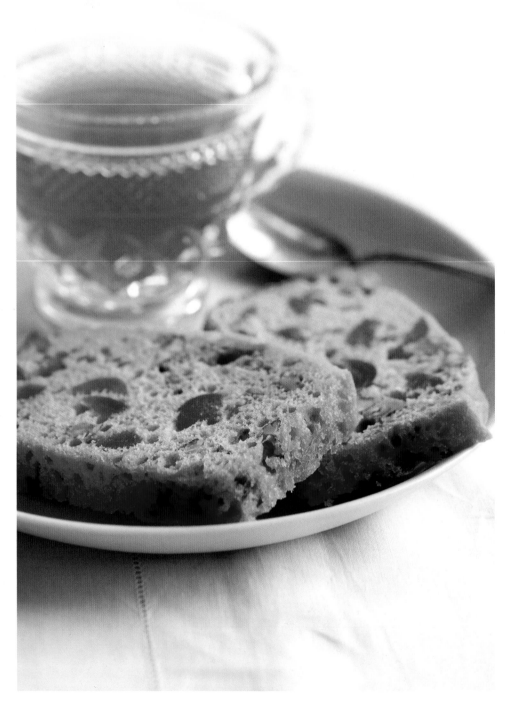

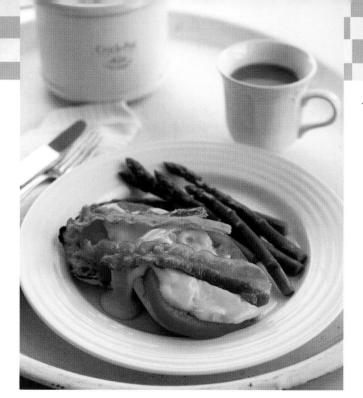

Welsh Rarebit ■ 318

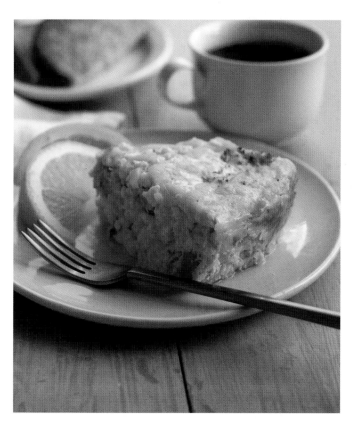

Egg and Broccoli
Casserole ■ 320

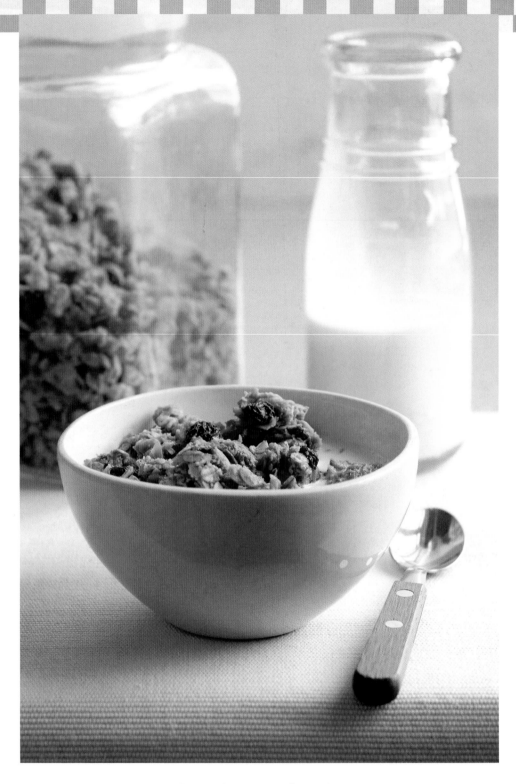

Confetti Scalloped Corn

Rhoda Atzeff • Harrisburg, PA

Makes 12 servings (Ideal slow cooker size: 4-quart)

2 eggs, beaten

1 cup fat-free sour cream

2 Tbsp. light, soft tub margarine, melted

1 small onion, finely chopped, or 2 Tbsp. dried chopped onion

11-oz. can Mexicorn, drained

14-oz. can cream-style corn

2-3 Tbsp. green jalapeno salsa, regular salsa, or chopped green chilies

8½-oz. pkg. corn bread mix

1. Combine all ingredients. Pour into lightly greased slow cooker.

2. Cover. Bake on High 2–2½ hours, or until corn is fully cooked.

Exchange List Values: Starch 2.0

Basic Nutritional Values: Calories 147 (Calories from Fat 32), Total Fat 4 gm (Saturated Fat 1.1 gm, Polyunsat Fat 0.6 gm, Monounsat Fat 1.2 gm, Cholesterol 37 mg), Sodium 408 mg, Total Carbohydrate 29 gm, Dietary Fiber 1 gm, Sugars 10 gm, Protein 4 gm

Corn Bread Casserole

Arlene Groff • Lewistown, PA

Makes 16 servings (Ideal slow cooker size: 4-quart)

1 qt. frozen whole-kernel corn, thawed

1 qt. creamed corn

8½-oz. pkg. corn muffin mix

1 egg

2 Tbsp. light, soft tub margarine

¼ tsp. garlic powder

2 Tbsp. sugar

¼ cup fat-free milk

½ tsp. salt

¼ tsp. pepper

1. Combine ingredients in greased slow cooker.

2. Cover. Cook on Low 3½–4 hours, stirring once halfway through.

Exchange List Values: Starch 2.0

Basic Nutritional Values: Calories 141 (Calories from Fat 23), Total Fat 3 gm (Saturated Fat 0.7 gm, Polyunsat Fat 0.5 gm, Monounsat Fat 0.8 gm, Cholesterol 13 mg), Sodium 412 mg, Total Carbohydrate 31 gm, Dietary Fiber 2 gm, Sugars 10 gm, Protein 3 gm

Slow Cooker Rice

Dorothy Horst • Tiskilwa, IL

Makes 20 servings (Ideal slow cooker size: 5–6-quart)

1 Tbsp. margarine, melted

4 cups converted long-grain rice, uncooked

10 cups water

2 tsp. salt

1. Pour margarine, rice, water, and salt into greased slow cooker.

2. Cover. Cook on High 2–3 hours, or until rice is tender, but not overcooked. Stir occasionally.

Exchange List Values: Starch 2.0

Basic Nutritional Values: Calories 140 (Calories from Fat 7), Total Fat 1 gm (Saturated Fat 0.1 gm, Polyunsat Fat 0.2 gm, Monounsat Fat 0.3 gm, Cholesterol 0 mg), Sodium 241 mg, Total Carbohydrate 30 gm, Dietary Fiber 0 gm, Sugars 0 gm, Protein 3 gm

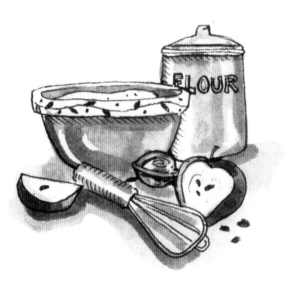

Fruited Wild Rice with Pecans

Dottie Schmidt • Kansas City, MO

Makes 8 servings (Ideal slow cooker size: 4-quart)

½ cup chopped onions

1 Tbsp. canola oil

6-oz. pkg. long-grain and wild rice

seasoning packet from wild rice package

1½ cups hot water

⅔ cup apple juice

1 large tart apple, chopped

¼ cup raisins

¼ cup coarsely chopped pecans

1. Combine all ingredients except pecans in slow cooker sprayed with non-fat cooking spray.

2. Cover. Cook on High 2–2½ hours.

3. Stir in pecans. Serve.

Exchange List Values: Starch 1.0, Fruit 1.0, Fat 0.5

Basic Nutritional Values: Calories 154 (Calories from Fat 43), Total Fat 5 gm (Saturated Fat 0.4 gm, Polyunsat Fat 1.3 gm, Monounsat Fat 2.7 gm, Cholesterol 0 mg), Sodium 237 mg, Total Carbohydrate 27 gm, Dietary Fiber 2 gm, Sugars 9 gm, Protein 3 gm

Mjeddrah

Dianna Milhizer • Brighton, MI

Makes 24 servings (Ideal slow cooker size: 5-quart)

10 cups water

4 cups dried lentils, rinsed

2 cups uncooked brown rice

$\frac{1}{4}$ cup olive oil

2 tsp. salt

1. Combine ingredients in large slow cooker.

2. Cover. Cook on High 8 hours, then on Low 2 hours. Add 2 more cups water, if needed, to allow rice to cook and to prevent dish from drying out.

3. This is traditionally eaten with a salad with an oil-and-vinegar dressing over the lentil-rice mixture, similar to a tostada without the tortilla.

Exchange List Values: Starch 2.0, Fat 0.5

Basic Nutritional Values: Calories 173 (Calories from Fat 27), Total Fat 3 gm (Saturated Fat 0.4 gm, Polyunsat Fat 0.5 gm, Monounsat Fat 1.9 gm, Cholesterol 0 mg), Sodium 196 mg, Total Carbohydrate 29 gm, Dietary Fiber 7 gm, Sugars 2 gm, Protein 9 gm

Risi Bisi (Peas and Rice)

Cyndie Marrara • Port Matilda, PA

Makes 8 servings (Ideal slow cooker size: 4-quart)

$1\frac{1}{2}$ cups converted long-grain white rice, uncooked

$\frac{3}{4}$ cup chopped onions

2 cloves garlic, minced

2 14$\frac{1}{2}$-oz. cans reduced-sodium chicken broth

$\frac{1}{3}$ cup water

$\frac{3}{4}$ tsp. Italian Seasoning Mix (see recipe on page 333)

$\frac{1}{2}$ tsp. dried basil leaves

$\frac{1}{2}$ cup frozen baby peas, thawed

$\frac{1}{4}$ cup freshly grated Parmesan cheese

1. Combine rice, onions, and garlic in slow cooker.

2. In saucepan, mix together chicken broth and water. Bring to boil. Add Italian seasoning and basil leaves. Stir into rice mixture.

3. Cover. Cook on Low 2–3 hours, or until liquid is absorbed.

4. Stir in peas. Cover. Cook 30 minutes. Stir in cheese.

Exchange List Values: Starch 2.0

Basic Nutritional Values: Calories 165 (Calories from Fat 11), Total Fat 1 gm (Saturated Fat 0.5 gm, Polyunsat Fat 0.1 gm, Monounsat Fat 0.4 gm, Cholesterol 3 mg), Sodium 409 mg, Total Carbohydrate 32 gm, Dietary Fiber 1 gm, Sugars 2 gm, Protein 6 gm

Green Rice Casserole

Ruth Hofstetter • Versailles, Missouri

Makes 6 servings (Ideal slow cooker size: 4-quart)

1⅓ cups fat-free evaporated milk

2 Tbsp. vegetable oil

3 eggs

one-fourth of a small onion, minced

half a small carrot, minced, optional

2 cups minced fresh parsley, or 10-oz. pkg. frozen chopped spinach, thawed and drained

¼ tsp. salt

¼ tsp. pepper

1 cup shredded fat-free sharp cheddar cheese

3 cups cooked long-grain rice

1. Beat together milk, oil, and eggs until well combined.

2. Stir in remaining ingredients. Mix well. Pour into greased slow cooker.

3. Cover. Cook on High 1 hour. Stir. Reduce heat to Low and cook 4–6 hours.

Exchange List Values: Starch 1.5, Milk, fat-free 0.5, Meat, medium fat 1.0, Fat 1.0

Basic Nutritional Values: Calories 264 (Calories from Fat 67), Total Fat 7 gm (Saturated Fat 1.4 gm, Polyunsat Fat 1.8 gm, Monounsat Fat 3.8 gm, Cholesterol 109 mg), Sodium 345 mg, Total Carbohydrate 32 gm, Dietary Fiber 1 gm, Sugars 7 gm, Protein 16 gm

Wild Rice

Ruth S. Weaver • Reinholds, PA

Makes 4–5 servings (Ideal slow cooker size: 3-4-quart)

1 cup wild rice, or wild rice mixture, uncooked

½ cup sliced mushrooms

½ cup diced onions

½ cup diced green, or red, peppers

1 Tbsp. oil

¼ tsp. salt

¼ tsp. pepper

2½ cups 98%-fat-free, reduced-sodium chicken broth

1. Layer rice and vegetables in slow cooker. Pour oil, salt, and pepper over vegetables. Stir.

2. Heat chicken broth. Pour over ingredients in slow cooker.

3. Cover. Cook on High 2½–3 hours, or until rice is soft and liquid is absorbed.

Exchange List Values: Starch 2.0

Basic Nutritional Values: Calories 157 (Calories from Fat 28), Total Fat 3 gm (Saturated Fat 0.2 gm, Polyunsat Fat 1.0 gm, Monounsat Fat 1.7 gm, Cholesterol 0 mg), Sodium 370 mg, Total Carbohydrate 27 gm, Dietary Fiber 3 gm, Sugars 3 gm, Protein 6 gm

Baked Potatoes

Lucille Metzler • Wellsboro, PA / Elizabeth Yutzy • Wauseon, OH / Glenda S. Weaver • Manheim, PA / Mary Jane Musser • Manheim, PA / Esther Becker • Gordonville, PA

Makes 6 servings (Ideal slow cooker size: 4-quart)

6 medium (5¾ ozs.) baking potatoes

1 Tbsp. margarine

1. Prick potatoes with fork. Rub each with margarine. Place in slow cooker.

2. Cover. Cook on High 3–5 hours, or Low 6–10 hours.

Exchange List Values: Starch 2.0

Basic Nutritional Values: Calories 147 (Calories from Fat 17), Total Fat 2 gm (Saturated Fat 0.3 gm, Polyunsat Fat 0.7 gm, Monounsat Fat 0.8 gm, Cholesterol 0 mg), Sodium 34 mg, Total Carbohydrate 29 gm, Dietary Fiber 3 gm, Sugars 3 gm, Protein 4 gm

Good snack choices include grains, fruits, and vegetables.

Pizza Potatoes

Margaret Wenger Johnson • Keezletown, VA

Makes 8 servings (Ideal slow cooker size: 4-quart)

6 (5¾ ozs.) medium potatoes, sliced

1 large onion, thinly sliced

2 Tbsp. olive oil

6 ozs. (1½ cups) grated fat-free mozzarella cheese

2 ozs. sliced turkey pepperoni

8-oz. can pizza sauce

1. Saute potato and onion slices in oil in skillet until onions appear transparent. Drain well.

2. In slow cooker, combine potatoes, onions, cheese, and pepperoni.

3. Pour pizza sauce over top.

4. Cover. Cook on Low 6–10 hours, or until potatoes are soft.

Exchange List Values: Starch 2.0, Meat, lean 1.0

Basic Nutritional Values: Calories 205 (Calories from Fat 43), Total Fat 5 gm (Saturated Fat 0.9 gm, Polyunsat Fat 0.8 gm, Monounsat Fat 2.9 gm, Cholesterol 12 mg), Sodium 417 mg, Total Carbohydrate 27 gm, Dietary Fiber 3 gm, Sugars 6 gm, Protein 13 gm

Potatoes O'Brien

Rebecca Meyerkorth • Wamego, KS

Makes 8 servings (Ideal slow cooker size: 4-quart)

32-oz. pkg. shredded potatoes

¼ cup chopped onions

¼ cup chopped green peppers

¼ tsp. salt

¼ tsp. pepper

2 Tbsp. margarine

3 Tbsp. flour

½ cup fat-free milk

10¾-oz. can 98%-fat-free, reduced-sodium cream of mushroom soup

1 cup shredded fat-free cheddar cheese, divided

1. Place potatoes, onions, and green peppers in slow cooker. Sprinkle with salt and pepper.

2. Melt margarine in saucepan. Stir in flour; then add half of milk. Stir rapidly to remove all lumps. Stir in remaining milk. Stir in mushroom soup and ½ cup cheese. Pour over potatoes.

3. Cover. Cook on Low 4–5 hours. Sprinkle remaining cheese on top about ½ hour before serving.

Exchange List Values: Starch 2.0, Fat 0.5

Basic Nutritional Values: Calories 193 (Calories from Fat 38), Total Fat 4 gm (Saturated Fat 1.0 gm, Polyunsat Fat 1.4 gm, Monounsat Fat 1.5 gm, Cholesterol 2 mg), Sodium 379 mg, Total Carbohydrate 30 gm, Dietary Fiber 2 gm, Sugars 3 gm, Protein 9 gm

VARIATION: Add to Step 1: 2 Tbsp. chopped pimento and 1 cup chopped ham.

Garlic Mashed Potatoes

Katrine Rose • Woodbridge, VA

Makes 6 servings (Ideal slow cooker size: 4-quart)

2 lbs. baking potatoes, unpeeled and cut into ½" cubes

¼ cup water

3 Tbsp. light, soft tub margarine

¾ tsp. salt

¾ tsp. garlic powder

¼ tsp. black pepper

1 cup 2% milk

1. Combine all ingredients, except milk, in slow cooker. Toss to combine.

2. Cover. Cook on Low 7 hours, or on High 4 hours.

3. Add milk to potatoes during last 30 minutes of cooking time.

4. Mash potatoes with potato masher or electric mixer until fairly smooth.

Exchange List Values: Starch 2.0, Fat 0.5

Basic Nutritional Values: Calories 167 (Calories from Fat 29), Total Fat 3 gm (Saturated Fat 0.4 gm, Polyunsat Fat 0.6 gm, Monounsat Fat 1.6 gm, Cholesterol 3 mg), Sodium 361 mg, Total Carbohydrate 31 gm, Dietary Fiber 3 gm, Sugars 4 gm, Protein 4 gm

Company Mashed Potatoes

Eileen Eash • Carlsbad, NM

Makes 12 servings (Ideal slow cooker size: 6-quart)

15 (5 lbs. total) medium-sized potatoes

1 cup reduced-fat sour cream

1 small onion, diced fine

1 tsp. salt

⅛–¼ tsp. pepper, according to your taste preference

1 cup buttermilk

1 cup fresh, chopped spinach, optional

1 cup grated Colby or cheddar cheese, optional

1. Peel and quarter potatoes. Place in slow cooker. Barely cover with water.

2. Cover. Cook on Low 8–10 hours. Drain water.

3. Mash potatoes. Add remaining ingredients except cheese.

4. Cover. Heat on Low 4–6 hours.

5. Sprinkle with cheese 5 minutes before serving.

Exchange List Values: Starch 2.0

Basic Nutritional Values: Calories 160 (Calories from Fat 18), Total Fat 2 gm (Saturated Fat 1.1 gm, Polyunsat Fat 0.1 gm, Monounsat Fat 0.5 gm, Cholesterol 7 mg), Sodium 236 mg, Total Carbohydrate 32 gm, Dietary Fiber 3 gm, Sugars 5 gm, Protein 5 gm

Notes:

1. Buttermilk gives mashed potatoes a unique flavor that most people enjoy. I often serve variations of this recipe for guests and they always ask what I put in the potatoes.

2. I save the water drained from cooking the potatoes and use it to make gravy or a soup base.

3. Small amounts of leftovers from this recipe add a special flavor to vegetable or noodle soup for another meal.

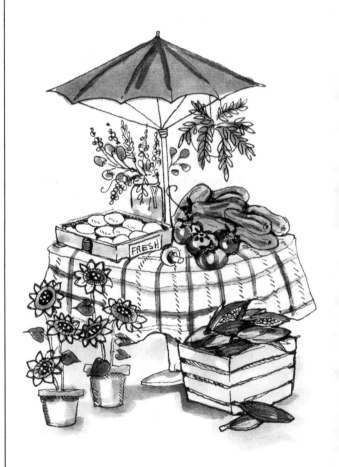

Creamy Mashed Potatoes

Brenda S. Burkholder • Port Republic, VA

Makes 10–12 servings (Ideal slow cooker size: 5-quart)

1 tsp. salt

4 Tbsp. margarine, melted

2¼ cups fat-free milk

6⅞ cups potato flakes

6 cups water

4 ozs. (approximately half of large pkg.) fat-free cream cheese, softened

1 cup fat-free sour cream

1. Combine first five ingredients as directed on potato box.

2. Whip cream cheese with electric mixer until creamy. Blend in sour cream.

3. Fold potatoes into cheese and sour cream. Beat well. Place in slow cooker.

4. Cover. Cook on Low 3–5 hours.

Exchange List Values: Starch 2.0, Fat 0.5

Basic Nutritional Values: Calories 173 (Calories from Fat 36), Total Fat 4 gm (Saturated Fat 0.8 gm, Polyunsat Fat 1.2 gm, Monounsat Fat 1.7 gm, Cholesterol 3 mg), Sodium 361 mg, Total Carbohydrate 29 gm, Dietary Fiber 2 gm, Sugars 4 gm, Protein 6 gm

Herbed Potatoes

Jo Haberkamp • Fairbank, IA

Recipe photo appears in color section.

Makes 6 servings (Ideal slow cooker size: 4-quart)

1½ lbs. small new potatoes

¼ cup water

¼ cup light, soft tub margarine, melted

3 Tbsp. chopped fresh parsley

1 Tbsp. lemon juice

1 Tbsp. chopped fresh chives

1 Tbsp. dill weed

¼-½ tsp. salt, according to your taste preference

⅛-¼ tsp. pepper, according to your taste preference

1. Wash potatoes. Peel a strip around the center of each potato. Place in slow cooker.

2. Add water.

3. Cover. Cook on High 2½–3 hours. Drain well.

4. In saucepan, heat margarine, parsley, lemon juice, chives, dill, salt, and pepper. Pour over potatoes.

5. Serve with ham or any meat dish that does not make gravy.

Exchange List Values: Starch 1.5, Fat 0.5

Basic Nutritional Values: Calories 122 (Calories from Fat 28), Total Fat 3 gm (Saturated Fat 0 gm, Polyunsat Fat 0.7 gm, Monounsat Fat 1.7 gm, Cholesterol 0 mg), Sodium 163 mg, Total Carbohydrate 22 gm, Dietary Fiber 2 gm, Sugars 2 gm, Protein 2 gm

Onion Potatoes

Donna Lantgen • Rapid City, SD

Makes 6 servings (Ideal slow cooker size: 4-quart)

6 medium potatoes, diced

1/3 cup olive oil

1 pkg. dry onion soup mix

1. Combine potatoes and olive oil in plastic bag. Shake well.

2. Add onion soup mix. Shake well.

3. Pour into slow cooker.

4. Cover. Cook on Low 6 hours, or High 3 hours.

Exchange List Values: Starch 2.0, Fat 2.0

Basic Nutritional Values: Calories 252 (Calories from Fat 110), Total Fat 12 gm (Saturated Fat 1.6 gm, Polyunsat Fat 1.1 gm, Monounsat Fat 8.9 gm, Cholesterol 0 mg), Sodium 465 mg, Total Carbohydrate 32 gm, Dietary Fiber 4 gm, Sugars 5 gm, Protein 5 gm

VARIATIONS: Add more zest to the potatoes by stirring in 1 small onion, chopped; 1 bell pepper, chopped; 1/2 tsp. salt; and 1/4 tsp. black pepper, after pouring the potatoes into the slow cooker. Continue with Step 4.

Potatoes Perfect

Naomi Ressler • Harrisonburg, VA

Makes 4-6 servings (Ideal slow cooker size: 4-quart)

1/4 lb. bacon, diced and browned until crisp

2 medium-sized onions, thinly sliced

6-8 medium-sized potatoes, thinly sliced

4 ozs. fat-free cheddar cheese, thinly sliced

salt to taste

pepper to taste

2 Tbsp. light, soft tub margarine

1. Layer half of bacon, onions, potatoes, and cheese in greased slow cooker. Season to taste.

2. Dot with margarine. Repeat layers.

3. Cover. Cook on Low 8–10 hours, or on High 3–4 hours, or until potatoes are soft.

Exchange List Values: Starch 2.0, Vegetable 1.0, Fat 1.0

Basic Nutritional Values: Calories 224 (Calories from Fat 38), Total Fat 4 gm (Saturated Fat 0.9 gm, Polyunsat Fat 0.7 gm, Monounsat Fat 2.1 gm, Cholesterol 6 mg), Sodium 262 mg, Total Carbohydrate 35 gm, Dietary Fiber 4 gm, Sugars 7 gm, Protein 12 gm

Lotsa Scalloped Potatoes

Fannie Miller • Hutchinson, KS

Makes 20–25 servings (Ideal slow cooker size: 6–7-quart, or 2 4–5-quart cookers)

5 lbs. potatoes, cooked and sliced

2 lbs. extra-lean, lower-sodium cooked ham, cubed

1/4 lb. light, soft tub margarine

1/2 cup flour

2 cups fat-free half-and-half

1/4 lb. reduced-fat mild cheese (your favorite), shredded

1/4–1/2 tsp. pepper

1. Place layers of sliced potatoes and ham in very large (or two smaller) slow cooker(s).

2. Melt margarine in saucepan on stove. Stir in flour. Gradually add half-and-half to make a white sauce, stirring constantly until smooth and thickened.

3. Stir in cheese and pepper. Stir until cheese is melted. Pour over potatoes and ham.

4. Cover. Cook on Low 2–3 hours.

Exchange List Values: Starch 1.0, Meat, lean 1.0

Basic Nutritional Values: Calories 136 (Calories from Fat 24), Total Fat 3 gm (Saturated Fat 1.0 gm, Polyunsat Fat 0.4 gm, Monounsat Fat 0.9 gm, Cholesterol 21 mg), Sodium 379 mg, Total Carbohydrate 19 gm, Dietary Fiber 1 gm, Sugars 4 gm, Protein 10 gm

Note: A great way to free up oven space.

Cheese Potatoes

Joyce Shackelford • Green Bay, WI

Makes 10 servings (Ideal slow cooker size: 5-quart)

6 potatoes, peeled and cut into 1/4" strips

3 ozs. reduced-fat sharp cheddar cheese, shredded

10 3/4-oz. can 98%-fat-free, reduced-sodium cream of chicken soup

1 small onion, chopped

4 Tbsp. margarine, melted

1 tsp. salt

1 tsp. pepper

1 cup sour cream

2 cups seasoned stuffing cubes

3 Tbsp. margarine, melted

1. Toss together potatoes and cheese. Place in slow cooker.

2. Combine soup, onion, 4 Tbsp. margarine, salt, and pepper. Pour over potatoes.

3. Cover. Cook on Low 8 hours.

4. Stir in sour cream. Cover and heat for 10 more minutes.

5. Meanwhile, toss together stuffing cubes and 3 Tbsp. margarine. Sprinkle over potatoes just before serving.

Exchange List Values: Starch 2.0, Fat 1.0

Basic Nutritional Values: Calories 190 (Calories from Fat 54), Total Fat 6 gm (Saturated Fat 1.5 gm, Polyunsat Fat 1.2 gm, Monounsat Fat 2.5 gm, Cholesterol 10 mg), Sodium 390 mg, Total Carbohydrate 29 gm, Dietary Fiber 2 gm, Sugars 5 gm, Protein 7 gm

Surround yourself with people who care about you and your diabetes. They are your very own support network.

Hot German Potato Salad

Judi Manos • West Islip, NY

Makes 7 servings (Ideal slow cooker size: 4–5-quart)

5 medium potatoes, cut $\frac{1}{4}$" thick

1 large onion, chopped

$\frac{1}{3}$ cup water

$\frac{1}{3}$ cup vinegar

2 Tbsp. flour

2 Tbsp. sugar

1 tsp. salt

$\frac{1}{2}$ tsp. celery seed

$\frac{1}{4}$ tsp. pepper

4 slices bacon, cooked crisp and crumbled

chopped fresh parsley

1. Combine potatoes and onions in slow cooker.

2. Combine remaining ingredients, except bacon and parsley. Pour over potatoes.

3. Cover. Cook on Low 8–10 hours.

4. Stir in bacon and parsley.

5. Serve warm or at room temperature with grilled bratwurst or Polish sausage, dilled pickles, pickled beets, and apples.

Exchange List Values: Starch 2.0

Basic Nutritional Values: Calories 149 (Calories from Fat 17), Total Fat 2 gm (Saturated Fat 0.6 gm, Polyunsat Fat 0.3 gm, Monounsat Fat 0.8 gm, Cholesterol 3 mg), Sodium 397 mg, Total Carbohydrate 30 gm, Dietary Fiber 3 gm, Sugars 8 gm, Protein 4 gm

Creamy Hash Browns

Judy Buller • Bluffton, OH /
Elaine Patton • West Middletown, PA /
Melissa Raber • Millersburg, OH

Makes 14 servings (Ideal slow cooker size: 4–5-quart)

2-lb. pkg. frozen, cubed hash brown potatoes

2 cups cubed, or shredded, fat-free American cheese

12 ozs. fat-free sour cream

$10\frac{3}{4}$-oz. can cream of celery soup

$10\frac{3}{4}$-oz. can 98%-fat-free, reduced-sodium cream of chicken soup

$\frac{1}{4}$ lb. sliced bacon, cooked and crumbled

1 medium onion, chopped

2 Tbsp. margarine, melted

$\frac{1}{4}$ tsp. pepper

1. Place potatoes in slow cooker. Combine remaining ingredients and pour over potatoes. Mix well.

2. Cover. Cook on Low 4–5 hours, or until potatoes are tender.

Exchange List Values: Starch 1.0, Carbohydrate 0.5, Fat 1.0

Basic Nutritional Values: Calories 167 (Calories from Fat 44), Total Fat 5 gm (Saturated Fat 1.4 gm, Polyunsat Fat 1.5 gm, Monounsat Fat 1.6 gm, Cholesterol 9 mg), Sodium 578 mg, Total Carbohydrate 23 gm, Dietary Fiber 2 gm, Sugars 4 gm, Protein 8 gm

Candied Sweet Potatoes

Julie Weaver • Reinholds, PA

Makes 8 servings (Ideal slow cooker size: 4-quart)

6–8 medium (6½ ozs. each) sweet potatoes

½ tsp. salt

2 Tbsp. margarine, melted

20-oz. can crushed pineapples, undrained

2 Tbsp. brown sugar

brown sugar substitute to equal 1 Tbsp.

1 tsp. nutmeg

1 tsp. cinnamon

1. Cook sweet potatoes until soft. Peel. Slice and place in slow cooker.

2. Combine remaining ingredients. Pour over sweet potatoes.

3. Cover. Cook on High 4 hours.

Exchange List Values: Starch 1.5, Fruit 1.0, Fat 0.5

Basic Nutritional Values: Calories 186 (Calories from Fat 30), Total Fat 3 gm (Saturated Fat 0.7 gm, Polyunsat Fat 1.1 gm, Monounsat Fat 1.3 gm, Cholesterol 0 mg), Sodium 193 mg, Total Carbohydrate 39 gm, Dietary Fiber 3 gm, Sugars 19 gm, Protein 2 gm

Sweet Potato Casserole

Jean Butzer • Batavia, NY

Makes 10 servings (Ideal slow cooker size: 4–5-quart)

2 29-oz. cans no-sugar-added sweet potatoes, drained and mashed

2½ Tbsp. light, soft tub margarine

1 Tbsp. sugar

1 Tbsp. brown sugar

brown sugar substitute to equal ½ tsp.

1 Tbsp. orange juice

2 eggs, beaten

½ cup fat-free milk

⅓ cup chopped pecans

2 Tbsp. brown sugar

brown sugar substitute to equal 1½ Tbsp.

2 Tbsp. flour

2 tsp. light, soft tub margarine, melted

1. Combine sweet potatoes, 2½ Tbsp. margarine, 1 Tbsp. sugar, 1 Tbsp. brown sugar, and sugar substitute to equal ½ tsp.

2. Beat in orange juice, eggs, and milk. Transfer to greased slow cooker.

3. Combine pecans, 2 Tbsp. brown sugar, sugar substitute to equal 1½ Tbsp., flour, and 2 tsp. margarine. Spread over sweet potatoes.

4. Cover. Cook on High 3–4 hours.

Exchange List Values: Starch 2.0, Carbohydrate 0.5, Fat 0.5

Basic Nutritional Values: Calories 218 (Calories from Fat 51), Total Fat 6 gm (Saturated Fat 0.7 gm, Polyunsat Fat 1.4 gm, Monounsat Fat 2.9 gm, Cholesterol 43 mg), Sodium 64 mg, Total Carbohydrate 40 gm, Dietary Fiber 5 gm, Sugars 24 gm, Protein 5 gm

Glazed Sweet Potatoes

Martha Hershey • Ronks, PA

Makes 10 servings (Ideal slow cooker size: 4-5-quart)

10 medium (6⅓ ozs. each) sweet potatoes

¼ cup light, soft tub margarine, melted

2 Tbsp. brown sugar

brown sugar substitute to equal 1 Tbsp.

½ cup orange juice

½ tsp. salt

1. Cook sweet potatoes until just soft. Peel and cut in half.

2. Combine remaining ingredients. Pour over potatoes.

3. Cover. Cook on High 2½–3 hours, or until tender but not mushy.

Exchange List Values: Starch 2.0, Carbohydrate 0.5

Basic Nutritional Values: Calories 169 (Calories from Fat 20), Total Fat 2 gm (Saturated Fat 0.1 gm, Polyunsat Fat 0.6 gm, Monounsat Fat 1.0 gm, Cholesterol 0 mg), Sodium 171 mg, Total Carbohydrate 36 gm, Dietary Fiber 2 gm, Sugars 11 gm, Protein 2 gm

Note: The sweet potatoes can be cooked and peeled ahead of time, and frozen in a single layer. Defrost before putting in slow cooker.

These are great to serve with Thanksgiving dinner.

Orange Yams

Gladys Longacre • Susquehanna, PA

Makes 6-8 servings (Ideal slow cooker size: 4-5-quart)

40-oz. can no-sugar-added yams, drained

2 apples, cored, peeled, thinly sliced

1½ Tbsp. light, soft tub margarine, melted

2 tsp. orange peel

1 cup orange juice

2 Tbsp. cornstarch

¼ cup brown sugar

brown sugar substitute to equal 2 Tbsp.

1 tsp. salt

dash ground cinnamon and/or nutmeg

1. Place yams and apples in slow cooker.

2. Add margarine and orange peel.

3. Combine remaining ingredients and pour over yams.

4. Cover. Cook on High 1 hour, and then on Low 2 hours, or until apples are tender.

Exchange List Values: Starch 2.0, Carbohydrate 1.0

Basic Nutritional Values: Calories 199 (Calories from Fat 11), Total Fat 1 gm (Saturated Fat 0.1 gm, Polyunsat Fat 0.4 gm, Monounsat Fat 0.5 gm, Cholesterol 0 mg), Sodium 324 mg, Total Carbohydrate 48 gm, Dietary Fiber 4 gm, Sugars 32 gm, Protein 3 gm

VARIATION: Substitute 6-8 medium-sized cooked sweet potatoes, or approximately 4 cups cubed butternut squash, for yams.

Sweet Potatoes and Apples

Bernita Boyts • Shawnee Mission, KS

Makes 8 servings (Ideal slow cooker size: 4-quart)

3 large sweet potatoes, peeled and cubed

3 large tart and firm apples, peeled and sliced

½ tsp. salt

⅛–¼ tsp. pepper

1 tsp. sage

1 tsp. ground cinnamon

4 Tbsp. light, soft tub margarine, melted

2 Tbsp. maple syrup

4 Tbsp. brown sugar

brown sugar substitute to equal 1 Tbsp.

toasted sliced almonds or chopped pecans, optional

1. Place half the sweet potatoes in slow cooker. Layer in half the apple slices.

2. Mix together dry seasonings. Sprinkle half over apples.

3. Mix together margarine, maple syrup, brown sugar, and sugar substitute. Spoon half over seasonings.

4. Repeat layers.

5. Cover. Cook on Low 6–8 hours, or until potatoes are soft, stirring occasionally.

6. To add a bit of crunch, sprinkle with toasted almonds or pecans when serving.

7. Serve with pork or poultry.

Exchange List Values: Starch 1.0, Fruit 1.0, Fat 0.5

Basic Nutritional Values: Calories 152 (Calories from Fat 24), Total Fat 3 gm (Saturated Fat 0.1 gm, Polyunsat Fat 0.7 gm, Monounsat Fat 1.3 gm, Cholesterol 0 mg), Sodium 201 mg, Total Carbohydrate 32 gm, Dietary Fiber 3 gm, Sugars 17 gm, Protein 1 gm

Sweet Potatoes with Applesauce

Judi Manos • West Islip, NY

Makes 6-8 servings (Ideal slow cooker size: 4-quart)

6 medium-sized sweet potatoes or yams

1½ cups unsweetened applesauce

¼ cup packed brown sugar

brown sugar substitute to equal 2 Tbsp.

2 Tbsp. light, soft tub margarine, melted

1 tsp. ground cinnamon

½ cup chopped pecans

1. Peel sweet potatoes and cut into ½" cubes. Place in slow cooker.

2. Combine remaining ingredients, except nuts. Spoon over potatoes.

3. Cover. Cook on Low 6–7 hours, or until potatoes are very tender.

4. Sprinkle with nuts.

Exchange List Values: Starch 1.5, Fruit 1.0, Fat 1.0

Basic Nutritional Values: Calories 213 (Calories from Fat 63), Total Fat 7 gm (Saturated Fat 0.5 gm, Polyunsat Fat 1.9 gm, Monounsat Fat 3.9 gm, Cholesterol 0 mg), Sodium 40 mg, Total Carbohydrate 37 gm, Dietary Fiber 3 gm, Sugars 17 gm, Protein 2 gm

Exercise can drop blood sugar too low, so carry a source of sugar with you to treat hypoglycemia.

Barbecued Black Beans with Sweet Potatoes

Barbara Jean Fabel • Wausau, WI

Makes 8 servings (Ideal slow cooker size: 4-quart)

4 large (10 ozs. each) sweet potatoes, peeled and cut into 8 chunks each

15-oz. can black beans, rinsed and drained

1 medium onion, diced

2 ribs celery, sliced

9 ozs. Sweet Baby Ray's Barbecue Sauce

1. Place sweet potatoes in slow cooker.

2. Combine remaining ingredients. Pour over sweet potatoes.

3. Cover. Cook on High 2–3 hours, or on Low 4 hours.

Exchange List Values: Starch 2.5

Basic Nutritional Values: Calories 180 (Calories from Fat 10), Total Fat 1 gm (Saturated Fat 0.2 gm, Polyunsat Fat 0.4 gm, Monounsat Fat 0.3 gm, Cholesterol 0 mg), Sodium 321 mg, Total Carbohydrate 38 gm, Dietary Fiber 5 gm, Sugars 11 gm, Protein 5 gm

Potato Filling

Miriam Nolt • New Holland, PA

Makes 32 servings (Ideal slow cooker size: 2 6-7-qt. cookers)

1 cup celery, chopped fine

1 medium onion, minced

2 Tbsp. light, soft tub margarine

2 Tbsp. canola oil

2 15-oz. pkgs. unseasoned bread cubes, toasted

3 eggs, beaten

4 egg whites

1 qt. fat-free milk

1 qt. mashed potatoes

2 pinches saffron

1 cup boiling water

1 tsp. pepper

1. Saute celery and onion in margarine and canola oil in skillet for about 15 minutes.

2. Combine sauteed mixture with bread cubes. Stir in remaining ingredients. Add more milk if mixture isn't very moist.

3. Pour into slow cookers. Cook on High 3 hours, stirring up from bottom every hour or so to make sure the filling isn't sticking.

Exchange List Values: Starch 1.5, Fat 0.5

Basic Nutritional Values: Calories 147 (Calories from Fat 36), Total Fat 4 gm (Saturated Fat 1.5 gm, Polyunsat Fat 1.1 gm, Monounsat Fat 1.2 gm, Cholesterol 22 mg), Sodium 280 mg, Total Carbohydrate 22 gm, Dietary Fiber 1 gm, Sugars 4 gm, Protein 5 gm

Moist Poultry Dressing

Virginia Bender • Dover, DE / Josie Boilman •
Maumee, OH / Sharon Brubaker •
Myerstown, PA / Joette Droz • Kalona, IA /
Jacqueline Stefl • E. Bethany, NY

Makes 14 servings (Ideal slow cooker size: 6-quart)

2 4½-oz. cans sliced mushrooms, drained

4 ribs celery, chopped (about 2 cups)

2 medium onions, chopped

¼ cup minced fresh parsley

¼ cup margarine

13 cups cubed day-old bread

¼ tsp. salt

1½ tsp. sage

1 tsp. poultry seasoning

1 tsp. dried thyme

½ tsp. pepper

2 eggs

14½-oz. can fat-free, lower-sodium chicken broth

1. In large skillet, sauté mushrooms, celery, onions, and parsley in margarine until vegetables are tender.

2. Toss together bread cubes, salt, sage, poultry seasoning, thyme, and pepper. Add mushroom mixture.

3. Combine eggs and broth and add to bread mixture. Mix well.

4. Pour into greased slow cooker. Cook on Low 5 hours, or until meat thermometer reaches 160°.

Exchange List Values: Starch 1.0, Vegetable 1.0, Fat 1.0

Basic Nutritional Values: Calories 151 (Calories from Fat 48), Total Fat 5 gm (Saturated Fat 1.1 gm, Polyunsat Fat 1.8 gm, Monounsat Fat 2.0 gm, Cholesterol 31 mg), Sodium 409 mg, Total Carbohydrate 20 gm, Dietary Fiber 2 gm, Sugars 3 gm, Protein 5 gm

VARIATIONS:

1. Use 2 bags bread cubes for stuffing. Make one mixed bread (white and wheat) and the other corn bread cubes.

2. Add ½ tsp. dried marjoram to Step 2.

Arlene Miller • Hutchinson, KS

Note: This is a good way to free up the oven when you're making a turkey.

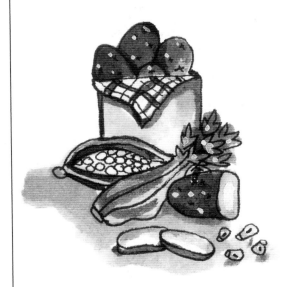

Mild Dressing

Jane Steiner • Orrville, OH

Makes 8 servings (Ideal slow cooker size: 4-quart)

16-oz. loaf homemade white bread

2 eggs, beaten

$\frac{1}{2}$ cup celery

$\frac{1}{4}$ cup diced onions

$\frac{1}{4}$ tsp. salt

$\frac{1}{2}$ tsp. pepper

1 cup giblets, cooked and cut up fine

1 cup fat-free milk

1. Set bread slices out to dry the day before using. Cut into small cubes.

2. Combine all ingredients except milk.

3. Moisten mixture with enough milk to make bread cubes soft but not soggy.

4. Pour into greased slow cooker. Cook on Low $3\frac{1}{2}$ hours, stirring every hour. When stirring, add a small amount of milk to sides of cooker—if needed—to keep dressing moist and to prevent sticking.

Exchange List Values: Starch 2.0, Meat, lean 1.0

Basic Nutritional Values: Calories 213 (Calories from Fat 37), Total Fat 4 gm (Saturated Fat 1.1 gm, Polyunsat Fat 1.4 gm, Monounsat Fat 1.1 gm, Cholesterol 135 mg), Sodium 427 mg, Total Carbohydrate 31 gm, Dietary Fiber 2 gm, Sugars 4 gm, Protein 12 gm

Slow Cooker Dressing

Marie Shank • Harrisonburg, VA

Makes 20 servings (Ideal slow cooker size: 6-quart)

2 ($8\frac{1}{2}$ ozs.) boxes Jiffy corn bread mix

8 slices day-old bread

3 eggs

1 onion, chopped

$\frac{1}{2}$ cup chopped celery

2 $10\frac{3}{4}$-oz. cans 98%-fat-free, reduced-sodium cream of chicken soup

2 tsp. sodium-free chicken bouillon powder, plus 2 cups water

$\frac{1}{2}$ tsp. pepper

$1\frac{1}{2}$ Tbsp. sage or poultry seasoning

1. Prepare corn bread according to package instructions.

2. Crumble corn bread and bread together.

3. In large bowl combine all ingredients and spoon into 6-qt. greased slow cooker, or 2 smaller cookers.

4. Cover. Cook on High 2–4 hours, or on Low 3–8 hours.

Exchange List Values: Starch 1.5, Fat 0.5

Basic Nutritional Values: Calories 133 (Calories from Fat 34), Total Fat 4 gm (Saturated Fat 1.5 gm, Polyunsat Fat 0.9 gm, Monounsat Fat 1.1 gm, Cholesterol 35 mg), Sodium 387 mg, Total Carbohydrate 26 gm, Dietary Fiber 1 gm, Sugars 6 gm, Protein 4 gm

VARIATIONS:

1. Prepare your favorite corn bread recipe in an 8"-square baking pan instead of using the corn bread mix.

2. Serve with roast chicken or turkey drumsticks.

Helen Kenagy • Carlsbad, NM

Slow Cooker Stuffing

Dede Peterson • Rapid City, SD

Makes 12 servings (Ideal slow cooker size: 6-quart)

12 cups toasted bread crumbs, or dressing mix

4 ozs. 50%-less-fat bulk sausage, browned and drained

1 cup, or more, finely chopped onions

1 cup, or more, finely chopped celery

2 Tbsp. canola oil

8-oz. can sliced mushrooms, with liquid

¼ cup chopped fresh parsley

2 tsp. poultry seasoning (omit if using dressing mix)

dash pepper

2 eggs, beaten

4 tsp. sodium-free bouillon powder

4 cups water

1. Combine bread crumbs and sausage.

2. Add onions and celery to oil in skillet and saute until tender. Stir in mushrooms and parsley. Add seasonings. Pour over bread crumbs and mix well.

3. Stir in eggs and bouillon mixed with water.

4. Pour into slow cooker and bake on High 1 hour, and on Low an additional 3 hours.

Exchange List Values: Starch 2.0, Fat 1.0

Basic Nutritional Values: Calories 209 (Calories from Fat 68), Total Fat 8 gm (Saturated Fat 1.5 gm, Polyunsat Fat 1.9 gm, Monounsat Fat 2.4 gm, Cholesterol 44 mg), Sodium 423 mg, Total Carbohydrate 28 gm, Dietary Fiber 2 gm, Sugars 4 gm, Protein 8 gm

VARIATIONS:

1. For a less spicy stuffing, reduce the poultry seasoning to ½ tsp.

   Dolores Metzler • Mechanicsburg, PA

2. Substitute 3½–4½ cups cooked and diced giblets in place of sausage. Add another can mushrooms and 2 tsp. sage in Step 2.

   Mrs. Don Martins • Fairbank, IA

Exercise with someone. It's more fun that way, and you can encourage each other when your motivation fails you.

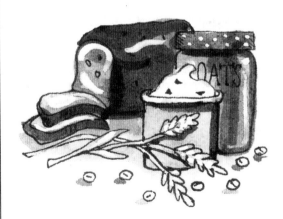

Mashed Potato Filling

Betty K. Drescher • Quakertown, PA

Makes 8–10 servings (Ideal slow cooker size: 6-quart)

½ cup diced onions

1 cup diced celery

2 Tbsp. canola oil

2½ cups fat-free milk

4 large eggs, beaten

8 ozs. unseasoned bread cubes, toasted

4 cups mashed potatoes

¾ tsp. salt

¼ tsp. pepper

1. Saute onions and celery in oil in skillet for 5–10 minutes, or until vegetables are tender.

2. Combine onions and celery, milk, and eggs. Pour over bread cubes. Mix lightly to absorb liquid.

3. Stir in potatoes and seasonings. Pour into greased slow cooker.

4. Cover. Cook on Low 4 hours.

Exchange List Values: Starch 2.0, Fat 1.0

Basic Nutritional Values: Calories 214 (Calories from Fat 54), Total Fat 6 gm (Saturated Fat 1.4 gm, Polyunsat Fat 1.6 gm, Monounsat Fat 2.7 gm, Cholesterol 88 mg), Sodium 382 mg, Total Carbohydrate 32 gm, Dietary Fiber 2 gm, Sugars 8 gm, Protein 8 gm

VARIATION: For more flavor, add the packet of seasoning from the bread cube package in Step 3.

Sweet Potato Stuffing

Tina Snyder • Manheim, PA

Makes 8 servings (Ideal slow cooker size: 4–5-quart)

½ cup chopped celery

½ cup chopped onions

1 Tbsp. canola oil

6 cups dry bread cubes

1 large sweet potato, cooked, peeled, and cubed

½ cup chicken broth

¼ cup chopped pecans

½ tsp. poultry seasoning

½ tsp. rubbed sage

¼ tsp. salt

¼ tsp. pepper

1. Saute celery and onion in skillet in oil until tender. Pour into greased slow cooker.

2. Add remaining ingredients. Toss gently.

3. Cover. Cook on Low 4 hours.

Exchange List Values: Starch 1.5, Fat 1.0

Basic Nutritional Values: Calories 146 (Calories from Fat 51), Total Fat 6 gm (Saturated Fat 0.5 gm, Polyunsat Fat 1.8 gm, Monounsat Fat 2.9 gm, Cholesterol 1 mg), Sodium 321 mg, Total Carbohydrate 21 gm, Dietary Fiber 2 gm, Sugars 3 gm, Protein 3 gm

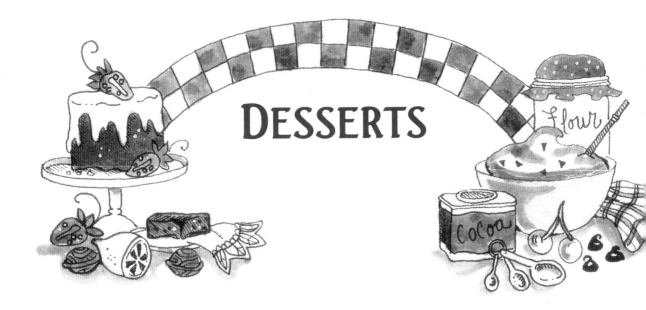

DESSERTS

Simple Bread Pudding

Melanie L. Thrower • McPherson, KS

Makes 8 servings (Ideal slow cooker size: 4-quart)

6–8 slices of bread, cubed

2 cups fat-free milk

2 eggs

¼ cup sugar

1 tsp. ground cinnamon

1 tsp. vanilla

SAUCE:

1 Tbsp. cornstarch

6-oz. can concentrated grape juice

1. Place bread in slow cooker.

2. Whisk together milk, eggs, sugar, cinnamon, and vanilla. Pour over bread.

3. Cover. Cook on High 2–2½ hours, or until mixture is set.

4. Combine cornstarch and concentrated juice in saucepan. Heat until boiling, stirring constantly, until sauce is thickened. Serve drizzled over bread pudding.

5. This is a fine dessert with a cold salad main dish.

Exchange List Values: Carbohydrate 2.5

Basic Nutritional Values: Calories 179 (Calories from Fat 19), Total Fat 2 gm (Saturated Fat 0.7 gm, Polyunsat Fat 0.6 gm, Monounsat Fat 0.6 gm, Cholesterol 55 mg), Sodium 153 mg, Total Carbohydrate 35 gm, Dietary Fiber 1 gm, Sugars 24 gm, Protein 5 gm

Bread Pudding

Winifred Ewy • Newton, KS / Helen King • Fairbank, IA / Elaine Patton, • West Middletown, PA

Makes 9 servings (Ideal slow cooker size: 4-quart)

8 slices bread (raisin bread is especially good), cubed

3 eggs

2 egg whites

2 cups fat-free half-and-half

2 Tbsp. sugar

sugar substitute to equal 1 Tbsp.

½ cup raisins (use only ¼ cup if using raisin bread)

½ tsp. cinnamon

SAUCE:

2 Tbsp. light, soft tub margarine

2 Tbsp. flour

1 cup water

6 Tbsp. sugar

sugar substitute to equal 3 Tbsp.

1 tsp. vanilla

1. Place bread cubes in greased slow cooker.

2. Beat together eggs, whites, and half-and-half. Stir in sugar, sugar substitute, raisins, and cinnamon. Pour over bread and stir.

3. Cover and cook on High 1 hour. Reduce heat to Low and cook 3–4 hours, or until thermometer reaches 160°.

4. Make sauce just before pudding is done baking. Begin by melting margarine in saucepan. Stir in flour until smooth. Gradually add water, sugar, sugar substitute, and vanilla. Bring to boil. Cook, stirring constantly for 2 minutes, or until thickened.

5. Serve sauce over warm bread pudding.

Exchange List Values: Carbohydrate 2.0, Fat 1.0

Basic Nutritional Values: Calories 200 (Calories from Fat 40), Total Fat 4 gm (Saturated Fat 1.4 gm, Polyunsat Fat 0.6 gm, Monounsat Fat 1.7 gm, Cholesterol 75 mg), Sodium 221 mg, Total Carbohydrate 34 gm, Dietary Fiber 1 gm, Sugars 21 gm, Protein 6 gm

VARIATIONS:

1. Use dried cherries instead of raisins. Use cherry flavoring in sauce instead of vanilla.

   Char Hagnes • Montague, MI

2. Use ¼ tsp. ground cinnamon and ¼ tsp. ground nutmeg, instead of ½ tsp. ground cinnamon in pudding.

3. Use 8 cups day-old unfrosted cinnamon rolls instead of the bread.

   Beatrice Orgist • Richardson, TX

4. Use ½ tsp. vanilla and ¼ tsp. ground nutmeg instead of ½ tsp. cinnamon.

   Nanci Keatley • Salem, OR

Apple-Nut Bread Pudding

Ruth Ann Hoover • New Holland, PA

Makes 10 servings (Ideal slow cooker size: 4-quart)

8 slices raisin bread, cubed

2 medium-sized tart apples, peeled and sliced

1 cup chopped pecans, toasted

$\frac{1}{2}$ cup sugar

sugar substitute to equal $\frac{1}{4}$ cup

1 tsp. ground cinnamon

$\frac{1}{2}$ tsp. ground nutmeg

1 egg, lightly beaten

3 egg whites, lightly beaten

2 cups fat-free half-and-half

$\frac{1}{4}$ cup apple juice

2 Tbsp. light, soft tub margarine, melted

1. Place bread cubes, apples, and pecans in greased slow cooker and mix together gently.

2. Combine sugar, sugar substitute, cinnamon, and nutmeg. Add remaining ingredients. Mix well. Pour over bread mixture.

3. Cover. Cook on Low 3–4 hours, or until knife inserted in center comes out clean.

4. Serve with ice cream, if diet allows.

Exchange List Values: Carbohydrate 2.0, Fat 2.0

Basic Nutritional Values: Calories 231 (Calories from Fat 87), Total Fat 10 gm (Saturated Fat 1.4 gm, Polyunsat Fat 2.3 gm, Monounsat Fat 5.1 gm, Cholesterol 25 mg), Sodium 191 mg, Total Carbohydrate 32 gm, Dietary Fiber 2 gm, Sugars 20 gm, Protein 6 gm

Mama's Rice Pudding

Donna Barnitz • Jenks, OK / Shari Jensen • Fountain, CO

Makes 8 servings (Ideal slow cooker size: 4-quart)

$\frac{1}{2}$ cup white rice, uncooked

$\frac{1}{4}$ cup sugar

sugar substitute to equal 2 Tbsp.

1 tsp. vanilla

1 tsp. lemon extract

1 cup plus 2 Tbsp. fat-free milk

1 tsp. butter

2 eggs, beaten

1 tsp. cinnamon

$\frac{1}{2}$ cup raisins

1 cup fat-free whipping cream, whipped

nutmeg

1. Combine all ingredients except whipped cream and nutmeg in slow cooker. Stir well.

2. Cover pot. Cook on Low 6–7 hours, until rice is tender and milk absorbed. Be sure to stir once every 2 hours during cooking.

3. Pour into bowl. Cover with plastic wrap and chill.

4. Before serving, fold in whipped cream and sprinkle with nutmeg.

Exchange List Values: Carbohydrate 2.0

Basic Nutritional Values: Calories 148 (Calories from Fat 17), Total Fat 2 gm (Saturated Fat 0.8 gm, Polyunsat Fat 0.2 gm, Monounsat Fat 0.7 gm, Cholesterol 55 mg), Sodium 43 mg, Total Carbohydrate 28 gm, Dietary Fiber 1 gm, Sugars 15 gm, Protein 4 gm

Deluxe Tapioca Pudding

Michelle Showalter • Bridgewater, VA

Makes 16 servings (Ideal slow cooker size: 5-quart)

2 qts. fat-free milk

3/4 cup dry small pearl tapioca

3/4 cup sugar

sugar substitute to equal 6 Tbsp.

4 eggs, beaten

2 tsp. vanilla

3 cups fat-free frozen whipped topping, thawed

chocolate candy bar, optional

1. Combine milk, tapioca, sugar, and sugar substitute in slow cooker.

2. Cook on High 3 hours.

3. Add a little of the hot milk to the eggs. Stir. Whisk eggs into milk mixture. Add vanilla.

4. Cover. Cook on High 20–30 minutes.

5. Cool. Chill in refrigerator. When fully chilled, beat with hand mixer to fluff the pudding.

6. Stir in whipped topping. Garnish with chopped candy bar.

Exchange List Values: Carbohydrate 2.0

Basic Nutritional Values: Calories 147 (Calories from Fat 12), Total Fat 1 gm (Saturated Fat 0.6 gm, Polyunsat Fat 0.2 gm, Monounsat Fat 0.5 gm, Cholesterol 56 mg), Sodium 77 mg, Total Carbohydrate 27 gm, Dietary Fiber 0 gm, Sugars 17 gm, Protein 6 gm

Slow Cooker Tapioca

Nancy W. Huber • Green Park, PA

Makes 10–12 servings (Ideal slow cooker size: 4-quart)

2 qts. fat-free milk

1 cup small pearl tapioca

1/2 cup sugar

sugar substitute to equal 1/4 cup

4 eggs, beaten

1 tsp. vanilla

1. Combine milk, tapioca, sugar, and sugar substitute in slow cooker. Cook on High 3 hours.

2. Mix together eggs, vanilla, and a little hot milk from slow cooker. Add to slow cooker. Cook on High 20 more minutes. Chill.

3. Serve with whipped cream or fruit.

Exchange List Values: Carbohydrate 2.0

Basic Nutritional Values: Calories 160 (Calories from Fat 16), Total Fat 2 gm (Saturated Fat 0.9 gm, Polyunsat Fat 0.2 gm, Monounsat Fat 0.7 gm, Cholesterol 74 mg), Sodium 93 mg, Total Carbohydrate 28 gm, Dietary Fiber 0 gm, Sugars 17 gm, Protein 8 gm

Blushing Apple Tapioca

Julie Weaver • Reinholds, PA

Makes 8-10 servings (Ideal slow cooker size: 4-quart)

8-10 medium tart apples

¼ cup sugar

sugar substitute to equal 2 Tbsp.

4 Tbsp. minute tapioca

4 Tbsp. red cinnamon candy

½ cup water

whipped topping, optional

1. Pare and core apples. Cut into eighths lengthwise and place in slow cooker.

2. Mix together sugar, sugar substitute, tapioca, candy, and water. Pour over apples.

3. Cook on High 3-4 hours.

4. Serve hot or cold. Top with whipped topping.

Exchange List Values: Carbohydrate 2.0

Basic Nutritional Values: Calories 117 (Calories from Fat 3), Total Fat 0 gm (Saturated Fat 0 gm, Polyunsat Fat 0.1 gm, Monounsat Fat 0 gm, Cholesterol 0 mg), Sodium 0 mg, Total Carbohydrate 30 gm, Dietary Fiber 2 gm, Sugars 23 gm, Protein 0 gm

Raisin Nut-Stuffed Apples

Margaret Rich • North Newton, KS

Makes 6 servings (Ideal slow cooker size: 4-quart)

6 medium baking apples, cored

1½ Tbsp. light, soft tub margarine, melted

2 Tbsp. packed brown sugar

brown sugar substitute to equal 1 Tbsp.

¾ cup raisins

3 Tbsp. chopped walnuts

½ cup water

1. Peel a strip around each apple about one-third of the way below the stem end to prevent splitting.

2. Mix together margarine, brown sugar, and sugar substitute. Stir in raisins and walnuts. Stuff into apple cavities.

3. Place apples in slow cooker. Add water.

4. Cover and cook on Low 6-8 hours.

Exchange List Values: Fruit 2.0, Carbohydrate 0.5, Fat 0.5

Basic Nutritional Values: Calories 187 (Calories from Fat 35), Total Fat 4 gm (Saturated Fat 0.4 gm, Polyunsat Fat 2.1 gm, Monounsat Fat 1.0 gm, Cholesterol 0 mg), Sodium 29 mg, Total Carbohydrate 41 gm, Dietary Fiber 5 gm, Sugars 32 gm, Protein 2 gm

Caramel Apples

Elaine Patton • West Middletown, PA /
Rhonda Lee Schmidt • Scranton, PA /
Renee Shirk • Mount Joy, PA

Makes 8 servings (Ideal slow cooker size: 4-quart)

4 very large tart apples, cored

1/2 cup apple juice

4 Tbsp. brown sugar

brown sugar substitute to equal 2 Tbsp.

12 hot cinnamon candies

4 Tbsp. light, soft tub margarine

8 caramel candies

1/4 tsp. ground cinnamon

whipped cream, optional

1. Remove 1/2"-wide strip of peel off the top of each apple and place apples in slow cooker.

2. Pour apple juice over apples.

3. Fill center of each apple with 1 Tbsp. brown sugar, 1/2 Tbsp. sugar substitute, 3 hot cinnamon candies, 1 Tbsp. margarine, and 2 caramel candies. Sprinkle with cinnamon.

4. Cover and cook on Low 4–6 hours, or until tender.

5. Serve hot with juice from bottom of slow cooker and whipped cream, if you wish.

Exchange List Values: Carbohydrate 2.0

Basic Nutritional Values: Calories 130 (Calories from Fat 26), Total Fat 3 gm (Saturated Fat 0.6 gm, Polyunsat Fat 0.6 gm, Monounsat Fat 1.3 gm, Cholesterol 0 mg), Sodium 63 mg, Total Carbohydrate 28 gm, Dietary Fiber 3 gm, Sugars 23 gm, Protein 1 gm

Cranberry Baked Apples

Judi Manos • West Islip, NY

Makes 8 servings (Ideal slow cooker size: 3-4-quart)

4 large cooking apples

1/3 cup packed brown sugar

1/4 cup dried cranberries

1/2 cup cranapple juice cocktail

2 Tbsp. light, soft tub margarine, melted

1/2 tsp. ground cinnamon

1/4 tsp. ground nutmeg

chopped nuts, optional

1. Core apples. Fill centers with brown sugar and cranberries. Place in slow cooker.

2. Combine cranapple juice and margarine. Pour over apples.

3. Sprinkle with cinnamon and nutmeg.

4. Cover. Cook on Low 4–6 hours.

5. To serve, spoon sauce over apples and sprinkle with nuts.

6. This is great with vanilla ice cream.

Exchange List Values: Carbohydrate 2.0

Basic Nutritional Values: Calories 121 (Calories from Fat 13), Total Fat 1 gm (Saturated Fat 0.1 gm, Polyunsat Fat 0.3 gm, Monounsat Fat 0.6 gm, Cholesterol 0 mg), Sodium 27 mg, Total Carbohydrate 29 gm, Dietary Fiber 3 gm, Sugars 25 gm, Protein 0 gm

This was one of our favorite recipes while growing up. When it's cooking, the house smells delicious. I'm suddenly full of memories of days gone by and a much more relaxing time. My mother passed away in October, and I re-found this recipe among her collection of favorites.

Fruit and Nut Baked Apples

Cyndie Marrara • Port Matilda, PA

Makes 4 servings (Ideal slow cooker size: 4-quart)

4 large firm baking apples

1 Tbsp. lemon juice

1/3 cup chopped dried apricots

1/3 cup chopped walnuts, or pecans

1 1/2 Tbsp. packed brown sugar

brown sugar substitute to equal 2 tsp.

1/2 tsp. cinnamon

1 1/2 Tbsp. light, soft tub margarine

1/2 cup water, or apple juice

4 pecan halves, optional

1. Scoop out centers of apples, creating a cavity 1 1/2" wide and stopping 1/2" from the bottom of each. Peel top of each apple down about 1". Brush edges with lemon juice.

2. Mix together apricots, nuts, brown sugar, sugar substitute, and cinnamon. Stir in margarine. Spoon mixture evenly into apples.

3. Put 1/2 cup water or juice in bottom of slow cooker. Put 2 apples in bottom, and 2 apples above, but not squarely on top of other apples. Cover and cook on Low 1 1/2–3 hours, or until tender.

4. Serve warm or at room temperature. Top each apple with a pecan half, if desired.

Exchange List Values: Fruit 2.0, Carbohydrate 0.5, Fat 1.5

Basic Nutritional Values: Calories 212 (Calories from Fat 77), Total Fat 9 gm (Saturated Fat 0.8 gm, Polyunsat Fat 5.2 gm, Monounsat Fat 1.9 gm, Cholesterol 0 mg), Sodium 40 mg, Total Carbohydrate 36 gm, Dietary Fiber 5 gm, Sugars 28 gm, Protein 2 gm

Wagon Master Apple-Cherry Sauce

Sharon Timpe • Mequon, WI

Makes 15 servings (Ideal slow cooker size: 4-quart)

2 21-oz. cans apple pie filling

2–3 cups frozen tart red cherries

1 Tbsp. butter or margarine

1/2 tsp. ground cinnamon

1/2 tsp. ground nutmeg

1/8 tsp. ground ginger

1/8 tsp. ground cloves

1. Combine all ingredients in slow cooker.

2. Cover. Heat on Low 3–4 hours, until hot and bubbly. Stir occasionally.

3. Serve warm over vanilla ice cream, pudding, pound cake, or shortcake biscuits. Top with whipped cream, if you wish.

Exchange List Values: Carbohydrate 1.5

Basic Nutritional Values: Calories 97 (Calories from Fat 9), Total Fat 1 gm (Saturated Fat 0.2 gm, Polyunsat Fat 0.3 gm, Monounsat Fat 0.4 gm, Cholesterol 0 mg), Sodium 44 mg, Total Carbohydrate 23 gm, Dietary Fiber 1 gm, Sugars 18 gm, Protein 0 gm

Apple Schnitz

Betty Hostetler • Allensville, PA

Makes 10 servings (Ideal slow cooker size: 3–4-quart)

1 qt. dried apples

3 cups water

1/4 cup sugar

sugar substitute to equal 4 Tbsp.

1 tsp. ground cinnamon

1 tsp. salt

1. Combine apples, water, sugar, sugar substitute, cinnamon, and salt in slow cooker.

2. Cover. Cook on Low 6 hours, or High 2½ hours.

3. Serve warm as a side dish with bean soup, or as filling for pies.

4. To use as pie filling, remove apples from slow cooker. Mash until smooth with potato masher or put through food mill. Cool.

Exchange List Values: Fruit 2.0

Basic Nutritional Values: Calories 105 (Calories from Fat 1), Total Fat 0 gm (Saturated Fat 0 gm, Polyunsat Fat 0 gm, Monounsat Fat 0 gm, Cholesterol 0 mg), Sodium 262 mg, Total Carbohydrate 28 gm, Dietary Fiber 3 gm, Sugars 21 gm, Protein 0 gm

Apple Crisp

Michelle Strite • Goshen, IN

Makes 12 servings (Ideal slow cooker size: 4-quart)

2/3 cup sugar

1¼ cups water

3 Tbsp. cornstarch

4 cups sliced, peeled apples

1/2 tsp. ground cinnamon

1/4 tsp. ground allspice

3/4 cup quick oatmeal

1/4 cup brown sugar

brown sugar substitute to equal 2 Tbsp.

1/2 cup flour

1/4 cup light, soft tub margarine, at room temperature

1. Combine 2/3 cup sugar, water, cornstarch, apples, cinnamon, and allspice. Place in cooker.

2. Combine remaining ingredients until crumbly. Sprinkle over apple filling.

3. Cover. Cook on Low 2–3 hours.

Exchange List Values: Carbohydrate 2.0

Basic Nutritional Values: Calories 134 (Calories from Fat 18), Total Fat 2 gm (Saturated Fat 0.2 gm, Polyunsat Fat 0.5 gm, Monounsat Fat 0.9 gm, Cholesterol 0 mg), Sodium 34 mg, Total Carbohydrate 29 gm, Dietary Fiber 2 gm, Sugars 15 gm, Protein 1 gm

Hot Fruit Salad

Sharon Miller • Holmesville, OH

Makes 16 servings (Ideal slow cooker size: 5-quart)

25-oz. jar chunky unsweetened applesauce

21-oz. can light cherry pie filling

20-oz. can pineapple chunks, packed in juice

15½-oz. can sliced peaches, packed in juice

15½-oz. can apricot halves, packed in juice

11-oz. can mandarin oranges, packed in juice

2 Tbsp. brown sugar

brown sugar substitute to equal 1 Tbsp.

1 tsp. ground cinnamon

1. Combine fruit in slow cooker, stirring gently.

2. Combine brown sugar, sugar substitute, and cinnamon. Sprinkle over mixture.

3. Cover. Bake on Low 3–4 hours.

Exchange List Values: Fruit 2.0

Basic Nutritional Values: Calories 105 (Calories from Fat 1), Total Fat 0 gm (Saturated Fat 0 gm, Polyunsat Fat 0.1 gm, Monounsat Fat 0.1 gm, Cholesterol 0 mg), Sodium 12 mg, Total Carbohydrate 27 gm, Dietary Fiber 2 gm, Sugars 24 gm, Protein 1 gm

Curried Fruit

Jane Meiser • Harrisonburg, VA

Makes 8–10 servings (Ideal slow cooker size: 4–5-quart)

16-oz. can peaches, undrained

16-oz. can apricots, undrained

16-oz. can pears, undrained

20-oz. can pineapple chunks, undrained

16-oz. can black cherries, undrained

2 Tbsp. brown sugar

brown sugar substitute to equal 1 Tbsp.

1 tsp. curry powder

3–4 Tbsp. quick-cooking tapioca, depending upon how thickened you'd like the finished dish to be

margarine, optional

1. Combine fruit. Let stand for at least 2 hours, or up to 8, to allow flavors to blend. Drain. Place in slow cooker.

2. Add remaining ingredients. Mix well. Top with margarine, if you want.

3. Cover. Cook on Low 8–10 hours.

4. Serve warm or at room temperature.

Exchange List Values: Fruit 2.0

Basic Nutritional Values: Calories 107 (Calories from Fat 1), Total Fat 0 gm (Saturated Fat 0 gm, Polyunsat Fat 0 gm, Monounsat Fat 0 gm, Cholesterol 0 mg), Sodium 7 mg, Total Carbohydrate 27 gm, Dietary Fiber 2 gm, Sugars 21 gm, Protein 1 gm

Fruit Dessert Topping

Lavina Hochstedler • Grand Blanc, MI

Makes 40 (2-Tbsp.) servings (Ideal slow cooker size: 4-quart)

3 tart apples, peeled and sliced

3 pears, peeled and sliced

1 Tbsp. lemon juice

2 Tbsp. brown sugar

brown sugar substitute to equal 1 Tbsp.

2 Tbsp. maple syrup

2 Tbsp. light, soft tub margarine, melted

½ cup chopped pecans

¼ cup raisins

2 cinnamon sticks

1 Tbsp. cornstarch

2 Tbsp. cold water

1. Toss apples and pears in lemon juice in slow cooker.

2. Combine brown sugar, sugar substitute, maple syrup, and margarine. Pour over fruit.

3. Stir in pecans, raisins, and cinnamon sticks.

4. Cover. Cook on Low 3–4 hours.

5. Combine cornstarch and water until smooth. Gradually stir into slow cooker.

6. Cover. Cook on High 30–40 minutes, or until thickened.

7. Discard cinnamon sticks. Serve over pound cake or ice cream.

Exchange List Values: Carbohydrate 0.5

Basic Nutritional Values: Calories 33 (Calories from Fat 13), Total Fat 1 gm (Saturated Fat 0.1 gm, Polyunsat Fat 0.4 gm, Monounsat Fat 0.8 gm, Cholesterol 0 mg), Sodium 5 mg, Total Carbohydrate 6 gm, Dietary Fiber 1 gm, Sugars 5 gm, Protein 0 gm

We also like this served along with pancakes or an egg casserole. We always use Fruit Dessert Topping for our breakfasts at church camp.

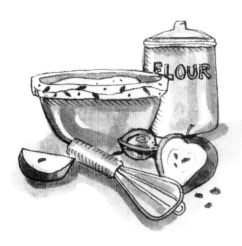

Rhubarb Sauce

Esther Porter • Minneapolis, MN

Makes 6 servings (Ideal slow cooker size: 3–4-quart)

1½ lbs. rhubarb

⅛ tsp. salt

½ cup water

½–⅔ cup sugar

1. Cut rhubarb into ½" slices.

2. Combine all ingredients in slow cooker. Cook on Low 4–5 hours.

3. Serve chilled.

Exchange List Values: Carbohydrate 1.0

Basic Nutritional Values: Calories 80 (Calories from Fat 1), Total Fat 0 gm (Saturated Fat 0 gm, Polyunsat Fat 0 gm, Monounsat Fat 0 gm, Cholesterol 0 mg), Sodium 54 mg, Total Carbohydrate 20 gm, Dietary Fiber 2 gm, Sugars 17 gm, Protein 1 gm

VARIATION: Add 1 pint sliced strawberries about 30 minutes before removing from heat.

Zesty Pears

Barbara Walker • Sturgis, SD

Makes 8 servings (Ideal slow cooker size: 3–4-quart)

6 fresh pears

½ cup raisins

¼ cup brown sugar

1 tsp. grated lemon peel

¼ cup brandy

½ cup sauterne wine

½ cup macaroon crumbs

1. Peel and core pears. Cut into thin slices.

2. Combine raisins, sugar, and lemon peel. Layer alternately with pear slices in slow cooker.

3. Pour brandy and wine over top.

4. Cover. Cook on Low 4–6 hours.

5. Spoon into serving dishes. Cool. Sprinkle with macaroons. Serve plain or topped with sour cream.

Exchange List Values: Carbohydrate 2.0

Basic Nutritional Values: Calories 140 (Calories from Fat 13), Total Fat 1 gm (Saturated Fat 0.9 gm, Polyunsat Fat 0.1 gm, Monounsat Fat 0.1 gm, Cholesterol 0 mg), Sodium 11 mg, Total Carbohydrate 33 gm, Dietary Fiber 3 gm, Sugars 28 gm, Protein 1 gm

Fruit Compote Dessert

Beatrice Orgish • Richardson, TX

Makes 8 servings (Ideal slow cooker size: 4-quart)

2 medium tart apples, peeled

2 medium fresh peaches, peeled and cubed

2 cups unsweetened pineapple chunks

1¼ cups unsweetened pineapple juice

¼ cup honey

2¼"-thick lemon slices

3½"-long cinnamon stick

1 medium firm banana, thinly sliced

whipped cream, optional

sliced almonds, optional

maraschino cherries, optional

1. Cut apples into ¼" slices and then in half horizontally. Place in slow cooker.

2. Add peaches, pineapple chunks, pineapple juice, honey, lemon, and cinnamon. Cover and cook on Low 3–4 hours.

3. Stir in banana slices just before serving. Garnish with whipped cream, sliced almonds, and cherries, if you wish.

Exchange List Values: Fruit 2.0

Basic Nutritional Values: Calories 117 (Calories from Fat 4), Total Fat 0 gm (Saturated Fat 0 gm, Polyunsat Fat 0.1 gm, Monounsat Fat 0.1 gm, Cholesterol 0 mg), Sodium 2 mg, Total Carbohydrate 31 gm, Dietary Fiber 2 gm, Sugars 27 gm, Protein 1 gm

Scandinavian Fruit Soup

Willard E. Roth • Elkhart, IN

Makes 14 servings (Ideal slow cooker size: 4-quart)

1 cup dried apricots

1 cup dried sliced apples

1 cup dried pitted plums

1 cup canned pitted red cherries

½ cup quick-cooking tapioca

1 cup grape juice, or red wine

3 cups water, or more

½ cup orange juice

¼ cup lemon juice

1 Tbsp. grated orange peel

2 Tbsp. brown sugar

brown sugar substitute to equal 1 Tbsp.

1. Combine apricots, apples, plums, cherries, tapioca, and grape juice in slow cooker. Cover with water.

2. Cook on Low for at least 8 hours.

3. Before serving, stir in remaining ingredients.

4. Serve warm or cold, as a soup or dessert. Delicious served chilled over vanilla ice cream or frozen yogurt.

Exchange List Values: Fruit 2.0

Basic Nutritional Values: Calories 120 (Calories from Fat 1), Total Fat 0 gm (Saturated Fat 0 gm, Polyunsat Fat 0 gm, Monounsat Fat 0.1 gm, Cholesterol 0 mg), Sodium 10 mg, Total Carbohydrate 31 gm, Dietary Fiber 2 gm, Sugars 21 gm, Protein 1 gm

Strawberry Rhubarb Sauce

Tina Snyder • Manheim, PA

Makes 8 servings (Ideal slow cooker size: 4-quart)

6 cups chopped rhubarb

1 cup sugar

1 cinnamon stick

½ cup white grape juice

2 cups sliced strawberries

1. Place rhubarb in slow cooker. Pour sugar over rhubarb. Add cinnamon stick and grape juice. Stir well.

2. Cover and cook on Low 5–6 hours, or until rhubarb is tender.

3. Stir in strawberries. Cook 1 hour longer.

4. Remove cinnamon stick. Chill.

5. Serve over cake or ice cream.

Exchange List Values: Carbohydrate 2.0

Basic Nutritional Values: Calories 132 (Calories from Fat 3), Total Fat 0 gm (Saturated Fat 0 gm, Polyunsat Fat 0.1 gm, Monounsat Fat 0 gm, Cholesterol 0 mg), Sodium 5 mg, Total Carbohydrate 33 gm, Dietary Fiber 3 gm, Sugars 29 gm, Protein 1 gm

Spiced Applesauce

Judi Manos • West Islip, NY

Makes 12 servings (Ideal slow cooker size: 4-quart)

12 cups cored, pared, thinly sliced, medium cooking apples

¼ cup sugar

sugar substitute to equal 2 Tbsp.

½ tsp. cinnamon

1 cup water

1 Tbsp. lemon juice

freshly grated nutmeg, optional

1. Place apples in slow cooker.

2. Combine sugar, sugar substitute, and cinnamon. Mix with apples. Stir in water and lemon juice, and nutmeg, if desired.

3. Cover. Cook on Low 5–7 hours, or High 2½–3½ hours.

4. Stir for a chunky sauce. Serve hot or cold.

Exchange List Values: Carbohydrate 1.0

Basic Nutritional Values: Calories 75 (Calories from Fat 3), Total Fat 0 gm (Saturated Fat 0 gm, Polyunsat Fat 0.1 gm, Monounsat Fat 0 gm, Cholesterol 0 mg), Sodium 0 mg, Total Carbohydrate 20 gm, Dietary Fiber 2 gm, Sugars 18 gm, Protein 0 gm

Physical activity is essential to weight control.

Quick Yummy Peaches

Willard E. Roth • Elkhart, IN

Makes 8 servings (Ideal slow cooker size: 4-quart)

1/3 cup buttermilk baking mix

2/3 cup dry quick oats

1/4 cup brown sugar

brown sugar substitute to equal 2 Tbsp.

1 tsp. cinnamon

4 cups sliced peaches (canned or fresh)

1/2 cup peach juice, or water

1. Mix together baking mix, oats, brown sugar, sugar substitute, and cinnamon in greased slow cooker.

2. Stir in peaches and peach juice.

3. Cook on Low at least 5 hours. (If you like a drier cobbler, remove lid for last 15–30 minutes of cooking.)

4. Serve with frozen yogurt or ice cream.

Exchange List Values: Carbohydrate 2.0

Basic Nutritional Values: Calories 131 (Calories from Fat 11), Total Fat 1 gm (Saturated Fat 0.1 gm, Polyunsat Fat 0.5 gm, Monounsat Fat 0.4 gm, Cholesterol 0 mg), Sodium 76 mg, Total Carbohydrate 29 gm, Dietary Fiber 3 gm, Sugars 20 gm, Protein 2 gm

Scalloped Pineapples

Shirley Hinh • Wayland, IA

Makes 8 servings (Ideal slow cooker size: 4-quart)

1/2 cup sugar

sugar substitute to equal 1/4 cup

3 eggs

1/4 cup light, soft tub margarine, melted

3/4 cup milk

20-oz. can crushed pineapple, drained

8 slices bread (crusts removed), cubed

1. Mix together all ingredients in slow cooker.

2. Cook on High 2 hours. Reduce heat to Low and cook 1 more hour.

3. Delicious served as a side dish to ham or poultry, or as a dessert served warm or cold. Eat hot or chilled with vanilla ice cream or frozen yogurt.

Exchange List Values: Carbohydrate 2.0, Fat 0.5

Basic Nutritional Values: Calories 181 (Calories from Fat 44), Total Fat 5 gm (Saturated Fat 1.1 gm, Polyunsat Fat 1.1 gm, Monounsat Fat 2.1 gm, Cholesterol 81 mg), Sodium 176 mg, Total Carbohydrate 30 gm, Dietary Fiber 1 gm, Sugars 21 gm, Protein 5 gm

Black and Blue Cobbler

Renee Shirk • Mount Joy, PA

Makes 12 servings (Ideal slow cooker size: 5-quart)

1 cup flour

6 Tbsp. sugar

sugar substitute to equal 3 Tbsp.

1 tsp. baking powder

¼ tsp. salt

¼ tsp. ground cinnamon

¼ tsp. ground nutmeg

2 eggs, beaten

2 Tbsp. milk

2 Tbsp. vegetable oil

2 cups fresh or frozen blueberries

2 cups fresh or frozen blackberries

¾ cup water

1 tsp. grated orange peel

6 Tbsp. sugar

sugar substitute to equal 3 Tbsp.

whipped topping, or ice cream, optional

1. Combine flour, 6 Tbsp. sugar, sugar substitute to equal 3 Tbsp., baking powder, salt, cinnamon, and nutmeg.

2. Combine eggs, milk, and oil. Stir into dry ingredients until moistened.

3. Spread the batter evenly over bottom of greased slow cooker.

4. In saucepan, combine berries, water, orange peel, 6 Tbsp. sugar, and sugar substitute to equal 3 Tbsp. Bring to boil. Remove from heat and pour over batter. Cover.

5. Cook on High 2–2½ hours, or until toothpick inserted into batter comes out clean. Turn off cooker.

6. Uncover and let stand 30 minutes before serving. Spoon from cooker and serve with whipped topping or ice cream, if desired.

Exchange List Values: Carbohydrate 2.0, Fat 0.5

Basic Nutritional Values: Calories 170 (Calories from Fat 31), Total Fat 3 gm (Saturated Fat 0.5 gm, Polyunsat Fat 0.9 gm, Monounsat Fat 1.7 gm, Cholesterol 36 mg), Sodium 92 mg, Total Carbohydrate 34 gm, Dietary Fiber 2 gm, Sugars 23 gm, Protein 3 gm

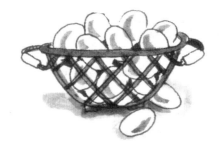

Cranberry Pudding

Margaret Wheeler • North Bend, OR

Makes 12 servings (Ideal slow cooker size: 4–5-quart)

PUDDING:

1⅓ cups flour

½ tsp. salt

2 tsp. baking soda

⅓ cup boiling water

6 Tbsp. dark molasses

2 cups whole cranberries

½ cup chopped walnuts

½ cup water

BUTTER SAUCE:

1 cup confectioners' sugar

½ cup fat-free half-and-half

4 Tbsp. light, soft tub margarine

1 tsp. vanilla

1. Mix together flour and salt.

2. Dissolve soda in boiling water. Add to flour and salt.

3. Stir in molasses. Blend well.

4. Fold in cranberries and nuts.

5. Pour into well-greased and floured bread or cake pan that will sit in your cooker. Cover with greased tinfoil.

6. Pour ½ cup water into cooker. Place foil-covered pan in cooker. Cover with cooker lid and steam on High 3–4 hours, or until pudding tests done with a wooden pick.

7. Remove pan and uncover. Let stand 5 minutes, then unmold.

8. To make butter sauce, mix together all ingredients in saucepan. Cook, stirring over medium heat, until sugar dissolves.

9. Serve warm butter sauce over warm cranberry pudding.

Exchange List Values: Carbohydrate 2.0, Fat 0.5

Basic Nutritional Values: Calories 177 (Calories from Fat 46), Total Fat 5 gm (Saturated Fat 0.5 gm, Polyunsat Fat 2.7 gm, Monounsat Fat 1.3 gm, Cholesterol 1 mg), Sodium 355 mg, Total Carbohydrate 31 gm, Dietary Fiber 1 gm, Sugars 18 gm, Protein 3 gm

Slow Cooker Pumpkin Pie Pudding

Joette Droz • Kalona, IA

Makes 8 servings (Ideal slow cooker size: 4-quart)

15-oz. can solid-pack pumpkin

12-oz. can fat-free evaporated milk

½ cup sugar

sugar substitute to equal 2 Tbsp.

½ cup buttermilk baking mix

2 eggs, beaten

2 Tbsp. light, soft tub margarine, melted

1 Tbsp. pumpkin pie spice

2 tsp. vanilla

1. Mix together all ingredients. Pour into greased slow cooker.

2. Cover and cook on Low 6–7 hours, or until thermometer reads 160°.

3. Serve in bowls topped with fat-free whipped topping, if you wish.

Exchange List Values: Carbohydrate 2.0, Fat 0.5

Basic Nutritional Values: Calories 171 (Calories from Fat 36), Total Fat 4 gm (Saturated Fat 0.7 gm, Polyunsat Fat 0.9 gm, Monounsat Fat 1.6 gm, Cholesterol 53 mg), Sodium 203 mg, Total Carbohydrate 28 gm, Dietary Fiber 2 gm, Sugars 19 gm, Protein 6 gm

Low-Fat Apple Cake

Sue Hamilton • Minooka, IL

Makes 10 servings (Ideal slow cooker size: 4-quart)

1 cup flour

¾ cup sugar

sugar substitute to equal 2 Tbsp.

2 tsp. baking powder

1 tsp. ground cinnamon

¼ tsp. salt

4 medium-sized cooking apples, chopped

2 eggs, beaten

2 tsp. vanilla

1. Combine flour, sugar, sugar substitute, baking powder, cinnamon, and salt.

2. Add apples, stirring lightly to coat.

3. Combine eggs and vanilla. Add to apple mixture. Stir until just moistened. Spoon into lightly greased slow cooker.

4. Cover. Bake on High 2½–3 hours.

5. Serve warm. Top with frozen whipped topping, thawed, or ice cream and a sprinkle of cinnamon, if you wish.

Exchange List Values: Carbohydrate 2.0

Basic Nutritional Values: Calories 152 (Calories from Fat 11), Total Fat 1 gm (Saturated Fat 0.4 gm, Polyunsat Fat 0.2 gm, Monounsat Fat 0.4 gm, Cholesterol 43 mg), Sodium 144 mg, Total Carbohydrate 33 gm, Dietary Fiber 2 gm, Sugars 22 gm, Protein 3 gm

VARIATION: Stir ½ cup broken English or black walnuts, or ½ cup raisins, into Step 2.

The slow cooker is great for baking desserts. Your guests will be pleasantly surprised to see a cake coming from your slow cooker.

Lemon Pudding Cake

Jean Butzer • Batavia, NY

Makes 6 servings (Ideal slow cooker size: 3-4-quart)

3 eggs, separated

1 tsp. grated lemon peel

1/4 cup lemon juice

1 Tbsp. light, soft tub margarine, melted

1 1/2 cups fat-free half-and-half

1/2 cup sugar

sugar substitute to equal 2 Tbsp.

1/4 cup flour

1/8 tsp. salt

1. Beat egg whites until stiff peaks form. Set aside.

2. Beat egg yolks. Blend in lemon peel, lemon juice, margarine, and half-and-half.

3. In separate bowl, combine sugar, sugar substitute, flour, and salt. Add to egg-lemon mixture, beating until smooth.

4. Fold into beaten egg whites.

5. Spoon into slow cooker.

6. Cover and cook on High 2-3 hours.

7. Serve from cooker.

Exchange List Values: Carbohydrate 2.0, Fat 0.5

Basic Nutritional Values: Calories 169 (Calories from Fat 37), Total Fat 4 gm (Saturated Fat 1.5 gm, Polyunsat Fat 0.5 gm, Monounsat Fat 1.4 gm, Cholesterol 111 mg), Sodium 185 mg, Total Carbohydrate 27 gm, Dietary Fiber 0 gm, Sugars 20 gm, Protein 5 gm

Dump Cake

Janice Muller • Derwood, MD

Makes 15 servings (Ideal slow cooker size: 4-5-quart)

20-oz. can crushed pineapple

21-oz. can light blueberry or cherry pie filling

18 1/2-oz. pkg. yellow cake mix

cinnamon

1/3 cup light, soft tub margarine

1/3 cup chopped walnuts

1. Grease bottom and sides of slow cooker.

2. Spread layers of pineapple, blueberry pie filling, and dry cake mix. Be careful not to mix the layers.

3. Sprinkle with cinnamon.

4. Top with thin layers of margarine chunks and nuts.

5. Cover. Cook on High 2-3 hours.

6. Serve with vanilla ice cream, if you wish.

Exchange List Values: Carbohydrate 2.5, Fat 1.0

Basic Nutritional Values: Calories 219 (Calories from Fat 57), Total Fat 6 gm (Saturated Fat 1.5 gm, Polyunsat Fat 2.4 gm, Monounsat Fat 2.2 gm, Cholesterol 0 mg), Sodium 250 mg, Total Carbohydrate 41 gm, Dietary Fiber 1 gm, Sugars 28 gm, Protein 2 gm

VARIATION: Use a pkg. of spice cake mix and apple pie filling.

Creamy Orange Cheesecake

Jeanette Oberholtzer • Manheim, PA

Recipe photo appears in color section.

Makes 10 servings (Ideal slow cooker size: 5–6-quart)

CRUST:

¾ cup graham cracker crumbs

2 Tbsp. sugar

3 Tbsp. light, soft tub margarine, melted

FILLING:

2 8-oz. pkgs. fat-free cream cheese, at room temperature

⅔ cup sugar

2 eggs

1 egg yolk

¼ cup frozen orange juice concentrate

1 tsp. orange peel

1 Tbsp. flour

½ tsp. vanilla

1. Combine crust ingredients. Pat into 7" or 9" springform pan, whichever size fits into your slow cooker.

2. Cream together cream cheese and sugar. Add eggs and yolk. Beat for 3 minutes.

3. Beat in juice, peel, flour, and vanilla. Beat 2 minutes.

4. Pour batter into crust. Place pan on rack in slow cooker.

5. Cover. Cook on High 2½–3 hours. Turn off and let stand for 1–2 hours, or until cool enough to remove from cooker.

6. Cool completely before removing sides of pan. Chill before serving.

7. Serve with thawed frozen whipped topping and fresh or mandarin orange slices, if you wish.

Exchange List Values: Carbohydrate 1.5, Meat, lean 1.0

Basic Nutritional Values: Calories 159 (Calories from Fat 23), Total Fat 3 gm (Saturated Fat 0.7 gm, Polyunsat Fat 0.6 gm, Monounsat Fat 1.1 gm, Cholesterol 69 mg), Sodium 300 mg, Total Carbohydrate 25 gm, Dietary Fiber 0 gm, Sugars 19 gm, Protein 9 gm

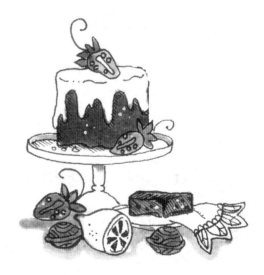

Carrot Cake

Colleen Heatwole • Burton, MI

Makes 10 servings (Ideal slow cooker size: 4–5-quart)

⅓ cup canola oil

2 eggs

1 Tbsp. hot water

½ cup grated raw carrots

¾ cup flour

¾ cup sugar

½ tsp. baking powder

⅛ tsp. salt

¼ tsp. ground allspice

½ tsp. ground cinnamon

⅛ tsp. ground cloves

½ cup chopped nuts

½ cup raisins or chopped dates

2 Tbsp. flour

1. In large bowl, beat oil, eggs, and water for 1 minute.

2. Add carrots. Mix well.

3. Stir together ¾ cup flour, sugar, baking powder, salt, allspice, cinnamon, and cloves. Add to creamed mixture.

4. Toss nuts and raisins in bowl with 2 Tbsp. flour. Add to creamed mixture. Mix well.

5. Pour into greased and floured 3-lb. shortening can or slow cooker baking insert. Place can or baking insert in slow cooker.

6. Cover insert with its lid, or cover can with 8 paper towels, folded down over edge of slow cooker to absorb moisture. Cover paper towels with cooker lid. Cook on High 3–4 hours.

7. Remove can or insert from cooker and allow to cool on rack for 10 minutes. Run knife around edge of cake. Invert onto serving plate.

Exchange List Values: Carbohydrate 2.0, Fat 3.0

Basic Nutritional Values: Calories 274 (Calories from Fat 147), Total Fat 16 gm (Saturated Fat 1.5 gm, Polyunsat Fat 6.4 gm, Monounsat Fat 7.6 gm, Cholesterol 43 mg), Sodium 66 mg, Total Carbohydrate 30 gm, Dietary Fiber 1 gm, Sugars 20 gm, Protein 4 gm

The key to weight loss is simple: Burn more calories than you eat.

Chocolate Peanut Butter Cake

Ruth Ann Gingrich • New Holland, PA

Makes 11 servings (Ideal slow cooker size: 4-quart)

2 cups (half a package) milk chocolate cake mix

$1/2$ cup water

$1/4$ cup peanut butter

1 egg

2 egg whites

6 Tbsp. chopped walnuts

1. Combine all ingredients. Beat 2 minutes in electric mixer.

2. Pour into greased and floured 3-lb. shortening can. Place can in slow cooker.

3. Cover top of can with 8 paper towels.

4. Cover cooker. Bake on High 2–3 hours.

5. Allow to cool for 10 minutes. Run knife around edge and invert cake onto serving plate. Cool completely before slicing and serving.

Exchange List Values: Carbohydrate 1.5, Fat 1.5

Basic Nutritional Values: Calories 165 (Calories from Fat 75), Total Fat 8 gm (Saturated Fat 1.5 gm, Polyunsat Fat 3.6 gm, Monounsat Fat 2.8 gm, Cholesterol 19 mg), Sodium 255 mg, Total Carbohydrate 20 gm, Dietary Fiber 1 gm, Sugars 11 gm, Protein 4 gm

Harvey Wallbanger Cake

Roseann Wilson • Albuquerque, NM

Makes 18 servings (Ideal slow cooker size: 4–5-quart)

CAKE:

16-oz. pkg. pound cake mix

$1/3$ cup vanilla instant pudding (reserve rest of pudding from 3-oz. pkg. for glaze)

2 Tbsp. canola oil

3 eggs

2 Tbsp. Galliano liqueur

$2/3$ cup orange juice

GLAZE:

remaining pudding mix

$2/3$ cup orange juice

1 Tbsp. Galliano liqueur

1. Mix together all ingredients for cake. Beat for 3 minutes. Pour batter into greased and floured bread or cake pan that will fit into your slow cooker. Cover pan.

2. Bake in covered slow cooker on High $2^1\!/_2$–$3^1\!/_2$ hours.

3. Invert cake onto serving platter.

4. Mix together glaze ingredients. Spoon over cake.

Exchange List Values: Carbohydrate 2.0, Fat 0.5

Basic Nutritional Values: Calories 165 (Calories from Fat 49), Total Fat 5 gm (Saturated Fat 1.5 gm, Polyunsat Fat 0.8 gm, Monounsat Fat 2.1 gm, Cholesterol 36 mg), Sodium 168 mg, Total Carbohydrate 28 gm, Dietary Fiber 0 gm, Sugars 19 gm, Protein 2 gm

Graham Cracker Cookies

Cassandra Ly • Carlisle, PA

Makes 96 1-cookie servings (Ideal slow cooker size: 4-quart)

12-oz. pkg. (2 cups) semisweet chocolate chips

2 1-oz. squares unsweetened baking chocolate, shaved

2 14-oz. cans fat-free sweetened condensed milk

3¾ cups crushed graham cracker crumbs, divided

1 cup finely chopped walnuts

1. Place chocolate in slow cooker.

2. Cover. Cook on High 1 hour, stirring every 15 minutes. Continue to cook on Low heat, stirring every 15 minutes, or until chocolate is melted (about 30 minutes).

3. Stir milk into melted chocolate.

4. Add 3 cups graham cracker crumbs, 1 cup at a time, stirring after each addition.

5. Stir in nuts. Mixture should be thick but not stiff.

6. Stir in remaining graham cracker crumbs to reach consistency of cookie dough.

7. Drop by heaping teaspoonfuls onto lightly greased cookie sheets. Keep remaining mixture warm by covering and turning the slow cooker to warm.

8. Bake at 325° for 7–9 minutes, or until tops of cookies begin to crack. Remove from oven. Cool 1–2 minutes before transferring to waxed paper.

Exchange List Values: Carbohydrate 0.5, Fat 0.5

Basic Nutritional Values: Calories 65 (Calories from Fat 23), Total Fat 3 gm (Saturated Fat 0.9 gm, Polyunsat Fat 0.8 gm, Monounsat Fat 0.9 gm, Cholesterol 0 mg), Sodium 29 mg, Total Carbohydrate 10 gm, Dietary Fiber 0 gm, Sugars 8 gm, Protein 1 gm

Note: These cookies freeze well.

This delectable fudge-like cookie is a family favorite. The original recipe (from my maternal grandmother) was so involved and yielded so few cookies that my mom and I would get together to make a couple of batches only at Christmastime. Adapting the recipe for using a slow cooker, rather than a double boiler, allows me to prepare a double batch without help.

Apple Peanut Crumble

Phyllis Attig • Reynolds, IL / Joan Becker • Dodge City, KS / Pam Hochstedler • Kalona, IA

Recipe photo appears in color section.

Makes 8 servings (Ideal slow cooker size: 4-quart)

4 medium cooking apples, peeled and sliced

⅓ cup packed brown sugar

brown sugar substitute to equal 3 Tbsp.

½ cup flour

½ cup quick-cooking dry oats

½ tsp. cinnamon

¼–½ tsp. nutmeg

¼ cup light, soft tub margarine, softened

2 Tbsp. peanut butter

ice cream, or whipped cream, optional

1. Place apple slices in slow cooker.

2. Combine brown sugar, sugar substitute, flour, oats, cinnamon, and nutmeg.

3. Cut in margarine and peanut butter. Sprinkle over apples.

4. Cover cooker and cook on Low 5–6 hours.

5. Serve warm or cold, plain or with ice cream or whipped cream.

Exchange List Values: Carbohydrate 2.0, Fat 0.5

Basic Nutritional Values: Calories 164 (Calories from Fat 45), Total Fat 5 gm (Saturated Fat 0.7 gm, Polyunsat Fat 1.3 gm, Monounsat Fat 2.4 gm, Cholesterol 0 mg), Sodium 71 mg, Total Carbohydrate 29 gm, Dietary Fiber 2 gm, Sugars 18 gm, Protein 3 gm

Cherry Delight

Anna Musser • Manheim, PA / Marianne J. Troyer • Millersburg, OH

Makes 10–12 servings (Ideal slow cooker size: 4-quart)

20-oz. can cherry pie filling, light

½ pkg. yellow cake mix

¼ cup light, soft tub margarine, melted

⅓ cup walnuts, optional

1. Place pie filling in greased slow cooker.

2. Combine dry cake mix and margarine (mixture will be crumbly). Sprinkle over filling. Sprinkle with walnuts, if desired.

3. Cover and cook on Low 4 hours, or on High 2 hours.

4. Allow to cool, then serve in bowls with dips of ice cream, if you wish.

Exchange List Values: Carbohydrate 2.0

Basic Nutritional Values: Calories 137 (Calories from Fat 33), Total Fat 4 gm (Saturated Fat 0.9 gm, Polyunsat Fat 0.9 gm, Monounsat Fat 1.6 gm, Cholesterol 0 mg), Sodium 174 mg, Total Carbohydrate 26 gm, Dietary Fiber 1 gm, Sugars 19 gm, Protein 1 gm

Hot Fudge Cake

Maricarol Magil • Freehold, NJ

Makes 10 servings (Ideal slow cooker size: 4-quart)

1/2 cup packed brown sugar

brown sugar substitute to equal 1/4 cup

1 cup flour

3 Tbsp. unsweetened cocoa powder

2 tsp. baking powder

1/2 tsp. salt

1/2 cup fat-free half-and-half

2 Tbsp. melted butter

1/2 tsp. vanilla

6 Tbsp. brown sugar

brown sugar substitute to equal 3 Tbsp.

1/4 cup unsweetened cocoa powder

1 3/4 cups boiling water

1. Mix together 1/2 cup brown sugar, brown sugar substitute to equal 1/4 cup, flour, 3 Tbsp. cocoa, baking powder, and salt.

2. Stir in half-and-half, butter, and vanilla. Spread over bottom of slow cooker.

3. Mix together 6 Tbsp. brown sugar, brown sugar substitute to equal 3 Tbsp., and 1/4 cup cocoa. Sprinkle over mixture in slow cooker.

4. Pour in boiling water. Do not stir.

5. Cover and cook on High 2–3 hours, or until toothpick inserted comes out clean.

6. Serve warm with vanilla ice cream, if diets allow.

Exchange List Values: Carbohydrate 2.0

Basic Nutritional Values: Calories 143 (Calories from Fat 11), Total Fat 1 gm (Saturated Fat 0.4 gm, Polyunsat Fat 0.2 gm, Monounsat Fat 0.4 gm, Cholesterol 1 mg), Sodium 226 mg, Total Carbohydrate 32 gm, Dietary Fiber 2 gm, Sugars 21 gm, Protein 2 gm

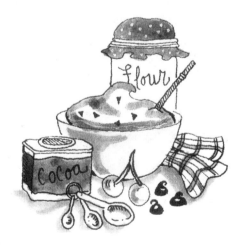

Chocolate Pudding Cake

Lee Ann Hazlett • Freeport, IL /
Della Yoder • Kalona, IA

Makes 24 servings (Ideal slow cooker size: 4–5-quart)

18½-oz. pkg. chocolate cake mix

3.9-oz. pkg. instant chocolate pudding mix

2 cups (16 ozs.) fat-free sour cream

4 eggs

1 cup water

½ cup canola oil

2 Tbsp. semisweet chocolate chips

1. Combine cake mix, pudding mix, sour cream, eggs, water, and oil in electric mixer bowl. Beat on medium speed for 2 minutes. Stir in chocolate chips.

2. Pour into greased slow cooker. Cover and cook on Low 6–7 hours, or on High 3–4 hours, or until toothpick inserted near center comes out with moist crumbs.

3. Serve with whipped cream, or ice cream, if you wish.

Exchange List Values: Carbohydrate 1.5, Fat 1.5

Basic Nutritional Values: Calories 186 (Calories from Fat 83), Total Fat 9 gm (Saturated Fat 1.5 gm, Polyunsat Fat 2.6 gm, Monounsat Fat 4.6 gm, Cholesterol 37 mg), Sodium 280 mg, Total Carbohydrate 24 gm, Dietary Fiber 1 gm, Sugars 13 gm, Protein 3 gm

Peanut Butter and Hot Fudge Pudding Cake

Sara Wilson • Blairstown, MO

Makes 6 servings (Ideal slow cooker size: 4-quart)

½ cup flour

¼ cup sugar

sugar substitute to equal 2 Tbsp.

¾ tsp. baking powder

⅓ cup fat-free milk

1 Tbsp. canola oil

½ tsp. vanilla

¼ cup peanut butter

¼ cup sugar

3 Tbsp. unsweetened cocoa powder

1 cup boiling water

1. Combine flour, ¼ cup sugar, sugar substitute, and baking powder. Add milk, oil, and vanilla. Mix until smooth. Stir in peanut butter. Pour into slow cooker.

2. Mix together ¼ cup sugar and cocoa powder. Gradually stir in boiling water. Pour mixture over batter in slow cooker. Do not stir.

3. Cover and cook on High 2–3 hours, or until toothpick inserted comes out clean.

4. Serve warm with ice cream, if you wish.

Exchange List Values: Carbohydrate 2.0, Fat 1.0

Basic Nutritional Values: Calories 197 (Calories from Fat 73), Total Fat 8 gm (Saturated Fat 1.1 gm, Polyunsat Fat 2.1 gm, Monounsat Fat 4.2 gm, Cholesterol 0 mg), Sodium 92 mg, Total Carbohydrate 29 gm, Dietary Fiber 2 gm, Sugars 18 gm, Protein 5 gm

Seven Layer Bars

Mary W. Stauffer • Ephrata, PA

Makes 18 servings (Ideal slow cooker size: 4–5-quart)

2 Tbsp. light, soft tub margarine, melted

$\frac{1}{2}$ cup graham cracker crumbs

$\frac{1}{4}$ cup chocolate chips

2 Tbsp. butterscotch chips

$\frac{1}{4}$ cup flaked coconut

$\frac{1}{2}$ cup chopped pecans

$\frac{1}{2}$ cup fat-free sweetened condensed milk

1. Layer ingredients in a bread or cake pan that fits in your slow cooker, in the order listed. Do not stir.

2. Cover and bake on High 2–3 hours, or until firm. Remove pan and uncover. Let stand 5 minutes.

3. Unmold carefully on plate and cool.

Exchange List Values: Carbohydrate 0.5, Fat 1.0

Basic Nutritional Values: Calories 87 (Calories from Fat 42), Total Fat 5 gm (Saturated Fat 1.4 gm, Polyunsat Fat 0.9 gm, Monounsat Fat 2.3 gm, Cholesterol 0 mg), Sodium 37 mg, Total Carbohydrate 11 gm, Dietary Fiber 1 gm, Sugars 9 gm, Protein 1 gm

Chocolate Rice Pudding

Michele Ruvola • Selden, NY

Recipe photo appears in color section.

Makes 12 servings (Ideal slow cooker size: 3–4-quart)

4 cups cooked white rice

$\frac{1}{2}$ cup sugar

sugar substitute to equal 2 Tbsp.

$\frac{1}{4}$ cup baking cocoa powder

2 Tbsp. light, soft tub margarine, melted

1 tsp. vanilla

2 12-oz. cans fat-free evaporated milk

whipped cream, optional

sliced toasted almonds, optional

maraschino cherries, optional

1. Combine first 7 ingredients in greased slow cooker.

2. Cover. Cook on Low $2\frac{1}{2}$–$3\frac{1}{2}$ hours, or until liquid is absorbed.

3. Serve warm or chilled. Top individual servings with a dollop of whipped cream, sliced toasted almonds, and a maraschino cherry, if you wish.

Exchange List Values: Carbohydrate 2.5

Basic Nutritional Values: Calories 180 (Calories from Fat 15), Total Fat 2 gm (Saturated Fat 0.3 gm, Polyunsat Fat 0.3 gm, Monounsat Fat 0.8 gm, Cholesterol 0 mg), Sodium 104 mg, Total Carbohydrate 35 gm, Dietary Fiber 1 gm, Sugars 18 gm, Protein 7 gm

Water is the best thing to drink when you're exercising for less than an hour.

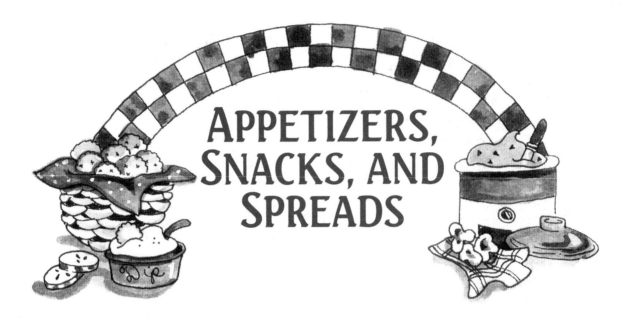

APPETIZERS, SNACKS, AND SPREADS

Quick and Easy Nacho Dip

Kristina Shull • Timberville, VA

Makes 20 servings (Ideal slow cooker size: 3-quart)

½ lb. 85%-lean ground beef

salt, optional

pepper, optional

onion powder, optional

2 cloves garlic, minced, optional

2 16-oz. jars salsa (as hot or mild as you like)

15-oz. can fat-free refried beans

1½ cups fat-free sour cream

1½ cups shredded reduced-fat sharp cheddar cheese, divided

1. Brown ground beef in skillet. Drain. Add salt, pepper, onion powder, and minced garlic.

2. Combine beef, salsa, beans, sour cream, and 1 cup cheese in slow cooker.

3. Cover. Heat on Low 2 hours. Just before serving, sprinkle with ½ cup cheese.

4. Serve with tortilla chips.

Exchange List Values: Carbohydrate 0.5, Meat, lean 1.0

Basic Nutritional Values: Calories 80 (Calories from Fat 27), Total Fat 3 gm (Saturated Fat 1.5 gm, Polyunsat Fat 0.2 gm, Monounsat Fat 1.0 gm, Cholesterol 14 mg), Sodium 298 mg, Total Carbohydrate 8 gm, Dietary Fiber 2 gm, Sugars 3 gm, Protein 6 gm

Red Pepper Cheese Dip

Ann Bender • Ft. Defiance, VA

Makes 12–15 servings (Ideal slow cooker size: 3–4-quart)

2 Tbsp. olive oil

4 large red peppers, cut into 1" squares

4 ozs. feta cheese

1. Pour oil into slow cooker. Stir in peppers.

2. Cover. Cook on Low 2 hours.

3. Serve with feta cheese on crackers.

Exchange List Values: Vegetable 1.0, Fat 0.5

Basic Nutritional Values: Calories 49 (Calories from Fat 32), Total Fat 4 gm (Saturated Fat 1.4 gm, Polyunsat Fat 0.3 gm, Monounsat Fat 1.7 gm, Cholesterol 7 mg), Sodium 86 mg, Total Carbohydrate 3 gm, Dietary Fiber 1 gm, Sugars 2 gm, Protein 2 gm

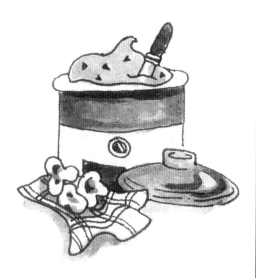

Hamburger Cheese Dip

Julia Lapp • New Holland, PA

Makes 20 servings (Ideal slow cooker size: 1-quart)

$\frac{3}{4}$ lb. ground beef, browned and crumbled into small pieces

$\frac{1}{8}$ tsp. salt

$\frac{1}{2}$ cup chopped green pepper

$\frac{3}{4}$ cup chopped onion

8-oz. can no-sugar-added tomato sauce

4-oz. can green chilies, chopped

1 Tbsp. Worcestershire sauce

1 Tbsp. brown sugar

8 ozs. Velveeta Light cheese, cubed

1 Tbsp. paprika

ground red pepper

1. Combine beef, salt, green pepper, onion, tomato sauce, green chilies, Worcestershire sauce, and brown sugar in slow cooker.

2. Cover. Cook on Low 2–3 hours. During the last hour stir in cheese, paprika, and red pepper.

3. Serve with tortilla chips.

Exchange List Values: Meat, lean 1.0

Basic Nutritional Values: Calories 64 (Calories from Fat 27), Total Fat 3 gm (Saturated Fat 1.5 gm, Polyunsat Fat 0.1 gm, Monounsat Fat 1.1 gm, Cholesterol 14 mg), Sodium 231 mg, Total Carbohydrate 4 gm, Dietary Fiber 1 gm, Sugars 3 gm, Protein 6 gm

VARIATION: Prepare recipe using only $\frac{1}{3}$–$\frac{1}{2}$ lb. ground beef.

Mexican Chip Dip Olé

Joy Sutter • Iowa City, IA

Makes 32 servings (Ideal slow cooker size: 3-quart)

1½ lbs. ground turkey

1 large onion, chopped

15-oz. can tomato sauce

4-oz. can green chilies, chopped

3-oz. can jalapeno peppers, chopped

1 lb. Velveeta Light cheese, cubed

1. Brown turkey and onion. Drain.

2. Add tomato sauce, chilies, jalapeno peppers, and cheese. Pour into slow cooker.

3. Cover. Cook on Low 4 hours, or High 2 hours.

4. Serve warm with tortilla chips.

Exchange List Values: Meat, medium fat 1.0

Basic Nutritional Values: Calories 75 (Calories from Fat 32), Total Fat 4 gm (Saturated Fat 1.5 gm, Polyunsat Fat 0.6 gm, Monounsat Fat 1.2 gm, Cholesterol 21 mg), Sodium 339 mg, Total Carbohydrate 3 gm, Dietary Fiber 0 gm, Sugars 3 gm, Protein 8 gm

Pizza Fondue

Lisa Warren • Parkesburg, PA

Makes 18 servings (Ideal slow cooker size: 3-quart)

½ lb. 85%-lean ground beef

2 15-oz. cans pizza sauce with cheese

4 ozs. grated fat-free cheddar cheese

4 ozs. grated reduced-fat mozzarella cheese

1 tsp. dried oregano

½ tsp. fennel seed, optional

1 Tbsp. cornstarch

1. Brown beef, crumble fine, and drain.

2. Combine all ingredients in slow cooker.

3. Cover. Heat on Low 2–3 hours.

4. Serve with tortilla chips.

Exchange List Values: Meat, medium fat 1.0

Basic Nutritional Values: Calories 76 (Calories from Fat 34), Total Fat 4 gm (Saturated Fat 1.4 gm, Polyunsat Fat 0.9 gm, Monounsat Fat 0.9 gm, Cholesterol 13 mg), Sodium 392 mg, Total Carbohydrate 4 gm, Dietary Fiber 0 gm, Sugars 3 gm, Protein 6 gm

Good 'n Hot Dip

Joyce B. Suiter • Garysburg, NC

Makes 40 servings (Ideal slow cooker size: 3-quart)

$^{3}/_{4}$ lb. ground beef

$^{3}/_{4}$ lb. bulk pork sausage

$10^{3}/_{4}$-oz. can 98%-fat-free, reduced-sodium cream of chicken soup

$10^{3}/_{4}$-oz. can cream of celery soup

24-oz. jar salsa (use hot for some zing)

10 ozs. Velveeta Light cheese, cubed

1. Brown beef and sausage, crumbling into small pieces. Drain.

2. Combine meat, soups, salsa, and cheese in slow cooker.

3. Cover. Cook on High 1 hour. Stir. Cook on Low until ready to serve.

4. Serve with chips.

Exchange List Values: Meat, lean 1.0

Basic Nutritional Values: Calories 60 (Calories from Fat 31), Total Fat 3 gm (Saturated Fat 1.5 gm, Polyunsat Fat 0.5 gm, Monounsat Fat 1.3 gm, Cholesterol 12 mg), Sodium 291 mg, Total Carbohydrate 3 gm, Dietary Fiber 0 gm, Sugars 1 gm, Protein 4 gm

Hot Cheese and Bacon Dip

Lee Ann Hazlett • Freeport, IL

Makes 25 servings (Ideal slow cooker size: 1-quart)

9 slices bacon, diced

2 8-oz. pkgs. fat-free cream cheese, cubed and softened

8 ozs. shredded reduced-fat mild cheddar cheese

1 cup fat-free half-and-half

2 tsp. Worcestershire sauce

1 tsp. dried minced onion

$^{1}/_{2}$ tsp. dry mustard

$^{1}/_{2}$ tsp. salt

2–3 drops Tabasco

1. Brown and drain bacon. Set aside.

2. Mix remaining ingredients in slow cooker.

3. Cover. Cook on Low 1 hour, stirring occasionally until cheese melts.

4. Stir in bacon.

5. Serve with fruit slices or French bread slices. (Dip fruit in lemon juice to prevent browning.)

Exchange List Values: Meat, lean 1.0

Basic Nutritional Values: Calories 54 (Calories from Fat 28), Total Fat 3 gm (Saturated Fat 1.5 gm, Polyunsat Fat 0.2 gm, Monounsat Fat 1.1 gm, Cholesterol 11 mg), Sodium 273 mg, Total Carbohydrate 2 gm, Dietary Fiber 0 gm, Sugars 1 gm, Protein 6 gm

Cheesy Hot Bean Dip

John D. Allen • Rye, CO

Makes 20 servings (Ideal slow cooker size: 3-quart)

16-oz. can refried beans

1 cup salsa

2 cups (8 ozs.) shredded reduced-fat Monterey Jack and reduced-fat cheddar cheeses, mixed

1 cup fat-free sour cream

3-oz. pkg. fat-free cream cheese, cubed

1 Tbsp. chili powder

¼ tsp. ground cumin

1. Combine all ingredients in slow cooker.

2. Cover. Cook on High 2 hours. Stir 2–3 times during cooking.

3. Serve warm from the cooker with chips.

Exchange List Values: Carbohydrate 0.5, Fat 0.5

Basic Nutritional Values: Calories 65 (Calories from Fat 22), Total Fat 2 gm (Saturated Fat 1.5 gm, Polyunsat Fat 0.1 gm, Monounsat Fat 0.7 gm, Cholesterol 11 mg), Sodium 275 mg, Total Carbohydrate 6 gm, Dietary Fiber 1 gm, Sugars 2 gm, Protein 6 gm

This bean dip is a favorite. Once you start on it, it's hard to leave it alone. We have been known to dip into it even when it's cold.

Refried Bean Dip

Maryann Markano • Wilmington, DE

Makes 12 servings (Ideal slow cooker size: 3-quart)

20-oz. can fat-free refried beans

1 cup shredded fat-free cheddar cheese

½ cup chopped green onions

2-4 Tbsp. bottled taco sauce (depending upon how spicy a dip you like)

1. Combine beans, cheese, onions, and taco sauce in slow cooker.

2. Cover. Cook on Low 2–2½ hours, or cook on High 30 minutes and then on Low 30 minutes.

3. Serve with tortilla chips.

Exchange List Values: Starch 0.5, Meat, very lean 1.0

Basic Nutritional Values: Calories 56 (Calories from Fat 0), Total Fat 0 gm (Saturated Fat 0 gm, Polyunsat Fat 0 gm, Monounsat Fat 0 gm, Cholesterol 1 mg), Sodium 270 mg, Total Carbohydrate 8 gm, Dietary Fiber 2 gm, Sugars 1 gm, Protein 5 gm

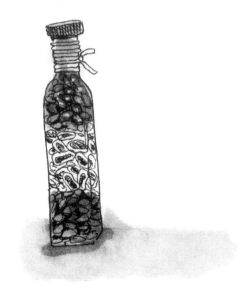

Short-Cut Fondue Dip

Jean Butzer • Batavia, NY

Makes 20 servings (Ideal slow cooker size: 1-quart)

2 10¾-oz. cans condensed cheese soup

3½ ozs. grated reduced-fat sharp cheddar cheese

1 Tbsp. Worcestershire sauce

1 tsp. lemon juice

2 Tbsp. dried chopped chives

celery sticks

cauliflower florets

corn chips

1. Combine soup, cheese, Worcestershire sauce, lemon juice, and chives in slow cooker.

2. Cover. Heat on Low 2–2½ hours. Stir until smooth and well blended.

3. Serve warm dip with celery sticks, cauliflower, and corn chips.

Exchange List Values: Fat 1.0

Basic Nutritional Values: Calories 44 (Calories from Fat 27), Total Fat 3 gm (Saturated Fat 1.5 gm, Polyunsat Fat 0.6 gm, Monounsat Fat 0.9 gm, Cholesterol 8 mg), Sodium 322 mg, Total Carbohydrate 3 gm, Dietary Fiber 0 gm, Sugars 1 gm, Protein 2 gm

Reuben Spread

Clarice Williams • Fairbank, IA /
Julie McKenzie • Punxsutawney, PA

Makes 52 servings (Ideal slow cooker size: 3-quart)

½-lb. corned beef, shredded or chopped, trimmed of fat

16-oz. can sauerkraut, well drained

1 cup shredded Swiss cheese

1 cup shredded cheddar cheese

1 cup mayonnaise

Thousand Island dressing, optional

1. Combine all ingredients except Thousand Island dressing in slow cooker. Mix well.

2. Cover. Cook on High 1–2 hours, until heated through, stirring occasionally.

3. Turn to Low, and keep warm in cooker while serving. Put spread on bread slices. Top individual servings with Thousand Island dressing, if desired.

Exchange List Values: Fat 1.0

Basic Nutritional Values: Calories 58 (Calories from Fat 49), Total Fat 5 gm (Saturated Fat 1.5 gm, Polyunsat Fat 1.9 gm, Monounsat Fat 1.6 gm, Cholesterol 10 mg), Sodium 113 mg, Total Carbohydrate 1 gm, Dietary Fiber 0 gm, Sugars 0 gm, Protein 2 gm

VARIATION: Use dried beef instead of traditional corned beef.

Note: Low-fat cheese and mayonnaise are not recommended for this spread.

TNT Dip

Sheila Plock • Boalsburg, PA

Makes 32 (¼ cup) servings (Ideal slow cooker size: 4-quart)

1¼ lbs. ground beef, browned

10¾-oz. can 98%-fat-free, reduced-sodium cream of mushroom soup

¼ cup light, soft tub margarine, melted

¾ lb. Velveeta Light, cubed

1 cup salsa

2 Tbsp. chili powder

1. Combine all ingredients in slow cooker.

2. Cover. Cook on High 1–1¼ hours, or until cheese is melted, stirring occasionally.

3. Serve with tortilla chips, corn chips, or party rye bread.

Exchange List Values: Meat, medium fat 1.0

Basic Nutritional Values: Calories 62 (Calories from Fat 32), Total Fat 4 gm (Saturated Fat 1.5 gm, Polyunsat Fat 0.3 gm, Monounsat Fat 1.4 gm, Cholesterol 14 mg), Sodium 215 mg, Total Carbohydrate 2 gm, Dietary Fiber 0 gm, Sugars 1 gm, Protein 5 gm

My son has hosted a Super Bowl party for his college friends at our house the past two years. He served this dip the first year, and the second year it was requested. His friends claim it's the best dip they've ever eaten. With a bunch of college kids it disappears quickly.

Hearty Beef Dip Fondue

Ann Bender • Ft. Defiance, VA / Charlotte Shaffer • East Earl, PA

Makes 10 (¼ cup) servings (Ideal slow cooker size: 3-quart)

1 cup fat-free milk

¾ cup fat-free half-and-half

2 8-oz. pkgs. fat-free cream cheese, cubed

2 tsp. dry mustard

¼ cup chopped green onions

2½ ozs. sliced dried beef, shredded or torn into small pieces

1. Heat milk and half-and-half in slow cooker on High.

2. Add cheese. Stir until melted.

3. Add mustard, green onions, and dried beef. Stir well.

4. Cover. Cook on Low for up to 6 hours.

5. Serve by dipping toasted bread pieces on long forks into mixture.

Exchange List Values: Carbohydrate 0.5, Meat, very lean 1.0

Basic Nutritional Values: Calories 72 (Calories from Fat 6), Total Fat 1 gm (Saturated Fat 0.1 gm, Polyunsat Fat 0 gm, Monounsat Fat 0.1 gm, Cholesterol 10 mg), Sodium 508 mg, Total Carbohydrate 6 gm, Dietary Fiber 0 gm, Sugars 4 gm, Protein 10 gm

VARIATIONS: Add ½ cup chopped pecans, 2 Tbsp. chopped olives, or 1 tsp. minced onion in Step 3.

Note: I make this on cold winter evenings, and we sit around the table playing games.

Hot Crab Dip

Cassandra Ly • Carlisle, PA /
Miriam Nolt • New Holland, PA

Makes 15–20 servings (Ideal slow cooker size: 3–4-quart)

½ cup milk

⅓ cup salsa

3 8-oz. pkgs. fat-free cream cheese, cubed

2 8-oz. pkgs. imitation crabmeat, flaked

1 cup thinly sliced green onions

4-oz. can chopped green chilies

1. Combine milk and salsa. Transfer to greased slow cooker.

2. Stir in cream cheese, crabmeat, onions, and chilies.

3. Cover. Cook on Low 3–4 hours, stirring every 30 minutes.

4. Serve with crackers or bread.

Exchange List Values: Carbohydrate 0.5, Meat, very lean 1.0

Basic Nutritional Values: Calories 60 (Calories from Fat 4), Total Fat 0 gm (Saturated Fat 0.1 gm, Polyunsat Fat 0.2 gm, Monounsat Fat 0.1 gm, Cholesterol 9 mg), Sodium 410 mg, Total Carbohydrate 5 gm, Dietary Fiber 0 gm, Sugars 4 gm, Protein 8 gm

Don't wear new exercise shoes
for prolonged exercise.
Break them in gradually.

Liver Paté

Barbara Walker • Sturgis, SD

Makes 12 (2 Tbsp.) servings (Ideal slow cooker size: 3-quart)

1 lb. chicken livers

½ cup dry wine

1 tsp. instant chicken bouillon

1 tsp. minced parsley

1 Tbsp. instant minced onion

¼ tsp. ground ginger

½ tsp. seasoning salt

1 Tbsp. light soy sauce

¼ tsp. dry mustard

¼ cup light, soft tub margarine

1 Tbsp. brandy

1. In slow cooker, combine all ingredients except margarine and brandy.

2. Cover. Cook on Low 4–5 hours. Let stand in liquid until cool.

3. Drain. Place in blender or food grinder. Add margarine and brandy. Process until smooth.

4. Serve with crackers or toast.

Exchange List Values: Meat, lean 1.0

Basic Nutritional Values: Calories 61 (Calories from Fat 28), Total Fat 3 gm (Saturated Fat 0.6 gm, Polyunsat Fat 0.6 gm, Monounsat Fat 1.2 gm, Cholesterol 137 mg), Sodium 235 mg, Total Carbohydrate 1 gm, Dietary Fiber 0 gm, Sugars 0 gm, Protein 6 gm

Cheesy New Orleans Shrimp Dip

Kelly Evenson • Pittsboro, NC

Recipe photo appears in color section.

Makes 20 servings (Ideal slow cooker size: 1-quart)

1 slice bacon

3 medium onions, chopped

1 clove garlic, minced

4 jumbo shrimp, peeled and deveined

1 medium tomato, peeled and chopped

7 ozs. (1¾ cups) reduced-fat Monterey Jack cheese, shredded

4 drops Tabasco sauce

⅛ tsp. cayenne pepper

dash black pepper

1. Cook bacon until crisp. Drain on paper towel. Crumble.

2. Saute onion and garlic in skillet sprayed with non-fat cooking spray. Drain on paper towel.

3. Coarsely chop shrimp.

4. Combine all ingredients in slow cooker.

5. Cover. Cook on Low 1 hour, or until cheese is melted. Thin with milk if too thick. Serve with chips.

Exchange List Values: Meat, lean 1.0

Basic Nutritional Values: Calories 43 (Calories from Fat 18), Total Fat 2 gm (Saturated Fat 1.5 gm, Polyunsat Fat 0.1 gm, Monounsat Fat 0.6 gm, Cholesterol 13 mg), Sodium 90 mg, Total Carbohydrate 2 gm, Dietary Fiber 0 gm, Sugars 2 gm, Protein 4 gm

Roasted Pepper and Artichoke Spread

Sherril Bieberly • Salina, KS

Makes 24 servings (Ideal slow cooker size: 1-quart)

1 cup grated Parmesan cheese

½ cup reduced-fat mayonnaise

8-oz. pkg. fat-free cream cheese, softened

1 clove garlic, minced

14-oz. can artichoke hearts, drained and chopped finely

⅓ cup finely chopped roasted red bell peppers (from 7¼-oz. jar)

1. Combine Parmesan cheese, mayonnaise, cream cheese, and garlic in food processor. Process until smooth. Place mixture in slow cooker.

2. Add artichoke hearts and red bell peppers. Stir well.

3. Cover. Cook on Low 1 hour. Stir again.

4. Use as spread for crackers, cut-up fresh vegetables, or snack-bread slices.

Exchange List Values: Fat 1.0

Basic Nutritional Values: Calories 49 (Calories from Fat 29), Total Fat 3 gm (Saturated Fat 1.3 gm, Polyunsat Fat 0.7 gm, Monounsat Fat 0.9 gm, Cholesterol 8 mg), Sodium 209 mg, Total Carbohydrate 2 gm, Dietary Fiber 0 gm, Sugars 1 gm, Protein 4 gm

Broccoli Cheese Dip

Carla Koslowsky • Hillsboro, KS

Makes 24 servings (Ideal slow cooker size: 3-quart)

1 cup chopped celery

$\frac{1}{2}$ cup chopped onion

10-oz. pkg. frozen chopped broccoli, cooked

1 cup cooked rice

$10\frac{3}{4}$-oz. can 98%-fat-free, reduced-sodium cream of mushroom soup

15 slices fat-free American cheese, melted and mixed with $\frac{2}{3}$ cup fat-free half-and-half

1. Combine all ingredients in slow cooker.

2. Cover. Heat on Low 2 hours.

3. Serve with snack breads or crackers.

Exchange List Values: Carbohydrate 0.5

Basic Nutritional Values: Calories 44 (Calories from Fat 4), Total Fat 0 gm (Saturated Fat 0.2 gm, Polyunsat Fat 0.1 gm, Monounsat Fat 0.1 gm, Cholesterol 3 mg), Sodium 234 mg, Total Carbohydrate 6 gm, Dietary Fiber 1 gm, Sugars 2 gm, Protein 4 gm

Chili Nuts

Barbara Aston • Ashdown, AR

Makes 80 (1 Tbsp.) servings (Ideal slow cooker size: 3-quart)

$\frac{1}{4}$ cup melted butter

2 12-oz. cans cocktail peanuts

$1\frac{5}{8}$-oz. pkg. chili seasoning mix

1. Pour butter over nuts in slow cooker. Sprinkle in dry chili mix. Toss together.

2. Cover. Heat on Low $2-2\frac{1}{2}$ hours. Turn to High. Remove lid and cook 10–15 minutes.

3. Serve warm or cool.

Exchange List Values: Fat 1.0

Basic Nutritional Values: Calories 56 (Calories from Fat 43), Total Fat 5 gm (Saturated Fat 1.0 gm, Polyunsat Fat 1.4 gm, Monounsat Fat 2.3 gm, Cholesterol 2 mg), Sodium 104 mg, Total Carbohydrate 2 gm, Dietary Fiber 1 gm, Sugars 0 gm, Protein 2 gm

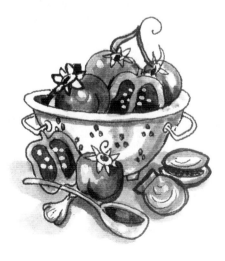

Baked Brie with Cranberry Chutney

Amymarlene Jensen • Fountain, CO

Makes 25 servings (Ideal slow cooker size: 1-quart)

1 cup fresh or dried cranberries

½ cup brown sugar

⅓ cup cider vinegar

2 Tbsp. water or orange juice

2 tsp. minced crystallized ginger

¼ tsp. cinnamon

⅛ tsp. ground cloves

oil

8-oz. round of Brie cheese

1 Tbsp. sliced almonds, toasted

1. Mix together cranberries, brown sugar, vinegar, water or juice, ginger, cinnamon, and cloves in slow cooker.

2. Cover. Cook on Low 4 hours. Stir once near the end to see if it is thickening. If not, remove top, turn heat to High and cook 30 minutes without lid.

3. Put cranberry chutney in covered container and chill for up to 2 weeks. When ready to serve, bring to room temperature.

4. Brush ovenproof plate with vegetable oil, place unpeeled Brie on plate, and bake uncovered at 350° for 9 minutes, until cheese is soft and partially melted. Remove from oven.

5. Top with half the chutney and garnish with almonds. Serve with crackers.

Exchange List Values: Fat 1.0

Basic Nutritional Values: Calories 38 (Calories from Fat 23), Total Fat 3 gm (Saturated Fat 1.5 gm, Polyunsat Fat 0.1 gm, Monounsat Fat 0.8 gm, Cholesterol 8 mg), Sodium 67 mg, Total Carbohydrate 3 gm, Dietary Fiber 0 gm, Sugars 3 gm, Protein 1 gm

Curried Almonds

Barbara Aston • Ashdown, AR

Makes 64 (1 Tbsp.) servings (Ideal slow cooker size: 3-quart)

2 Tbsp. melted butter

1 Tbsp. curry powder

½ tsp. seasoned salt

1 lb. blanched almonds

1. Combine butter with curry powder and seasoned salt.

2. Pour over almonds in slow cooker. Mix to coat well.

3. Cover. Cook on Low 2–3 hours. Turn to High. Uncover cooker and cook 1–1½ hours.

4. Serve hot or cold.

Exchange List Values: Fat 1.0

Basic Nutritional Values: Calories 45 (Calories from Fat 36), Total Fat 4 gm (Saturated Fat 0.5 gm, Polyunsat Fat 0.9 gm, Monounsat Fat 2.4 gm, Cholesterol 1 mg), Sodium 18 mg, Total Carbohydrate 1 gm, Dietary Fiber 1 gm, Sugars 0 gm, Protein 2 gm

Hot Artichoke Dip

Mary E. Wheatley • Mashpee, MA

Makes 30 (¼ cup) servings (Ideal slow cooker size: 4-quart)

2 14¾-oz. jars marinated artichoke hearts, drained

1 cup fat-free mayonnaise

1 cup fat-free sour cream

1 cup water chestnuts, chopped

2 cups freshly grated Parmesan cheese

¼ cup finely chopped green onions

1. Cut artichoke hearts into small pieces. Add mayonnaise, sour cream, water chestnuts, cheese, and green onions. Pour into slow cooker.

2. Cover. Cook on High 1–2 hours, or on Low 3–4 hours.

3. Serve with crackers or crusty French bread.

Exchange List Values: Carbohydrate 0.5, Fat 0.5

Basic Nutritional Values: Calories 57 (Calories from Fat 26), Total Fat 3 gm (Saturated Fat 1.2 gm, Polyunsat Fat 0.7 gm, Monounsat Fat 0.9 gm, Cholesterol 6 mg), Sodium 170 mg, Total Carbohydrate 5 gm, Dietary Fiber 0 gm, Sugars 2 gm, Protein 3 gm

Artichokes

Susan Yoder Graber • Eureka, IL

Makes 4 servings (Ideal slow cooker size: 3-quart)

4 artichokes

1 tsp. salt

2 Tbsp. lemon juice

1. Wash and trim artichokes by cutting off stems flush with bottoms of artichokes and by cutting ¾"–1" off the tops. Stand upright in slow cooker.

2. Mix together salt and lemon juice and pour over artichokes. Pour in water to cover ¾ of artichokes.

3. Cover. Cook on Low 8–10 hours, or High 2–4 hours.

4. Serve with melted butter. Pull off individual leaves and dip bottom of each into butter. Using your teeth, strip the individual leaf of the meaty portion at the bottom of each leaf.

Exchange List Values: Vegetable 3.0

Basic Nutritional Values: Calories 60 (Calories from Fat 2), Total Fat 0 gm (Saturated Fat 0 gm, Polyunsat Fat 0.1 gm, Monounsat Fat 0 gm, Cholesterol 0 mg), Sodium 397 mg, Total Carbohydrate 13 gm, Dietary Fiber 6 gm, Sugars 1 gm, Protein 4 gm

Note: *3 vegetable exchanges = 1 carbohydrate exchange*

All-American Snack

Doris M. Coyle-Zipp • South Ozone Park, NY /
Melissa Raber • Millersburg, OH / Ada Miller •
Sugarcreek, OH / Nanci Keatley • Salem, OR

Recipe photo appears in color section.

Makes 48 (¼ cup) servings (Ideal slow cooker size: 4-quart)

3 cups thin pretzel sticks

4 cups Wheat Chex

4 cups Cheerios

12-oz. can salted peanuts

¼ cup melted butter, or margarine

1 tsp. garlic powder

1 tsp. celery salt

½ tsp. seasoned salt

2 Tbsp. grated Parmesan cheese

1. Combine pretzels, cereal, and peanuts in large bowl.

2. Melt butter. Stir in garlic powder, celery salt, seasoned salt, and Parmesan cheese. Pour over pretzels and cereal. Toss until well mixed.

3. Pour into large slow cooker. Cover. Cook on Low 2½ hours, stirring every 30 minutes. Remove lid and cook another 30 minutes on Low.

4. Serve warm or at room temperature. Store in tightly covered container.

Exchange List Values: Starch 0.5, Fat 1.0

Basic Nutritional Values: Calories 77 (Calories from Fat 44), Total Fat 5 gm (Saturated Fat 1.2 gm, Polyunsat Fat 1.2 gm, Monounsat Fat 2.1 gm, Cholesterol 3 mg), Sodium 174 mg, Total Carbohydrate 7 gm, Dietary Fiber 1 gm, Sugars 1 gm, Protein 3 gm

VARIATIONS:

1. Use 3 cups Wheat Chex (instead of 4 cups) and 3 cups Cheerios (instead of 4 cups). Add 3 cups Corn Chex.

   Marcia S. Myer • Manheim, PA

2. Alter the amounts of pretzels, cereal, and peanuts to reflect your preferences.

Use moisturizing soaps instead of deodorant soaps to avoid drying out your skin.

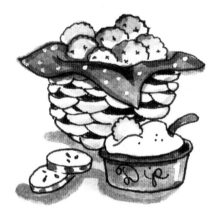

Snack Mix

Yvonne Boettger • Harrisonburg, VA

Makes 28 servings (Ideal slow cooker size: 5-quart)

8 cups Chex cereal, of any combination

6 cups from the following: pretzels, snack crackers, goldfish, Cheerios, nuts, bagel chips, toasted corn

6 Tbsp. light, soft tub margarine, melted

2 Tbsp. Worcestershire sauce

1 tsp. seasoning salt

½ tsp. garlic powder

½ tsp. onion salt

½ tsp. onion powder

1. Combine first two ingredients in slow cooker.

2. Combine margarine and seasonings. Pour over dry mixture. Toss until well mixed.

3. Cover. Cook on Low 2 hours, stirring every 30 minutes.

Exchange List Values: Starch 1.0, Fat 1.0

Basic Nutritional Values: Calories 110 (Calories from Fat 48), Total Fat 5 gm (Saturated Fat 1.3 gm, Polyunsat Fat 1.1 gm, Monounsat Fat 2.9 gm, Cholesterol 1 mg), Sodium 278 mg, Total Carbohydrate 14 gm, Dietary Fiber 2 gm, Sugars 2 gm, Protein 2 gm

Rhonda's Apple Butter

Rhonda Burgoon • Collingswood, NJ

Makes 24 (2 Tbsp.) servings (Ideal slow cooker size: 3-quart)

4 lbs. apples

2 tsp. cinnamon

½ tsp. ground cloves

1. Core, peel, and slice apples. Place in slow cooker.

2. Cover. Cook on High 2–3 hours. Reduce to Low and cook 8 hours. Apples should be a rich brown and be cooked down by half.

3. Stir in spices. Cook on High 2–3 hours with lid off. Stir until smooth.

4. Pour into freezer containers and freeze, or into sterilized jars and seal.

Exchange List Values: Fruit 0.5

Basic Nutritional Values: Calories 37 (Calories from Fat 2), Total Fat 0 gm (Saturated Fat 0 gm, Polyunsat Fat 0.1 gm, Monounsat Fat 0 gm, Cholesterol 0 mg), Sodium 0 mg, Total Carbohydrate 10 gm, Dietary Fiber 1 gm, Sugars 8 gm, Protein 0 gm

Shirley's Apple Butter

Shirley Sears • Tiskilwa, IL

Makes 96 (2 Tbsp.) servings (6 pints total) (Ideal slow cooker size: 6-quart)

4 qts. peeled tart apples, finely chopped

1½ cups sugar

sugar substitute to equal ¾ cup

2¾ tsp. cinnamon

¼ tsp. ground cloves

⅛ tsp. salt

1. Pour apples into slow cooker.

2. Combine remaining ingredients. Drizzle over apples.

3. Cover. Cook on High 3 hours, stirring well with a large spoon every hour. Reduce heat to Low and cook 10–12 hours, until butter becomes thick and dark in color. Stir occasionally with a strong wire whisk for smooth butter.

4. Freeze or pour into sterilized jars and seal.

Exchange List Values: Carbohydrate 0.5

Basic Nutritional Values: Calories 24 (Calories from Fat 1), Total Fat 0 gm (Saturated Fat 0 gm, Polyunsat Fat 0 gm, Monounsat Fat 0 gm, Cholesterol 0 mg), Sodium 3 mg, Total Carbohydrate 6 gm, Dietary Fiber 0 gm, Sugars 6 gm, Protein 0 gm

Ann's Apple Butter

Ann Bender • Ft. Defiance, VA

Makes 32 (2 Tbsp.) servings (Ideal slow cooker size: 3-quart)

7 cups unsweetened applesauce

1 cup sugar

sugar substitute to equal ½ cup

2 tsp. cinnamon

1 tsp. ground nutmeg

¼ tsp. allspice

1. Combine all ingredients in slow cooker.

2. Put a layer of paper towels under lid to prevent condensation from dripping into apple butter. Cook on High 8–10 hours. Remove lid during last hour. Stir occasionally.

Exchange List Values: Carbohydrate 1.0

Basic Nutritional Values: Calories 48 (Calories from Fat 1), Total Fat 0 gm (Saturated Fat 0 gm, Polyunsat Fat 0 gm, Monounsat Fat 0 gm, Cholesterol 0 mg), Sodium 1 mg, Total Carbohydrate 13 gm, Dietary Fiber 1 gm, Sugars 11 gm, Protein 0 gm

VARIATION: Use canned peaches, pears, or apricots in place of applesauce.

Pear Butter

Betty Moore • Plano, IL

Makes 40 (2 Tbsp.) servings (Ideal slow cooker size: 4-quart)

10 large pears (about 4 lbs.)

1 cup orange juice

1 cup sugar

sugar substitute to equal $1/2$ cup

1 tsp. ground cinnamon

1 tsp. ground cloves

$1/2$ tsp. ground allspice

1. Peel and quarter pears. Place in slow cooker.

2. Cover. Cook on Low 10–12 hours. Drain and then discard liquid.

3. Mash or puree pears. Add remaining ingredients. Mix well and return to slow cooker.

4. Cover. Cook on High 1 hour.

5. Place in hot, sterile jars and seal. Process in hot water bath for 10 minutes. Allow to cool undisturbed for 24 hours.

Exchange List Values: Carbohydrate 1.0

Basic Nutritional Values: Calories 56 (Calories from Fat 2), Total Fat 0 gm (Saturated Fat 0 gm, Polyunsat Fat 0 gm, Monounsat Fat 0 gm, Cholesterol 0 mg), Sodium 0 mg, Total Carbohydrate 14 gm, Dietary Fiber 1 gm, Sugars 13 gm, Protein 0 gm

Peach or Apricot Butter

Charlotte Shaffer • East Earl, PA

Makes 48 (2 Tbsp.) servings (Ideal slow cooker size: 4-quart)

4 1-lb. 13-oz. cans peaches or apricots

$1\frac{1}{2}$ cups sugar

sugar substitute to equal $3/4$ cup

2 tsp. cinnamon

1 tsp. ground cloves

1. Drain fruit. Remove pits. Puree in blender. Pour into slow cooker.

2. Stir in remaining ingredients.

3. Cover. Cook on High 8–10 hours. Remove cover during last half of cooking. Stir occasionally.

Exchange List Values: Carbohydrate 0.5

Basic Nutritional Values: Calories 39 (Calories from Fat 0), Total Fat 0 gm (Saturated Fat 0 gm, Polyunsat Fat 0 gm, Monounsat Fat 0 gm, Cholesterol 0 mg), Sodium 2 mg, Total Carbohydrate 10 gm, Dietary Fiber 1 gm, Sugars 10 gm, Protein 0 gm

Note: Spread on bread, or use as a topping for ice cream or toasted pound cake.

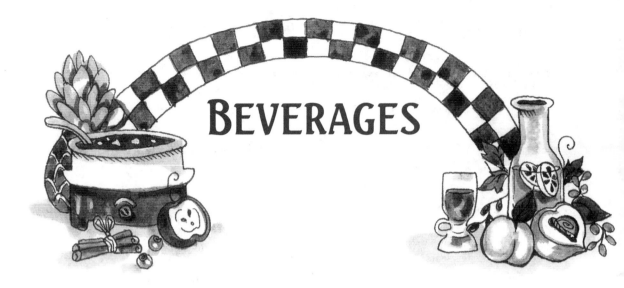

BEVERAGES

Hot Mulled Cider

Phyllis Attig • Reynolds, IL / Jean Butzer •
Batavia, NY / Doris G. Herr • Manheim, PA /
Mary E. Martin • Goshen, IN / Leona Miller •
Millersburg, OH / Marjora Miller • Archbold, OH /
Janet L. Roggie • Lowville, NY / Shirley Sears •
Tiskilwa, IL / Charlotte Shaffer • East Earl, PA /
Berenice M. Wagner • Dodge City, KS / Connie B.
Weaver • Bethlehem, PA / Maryann Westerberg •
Rosamond, CA / Carole Whaling • New Tripoli, PA

Makes 16 (½ cup) servings (Ideal slow cooker size: 4-quart)

¼ cup brown sugar

2 quarts apple cider

1 tsp. whole allspice

1½ tsp. whole cloves

2 cinnamon sticks

2 oranges, sliced, with peels on

1. Combine brown sugar and cider in slow cooker.

2. Put spices in tea strainer or tie in cheesecloth. Add to slow cooker. Stir in orange slices.

3. Cover and simmer on Low 2–8 hours.

Exchange List Values: Fruit 1.0

Basic Nutritional Values: Calories 76 (Calories from Fat 1), Total Fat 0 gm (Saturated Fat 0 gm, Polyunsat Fat 0 gm, Monounsat Fat 0 gm, Cholesterol 0 mg), Sodium 5 mg, Total Carbohydrate 19 gm, Dietary Fiber 0 gm, Sugars 18 gm, Protein 0 gm

VARIATION: Add a dash of ground nutmeg and salt.

Marsha Sabus • Fallbrook, CA

Cider Snap

Cathy Boshart • Lebanon, PA

Makes 16 servings (Ideal slow cooker size: 4-quart)

2 qts. apple cider, or apple juice

4 Tbsp. red cinnamon candies

at least 16 apple slices

at least 16 cinnamon sticks

1. Combine cider and cinnamon candies in slow cooker.

2. Cover. Cook on High for 2 hours, until candies dissolve and cider is hot.

3. Ladle into mugs and serve with apple slice floaters and cinnamon stick stirrers.

Exchange List Values: Fruit 1.5

Basic Nutritional Values: Calories 81 (Calories from Fat 1), Total Fat 0 gm (Saturated Fat 0 gm, Polyunsat Fat 0 gm, Monounsat Fat 0 gm, Cholesterol 0 mg), Sodium 4 mg, Total Carbohydrate 20 gm, Dietary Fiber 0 gm, Sugars 18, Protein 0 gm

This is a cold-winter-night luxury. Make it in the morning and keep it on Low throughout the day so its good fragrance fills the house.

Apple-Honey Tea

Jeanne Allen • Rye, CO

Makes 12 (1/2 cup) servings (Ideal slow cooker size: 3–4-quart)

12-oz. can frozen apple juice/cider concentrate

2 Tbsp. instant tea powder

1 Tbsp. honey

1/2 tsp. ground cinnamon

1. Reconstitute the apple juice/cider concentrate according to package directions. Pour into slow cooker.

2. Add tea powder, honey, and cinnamon. Stir to blend.

3. Heat on Low 1–2 hours. Stir well before serving, since cinnamon tends to settle on bottom.

Exchange List Values: Fruit 1.0

Basic Nutritional Values: Calories 66 (Calories from Fat 1), Total Fat 0 gm (Saturated Fat 0 gm, Polyunsat Fat 0 gm, Monounsat Fat 0 gm, Cholesterol 0 mg), Sodium 8 mg, Total Carbohydrate 16 gm, Dietary Fiber 0 gm, Sugars 16 gm, Protein 0 gm

Maple Mulled Cider

Leesa Lesenski • Wheately, MA

Makes 10 servings (Ideal slow cooker size: 4-quart)

½ gallon cider

3–4 cinnamon sticks

2 tsp. whole cloves

2 tsp. whole allspice

1–2 Tbsp. orange juice concentrate, optional

1 Tbsp. maple syrup, optional

1. Combine ingredients in slow cooker.

2. Cover. Heat on Low for 2 hours. Serve warm.

Exchange List Values: Fruit 1.5

Basic Nutritional Values: Calories 98 (Calories from Fat 1), Total Fat 0 gm (Saturated Fat 0 gm, Polyunsat Fat 0.1 gm, Monounsat Fat 0 gm, Cholesterol 0 mg), Sodium 7 mg, Total Carbohydrate 25 gm, Dietary Fiber 0 gm, Sugars 23 gm, Protein 0 gm

Serve at Halloween, Christmas caroling, or sledding parties.

Deep Red Apple Cider

Judi Manos • West Islip, NY

Makes 16 (½ cup) servings (Ideal slow cooker size: 4-quart)

5 cups apple cider

3 cups dry red wine

¼ cup brown sugar

½ tsp. whole cloves

¼ tsp. whole allspice

1 stick cinnamon

1. Combine all ingredients in slow cooker.

2. Cover. Cook on Low 3–4 hours.

3. Remove cloves, allspice, and cinnamon before serving.

Exchange List Values: Fruit 1.0

Basic Nutritional Values: Calories 58 (Calories from Fat 1), Total Fat 0 gm (Saturated Fat 0 gm, Polyunsat Fat 0 gm, Monounsat Fat 0 gm, Cholesterol 0 mg), Sodium 7 mg, Total Carbohydrate 14 gm, Dietary Fiber 0 gm, Sugars 14 gm, Protein 0 gm

VARIATION: You can use 8 cups apple cider and no red wine.

Try growing your own food—the closer to the ground it is, the better your food is going to be.

Hot Mulled Apple Tea

Barbara Tenney • Delta, PA

Makes 16 1-cup servings (Ideal slow cooker size: 5-quart)

$\frac{1}{2}$ gallon apple cider

$\frac{1}{2}$ gallon strong tea

1 sliced lemon

1 sliced orange

3 3" cinnamon sticks

1 Tbsp. whole cloves

1 Tbsp. allspice

1. Combine all in slow cooker.

2. Heat on Low 2 hours.

Exchange List Values: Fruit 1.0

Basic Nutritional Values: Calories 59 (Calories from Fat 1), Total Fat 0 gm (Saturated Fat 0 gm, Polyunsat Fat 0 gm, Monounsat Fat 0 gm, Cholesterol 0 mg), Sodium 7 mg, Total Carbohydrate 15 gm, Dietary Fiber 0 gm, Sugars 13 gm, Protein 0 gm

Spiced Apple Cider

Janice Muller • Derwood, MD

Makes 40 servings (Ideal slow cooker size: 5-6-quart)

2 sticks cinnamon

1 cup orange juice

1 tsp. cinnamon

1 tsp. ground cloves

$\frac{1}{4}$ cup lemon juice

2 tsp. whole cloves

1 gallon apple cider

2 tsp. ground nutmeg

$\frac{1}{2}$ cup pineapple juice

1 tsp. ginger

1 tsp. lemon peel

$\frac{1}{4}$ cup sugar

sugar substitute to equal $\frac{1}{4}$ cup

1. Mix all ingredients in 5-6-quart slow cooker.

2. Simmer on Low 4-6 hours.

Exchange List Values: Fruit 1.0

Basic Nutritional Values: Calories 58 (Calories from Fat 1), Total Fat 0 gm (Saturated Fat 0 gm, Polyunsat Fat 0 gm, Monounsat Fat 0 gm, Cholesterol 0 mg), Sodium 4 mg, Total Carbohydrate 14 gm, Dietary Fiber 0 gm, Sugars 13 gm, Protein 0 gm

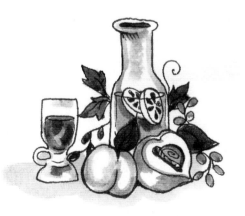

Hot Wassail Drink

Dale Peterson • Rapid City, SC

Makes 54 ($\frac{1}{2}$ cup) servings (Ideal slow cooker size: 6-quart)

12-oz. can frozen orange juice

12-oz. can frozen lemonade

2 qts. apple juice

1 cup sugar

sugar substitute to equal $\frac{1}{2}$ cup

3 Tbsp. whole cloves

2 Tbsp. ground ginger

4 tsp. ground cinnamon

10 cups hot water

6 cups strong tea

1. Mix juices, sugar, sugar substitute, and spices in slow cooker.

2. Add hot water and tea.

3. Heat on High until hot (1-2 hours), then on Low while serving.

Exchange List Values: Fruit 1.0

Basic Nutritional Values: Calories 61 (Calories from Fat 1), Total Fat 0 gm (Saturated Fat 0 gm, Polyunsat Fat 0 gm, Monounsat Fat 0 gm, Cholesterol 0 mg), Sodium 3 mg, Total Carbohydrate 16 gm, Dietary Fiber 0 gm, Sugars 15 gm, Protein 0 gm

Note: To garnish wassail with an orange, insert 10-12 whole cloves halfway into orange. Place studded orange in flat baking pan with $\frac{1}{4}$ cup water. Bake at 325°-350° for 30 minutes. Just before serving, float orange on top of wassail.

Orange Cider Punch

Naomi Ressler • Harrisonburg, VA

Makes 16 ($\frac{1}{2}$ cup) servings (Ideal slow cooker size: 4-quart)

$\frac{1}{2}$ cup sugar

sugar substitute to equal $\frac{1}{4}$ cup

2 cinnamon sticks

1 tsp. whole nutmeg

2 cups apple cider or apple juice

6 cups orange juice

fresh orange

1. Combine ingredients in slow cooker.

2. Cover. Cook on Low 4-10 hours, or High 2-3 hours.

3. Float thin slices of an orange in cooker before serving.

Exchange List Values: Fruit 1.5

Basic Nutritional Values: Calories 81 (Calories from Fat 2), Total Fat 0 gm (Saturated Fat 0 gm, Polyunsat Fat 0.1 gm, Monounsat Fat 0 gm, Cholesterol 0 mg), Sodium 2 mg, Total Carbohydrate 20 gm, Dietary Fiber 0 gm, Sugars 19 gm, Protein 1 gm

Hot Cranberry Cider

Kristi See • Weskan, KS

Makes 20 (½ cup) servings (Ideal slow cooker size: 4-quart)

2 qts. apple cider or apple juice

1 pt. cranberry juice cocktail

¼ cup sugar

2 cinnamon sticks

1 tsp. whole allspice

1 orange, studded with whole cloves

sweetener to equal 2 Tbsp.

1. Put all ingredients in slow cooker.

2. Cover. Cook on High 1 hour, then on Low 4–8 hours. Serve warm.

3. Serve with finger foods.

Exchange List Values: Fruit 1.0

Basic Nutritional Values: Calories 71 (Calories from Fat 1), Total Fat 0 gm (Saturated Fat 0 gm, Polyunsat Fat 0 gm, Monounsat Fat 0 gm, Cholesterol 0 mg), Sodium 4 mg, Total Carbohydrate 18 gm, Dietary Fiber 0 gm, Sugars 17 gm, Protein 0 gm

Note: I come from a family of eight children, and every Christmas we all get together. We eat dinner, and then sit around playing games and drinking Hot Cranberry Cider.

Fruity Wassail

Kelly Evenson • Pittsboro, NC

Makes 20 servings (Ideal slow cooker size: 6-quart)

6 cups apple cider

1 cinnamon stick

¼ tsp. ground nutmeg

¼ cup honey

3 Tbsp. lemon juice

1 tsp. grated lemon peel

46-oz. can pineapple juice

1. Combine ingredients in slow cooker.

2. Cover. Cook on Low 1–2 hours.

3. Serve warm from slow cooker.

Exchange List Values: Fruit 1.5

Basic Nutritional Values: Calories 85 (Calories from Fat 1), Total Fat 0 gm (Saturated Fat 0 gm, Polyunsat Fat 0 gm, Monounsat Fat 0 gm, Cholesterol 0 mg), Sodium 4 mg, Total Carbohydrate 21 gm, Dietary Fiber 0 gm, Sugars 20 gm, Protein 0 gm

VARIATION: Use 3 cups cranberry juice and reduce the amount of pineapple juice by 3 cups, to add more color and to change the flavor of the wassail.

Johnny Appleseed Tea

Sheila Plock • Boalsburg, PA

Makes 9 cups (Ideal slow cooker size: 4-quart)

2 qts. water, divided

6 tea bags, your favorite flavor

6 ozs. frozen apple juice, thawed

3 Tbsp. packed brown sugar

brown sugar substitute to equal 2 Tbsp.

1. Bring 1 quart water to boil. Add tea bags. Remove from heat. Cover and let steep 5 minutes. Pour into slow cooker.

2. Add remaining ingredients and mix well.

3. Cover. Heat on Low until hot. Continue on Low while serving from slow cooker.

Exchange List Values: Fruit 1.0

Basic Nutritional Values: Calories 60 (Calories from Fat 1), Total Fat 0 gm (Saturated Fat 0 gm, Polyunsat Fat 0 gm, Monounsat Fat 0 gm, Cholesterol 0 mg), Sodium 12 mg, Total Carbohydrate 15 gm, Dietary Fiber 0 gm, Sugars 14 gm, Protein 0 gm

I serve this wonderful hot beverage with cookies at our Open House Tea and Cookies afternoon, which I host at Christmastime for friends and neighbors.

Hot Fruit Tea

Kelly Evenson • Pittsboro, NC

Makes 20 servings (Ideal slow cooker size: 5-quart)

5–6 tea bags, fruit flavor of your choice

2 cups boiling water

¾ cup sugar

sugar substitute to equal ½ cup

2 cinnamon sticks

2½ qts. water

1¼ tsp. vanilla

1¼ tsp. almond extract

juice of 3 lemons

juice of 3 oranges

1. Steep tea bags in boiling water for 5 minutes.

2. Bring tea water, sugar, sugar substitute, cinnamon sticks, and 2½ qts. water to boil in saucepan. Remove from heat and add remaining ingredients.

3. Pour tea into slow cooker and keep warm there while serving.

Exchange List Values: Carbohydrate 0.5

Basic Nutritional Values: Calories 38 (Calories from Fat 0), Total Fat 0 gm (Saturated Fat 0 gm, Polyunsat Fat 0 gm, Monounsat Fat 0 gm, Cholesterol 0 mg), Sodium 4 mg, Total Carbohydrate 10 gm, Dietary Fiber 0 gm, Sugars 9 gm, Protein 0 gm

VARIATION: Float thinly cut fresh lemon and/or orange slices in tea.

Spicy Autumn Punch

Marlene Bogard • Newton, KS

Makes 16 servings (Ideal slow cooker size: 4-quart)

8 whole cloves

2 oranges

6 cups apple juice

1 cinnamon stick

1/4 tsp. ground nutmeg

3 Tbsp. lemon juice

1/4 cup honey

2 1/4 cups pineapple juice

1. Press cloves into oranges. Bake at 325°–350° for 30 minutes.

2. Meanwhile, combine apple juice and cinnamon stick in slow cooker.

3. Cover. Cook on High 1 hour.

4. Add remaining ingredients except oranges.

5. Cover. Cook on Low 2–3 hours. Add oranges at end, either whole or in quarters.

Exchange List Values: Fruit 1.5

Basic Nutritional Values: Calories 80 (Calories from Fat 1), Total Fat 0 gm (Saturated Fat 0 gm, Polyunsat Fat 0 gm, Monounsat Fat 0 gm, Cholesterol 0 mg), Sodium 4 mg, Total Carbohydrate 20 gm, Dietary Fiber 0 gm, Sugars 19 gm, Protein 0 gm

Hot Cranberry Tea

Sherrill Bieberly • Salina, KS

Makes 21 (2/3 cup) servings (Ideal slow cooker size: 4–5-quart)

1/2 cup sugar

sugar substitute to equal 1/4 cup

2 qts. water

3 cinnamon sticks

1 qt. cranberry juice

6-oz. can frozen orange juice

1 1/4 cups water

3 Tbsp. lemon juice

fresh lemon and/or orange slices

1. In saucepan, mix together sugar, sugar substitute, 2 quarts water, and cinnamon sticks. Bring to boil.

2. Pour into slow cooker along with remaining ingredients. Cover and cook on High 1 hour. Turn to Low. Serve warm.

Exchange List Values: Carbohydrate 1.0

Basic Nutritional Values: Calories 58 (Calories from Fat 1), Total Fat 0 gm (Saturated Fat 0 gm, Polyunsat Fat 0 gm, Monounsat Fat 0 gm, Cholesterol 0 mg), Sodium 1 mg, Total Carbohydrate 15 gm, Dietary Fiber 0 gm, Sugars 15 gm, Protein 0 gm

Hot Cranberry Punch

Janie Steele • Moore, OK

Makes 24 (²/₃ cup) servings (Ideal slow cooker size: 5-quart)

1 cup water

½ cup brown sugar

brown sugar substitute to equal ¼ cup

³/₈ tsp. salt

³/₈ tsp. nutmeg

³/₈ tsp. cinnamon

¾ tsp. allspice

1⅛ tsp. cloves

46-oz. can unsweetened pineapple juice

64-oz. bottle cranberry juice cocktail

rum flavoring, optional

red food coloring, optional

24 cinnamon sticks

1. Combine water, sugar, and sugar substitute in slow cooker. Bring to boil.

2. Place salt and spices in bag or tea ball. Add spice ball to cooker.

3. Cover. Cook on High 1 hour.

4. Add juices, and rum flavoring and food coloring, if desired.

5. Cover. Cook on High 2–3 hours, until hot.

6. Serve in cups, each with a cinnamon-stick stirrer.

Exchange List Values: Fruit 1.5

Basic Nutritional Values: Calories 92 (Calories from Fat 2), Total Fat 0 gm (Saturated Fat 0 gm, Polyunsat Fat 0.1 gm, Monounsat Fat 0 gm, Cholesterol 0 mg), Sodium 42 mg, Total Carbohydrate 23 gm, Dietary Fiber 0 gm, Sugars 22 gm, Protein 0 gm

Mulled Wine

Julie McKenzie • Punxsutawney, PA

Makes 8 1-cup servings (Ideal slow cooker size: 3-4-quart)

½ cup sugar

1½ cups boiling water

half a lemon, sliced thin

3 cinnamon sticks

3 whole cloves

1 bottle red dinner wine (burgundy or claret)

1. Dissolve sugar in boiling water in saucepan.

2. Add remaining ingredients.

3. Pour into slow cooker. Heat on Low for at least 1 hour, until wine is hot. Do not boil.

4. Serve from cooker into mugs.

Exchange List Values: Carbohydrate 1.0

Basic Nutritional Values: Calories 91 (Calories from Fat 1), Total Fat 0 gm (Saturated Fat 0 gm, Polyunsat Fat 0.1 gm, Monounsat Fat 0 gm, Cholesterol 0 mg), Sodium 6 mg, Total Carbohydrate 14 gm, Dietary Fiber 0 gm, Sugars 13 gm, Protein 0 gm

Christmas Wassail

Dottie Schmidt • Kansas City, MO

Makes 10 servings (Ideal slow cooker size: 4-quart)

2 cups cranberry juice cocktail

$3\frac{1}{4}$ cups hot water

3 Tbsp. sugar

sugar substitute to equal $1\frac{1}{2}$ Tbsp.

6-oz. can lemonade concentrate

1 stick cinnamon

5 whole cloves

2 oranges, cut in 10 thin slices

1. Combine all ingredients except oranges in slow cooker. Stir until sugar and sugar substitute are dissolved.

2. Cover. Cook on High 1 hour. Strain out spices.

3. Serve hot with an orange slice floating in each cup.

Exchange List Values: Carbohydrate 1.5

Basic Nutritional Values: Calories 90 (Calories from Fat 3), Total Fat 0 gm (Saturated Fat 0.1 gm, Polyunsat Fat 0.1 gm, Monounsat Fat 0 gm, Cholesterol 0 mg), Sodium 5 mg, Total Carbohydrate 24 gm, Dietary Fiber 0 gm, Sugars 22 gm, Protein 0 gm

Almond Tea

Frances Schrag • Newton, KS

Makes 12 1-cup servings (Ideal slow cooker size: 4-quart)

10 cups boiling water

1 Tbsp. instant tea

$\frac{2}{3}$ cup lemon juice

$\frac{1}{2}$ cup sugar

$\frac{1}{2}$ cup Splenda

1 tsp. vanilla

1 tsp. almond extract

1. Mix together all ingredients in slow cooker.

2. Turn to High and heat thoroughly (about 1 hour). Turn to Low while serving.

Exchange List Values: Carbohydrate 0.5

Basic Nutritional Values: Calories 40 (Calories from Fat 0), Total Fat 0 gm (Saturated Fat 0 gm, Polyunsat Fat 0 gm, Monounsat Fat 0 gm, Cholesterol 0 mg), Sodium 3 mg, Total Carbohydrate 10 gm, Dietary Fiber 0 gm, Sugars 9 gm, Protein 0 gm

Hot (Buttered) Lemonade

Janie Steele • Moore, OK

Makes 6 servings (Ideal slow cooker size: 4-quart)

4½ cups water

6 Tbsp. sugar

sugar substitute to equal 3 Tbsp.

1½ tsp. grated lemon peel

¾ cup lemon juice

2 Tbsp. light, soft tub margarine

6 cinnamon sticks

1. Combine water, sugar, sugar substitute, lemon peel, lemon juice, and margarine in slow cooker.

2. Cover. Cook on High for 2½ hours, or until well heated through.

3. Serve very hot with a cinnamon stick in each mug.

Exchange List Values: Carbohydrate 1.0

Basic Nutritional Values: Calories 69 (Calories from Fat 13), Total Fat 1 gm (Saturated Fat 0.1 gm, Polyunsat Fat 0.3 gm, Monounsat Fat 0.8 gm, Cholesterol 0 mg), Sodium 36 mg, Total Carbohydrate 15 gm, Dietary Fiber 0 gm, Sugars 14 gm, Protein 0 gm

Seek support from family, friends, and coworkers.

Hot Chocolate with Stir-Ins

Stacy Schmucker Stoltzfus • Enola, PA

Makes 12 servings (96 ozs.) (Ideal slow cooker size: 4–5-quart)

9½ cups water

1½ cups hot chocolate mix

STIR-INS:

    smooth peanut butter

    chocolate-mint candies, chopped

    candy canes, broken

    assorted flavored syrups: hazelnut, almond, raspberry, Irish creme

    instant coffee granules

    cinnamon

    nutmeg

whipped topping

candy sprinkles

1. Pour water into slow cooker. Heat on High 1–2 hours. (Or heat water in tea kettle and pour into slow cooker.) Turn cooker to Low to keep hot for hours.

2. Stir in hot chocolate mix until blended.

3. Arrange stir-ins in small bowls.

4. Instruct guests to place approximately 1 Tbsp. of desired stir-in in mug before ladling in hot chocolate. Stir well.

5. Top with whipped topping and candy sprinkles.

Exchange List Values: Carbohydrate 1.0

Basic Nutritional Values: Calories 63 (Calories from Fat 14), Total Fat 2 gm (Saturated Fat 0.3 gm, Polyunsat Fat 0.4 gm, Monounsat Fat 0.7 gm, Cholesterol 0 mg), Sodium 32 mg, Total Carbohydrate 12 gm, Dietary Fiber 0 gm, Sugars 3 gm, Protein 1 gm

Note: One serving of each stir-in was used in the nutritional analysis.

Crockery Cocoa

Betty Hostetler • Allensville, PA

**Makes 12 servings, depending on size of mugs
(Ideal slow cooker size: 4–5-quart)**

½ cup sugar

½ cup unsweetened cocoa powder

2 cups boiling water

3½ cups nonfat dry milk powder

6 cups water

1 tsp. vanilla

marshmallows, optional

1 tsp. ground cinnamon, optional

1. Combine sugar and cocoa powder in slow cooker. Add 2 cups boiling water. Stir well to dissolve.

2. Add dry milk powder, 6 cups water, and vanilla. Stir well to dissolve.

3. Cover. Cook on Low 4 hours, or High 1–1½ hours.

4. Before serving, beat with rotary beater to make frothy. Ladle into mugs. Top with marshmallows and sprinkle with cinnamon, if you wish.

Exchange List Values: Milk, fat-free 1.0, Carbohydrate 0.5

Basic Nutritional Values: Calories 111 (Calories from Fat 6), Total Fat 1 gm (Saturated Fat 0.3 gm, Polyunsat Fat 0 gm, Monounsat Fat 0.2 gm, Cholesterol 4 mg), Sodium 110 mg, Total Carbohydrate 21 gm, Dietary Fiber 1 gm, Sugars 19 gm, Protein 8 gm

VARIATIONS:

1. Add ⅛ tsp. ground nutmeg along with ground cinnamon in Step 4.

2. Mocha-style—Stir ¾ tsp. coffee crystals into each serving in Step 4.

3. Coffee-Cocoa—Pour half-cups of freshly brewed, high-quality coffee; top with half-cups of Crockery Cocoa.

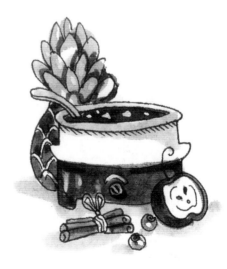

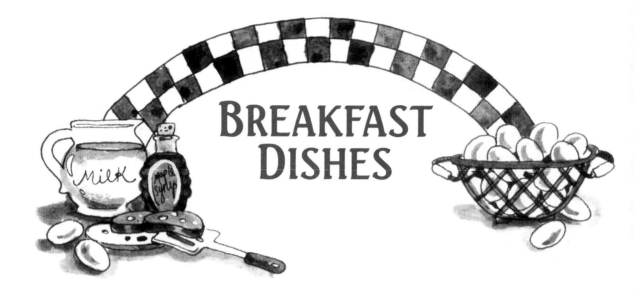

BREAKFAST DISHES

Welsh Rarebit

Sharon Timpe • Mequon, WI

Recipe photo appears in color section.

Makes 16 servings (Ideal slow cooker size: 3–4-quart)

12-oz. can beer

1 Tbsp. dry mustard

1 tsp. Worcestershire sauce

$\frac{1}{8}$ tsp. black or white pepper

8 ozs. reduced-fat American cheese, cubed

8 ozs. reduced-fat sharp cheddar cheese, cubed

English muffins or toast, optional

bacon, cooked until crisp, optional

tomato slices, optional

fresh steamed asparagus spears, optional

1. In slow cooker, combine beer, mustard, Worcestershire sauce, and pepper.

2. Cover and cook on High 1–2 hours, until mixture boils.

3. Add cheese, a little at a time, stirring constantly until all cheese melts.

4. Heat on High 20–30 minutes with cover off, stirring frequently.

5. Serve hot over toasted English muffins or over toasted bread cut into triangles. Garnish with strips of crisp bacon and tomato slices or asparagus spears.

Exchange List Values: Meat, medium fat 1.0

Basic Nutritional Values: Calories 69 (Calories from Fat 46), Total Fat 5 gm (Saturated Fat 3.0 gm, Polyunsat Fat 0.1 gm, Monounsat Fat 1.5 gm, Cholesterol 17 mg), Sodium 317 mg, Total Carbohydrate 2 gm, Dietary Fiber 0 gm, Sugars 2 gm, Protein 6 gm

Note: If Rarebit is left in slow cooker after it has cooked (Step 4), it will begin to curdle.

This is a good dish for brunch with fresh fruit, juice, and coffee. Also makes a great lunch or late-night light supper. Serve with a tossed green salad, especially fresh spinach and orange slices with a vinaigrette dressing.

Cheese Souffle Casserole

Iva Schmidt • Fergus Falls, MN

Makes 6 servings (Ideal slow cooker size: 3–4-quart)

8 slices bread (crusts removed), cubed or torn into squares

2 cups (8 ozs.) grated fat-free cheddar cheese

1 cup cooked, chopped extra-lean, lower-sodium ham

4 eggs

1 cup fat-free half-and-half

1 cup fat-free evaporated milk

1 Tbsp. parsley

paprika

1. Lightly grease slow cooker. Alternate layers of bread and cheese and ham.

2. Beat together eggs, half-and-half, milk, and parsley. Pour over bread in slow cooker.

3. Sprinkle with paprika.

4. Cover and cook on Low 3–4 hours. (The longer cooking time yields a firmer, dryer dish.)

5. About 30 minutes before finish, increase temperature to High and remove lid.

Exchange List Values: Starch 1.0, Milk, fat-free 0.5, Meat, lean 2.0

Basic Nutritional Values: Calories 233 (Calories from Fat 46), Total Fat 5 gm (Saturated Fat 1.9 gm, Polyunsat Fat 0.9 gm, Monounsat Fat 1.6 gm, Cholesterol 159 mg), Sodium 650 mg, Total Carbohydrate 22 gm, Dietary Fiber 0 gm, Sugars 9 gm, Protein 23 gm

Breakfast Casserole

Shirley Hinh • Wayland, IA

Makes 10 servings (Ideal slow cooker size: 4-quart)

4 eggs, beaten

4 egg whites, lightly beaten

$\frac{1}{3}$ lb. little smokies (cocktail wieners)

$1\frac{1}{2}$ cups fat-free milk

1 cup shredded fat-free cheddar cheese

8 slices bread, torn into pieces

$\frac{1}{2}$ tsp. dry mustard

1 cup shredded reduced-fat mozzarella cheese

1. Mix together all ingredients except mozzarella cheese. Pour into greased slow cooker.

2. Sprinkle mozzarella cheese over top.

3. Cover and cook 2 hours on High, and then 1 hour on Low.

Exchange List Values: Starch 1.0, Meat, medium fat 1.0, Fat 1.0

Basic Nutritional Values: Calories 194 (Calories from Fat 76), Total Fat 8 gm (Saturated Fat 3.4 gm, Polyunsat Fat 1.2 gm, Monounsat Fat 3.1 gm, Cholesterol 103 mg), Sodium 485 mg, Total Carbohydrate 13 gm, Dietary Fiber 0 gm, Sugars 4 gm, Protein 15 gm

Egg and Cheese Bake

Evie Hershey • Atglen, PA

Makes 6 servings (Ideal slow cooker size: 4-quart)

3 cups toasted bread cubes

1½ cups shredded reduced-fat sharp cheddar
   cheese

fried, crumbled bacon, or ham chunks, optional

4 eggs, beaten

4 egg whites

3 cups fat-free milk

¼ tsp. pepper

1. Combine bread cubes, cheese, and meat
   in greased slow cooker.

2. Mix together eggs, milk, and pepper.
   Pour over bread.

3. Cook on Low 4–6 hours.

**Exchange List Values: Starch 1.0, Milk,
fat-free 0.5, Meat, medium fat 1.0**

Basic Nutritional Values: Calories 193 (Calories
from Fat 65), Total Fat 7 gm (Saturated Fat 3.3 gm,
Polyunsat Fat 1.0 gm, Monounsat Fat 2.3 gm,
Cholesterol 155 mg), Sodium 377 mg, Total
Carbohydrate 18 gm, Dietary Fiber 1 gm, Sugars
8 gm, Protein 16 gm

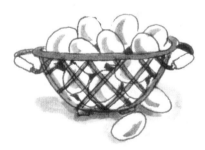

Egg and Broccoli Casserole

Joette Droz • Kalona, IA

Recipe photo appears in color section.

Makes 8 servings (Ideal slow cooker size: 4-quart)

24-oz. carton small-curd low-fat (1% milkfat)
   cottage cheese

10-oz. pkg. frozen chopped broccoli, thawed
   and drained

1½ cups (6 ozs.) shredded cheddar cheese

6 eggs, beaten

⅓ cup flour

2 Tbsp. canola oil

3 Tbsp. finely chopped onion

shredded cheese, optional

1. Combine first 7 ingredients. Pour into
   greased slow cooker.

2. Cover and cook on High 1 hour. Stir.
   Reduce heat to Low. Cover and cook
   2½–3 hours, or until temperature
   reaches 160° and eggs are set.

3. Sprinkle with cheese, if you wish,
   and serve.

**Exchange List Values: Carbohydrate 0.5,
Meat, lean 3.0**

Basic Nutritional Values: Calories 211 (Calories
from Fat 74), Total Fat 8 gm (Saturated Fat 2.3 gm,
Polyunsat Fat 1.6 gm, Monounsat Fat 3.7 gm,
Cholesterol 165 mg), Sodium 550 mg, Total
Carbohydrate 10 gm, Dietary Fiber 1 gm, Sugars
5 gm, Protein 23 gm

Breakfast Skillet

Sue Hamilton • Minooka, IL

Makes 6 servings (Ideal slow cooker size: 4-quart)

3 cups non-fat milk

5$\frac{1}{2}$-oz. box au gratin potatoes

1 tsp. hot sauce

5 eggs, lightly beaten

1 Tbsp. prepared mustard

4-oz. can sliced mushrooms

4 slices bacon, fried and crumbled

1 cup shredded fat-free cheddar cheese

1. Combine milk, au gratin sauce packet, hot sauce, eggs, and mustard.

2. Stir in dried potatoes, mushrooms, and bacon.

3. Cover. Cook on High 2$\frac{1}{2}$–3 hours, or on Low 5–6 hours.

4. Sprinkle cheese over top. Cover until cheese melts.

Exchange List Values: Starch 1.5, Milk, fat-free 0.5, Meat, lean 2.0

Basic Nutritional Values: Calories 251 (Calories from Fat 67), Total Fat 7 gm (Saturated Fat 3.1 gm, Polyunsat Fat 0.9 gm, Monounsat Fat 2.9 gm, Cholesterol 185 mg), Sodium 941 mg, Total Carbohydrate 29 gm, Dietary Fiber 2 gm, Sugars 9 gm, Protein 20 gm

Get plenty of sleep—it revitalizes your body and your mind.

Western Omelet Casserole

Mary Louise Martin • Boyd, WI

Makes 10 servings (Ideal slow cooker size: 4–5-quart)

32-oz. bag frozen hash brown potatoes

8 ozs. extra-lean, lower-sodium cooked ham, cubed

1 medium onion, diced

1$\frac{1}{2}$ cups shredded fat-free cheddar cheese

12 eggs

1 cup fat-free milk

$\frac{1}{2}$ tsp. salt

1 tsp. pepper

1. Layer one-third each of frozen potatoes, ham, onions, and cheese in bottom of slow cooker. Repeat 2 times.

2. Beat together eggs, milk, salt, and pepper. Pour over mixture in slow cooker.

3. Cover. Cook on Low 8–9 hours.

4. Serve with orange juice and fresh fruit.

Exchange List Values: Starch 1.5, Meat, lean 2.0

Basic Nutritional Values: Calories 237 (Calories from Fat 63), Total Fat 7 gm (Saturated Fat 2.7 gm, Polyunsat Fat 1.2 gm, Monounsat Fat 2.5 gm, Cholesterol 268 mg), Sodium 563 mg, Total Carbohydrate 24 gm, Dietary Fiber 2 gm, Sugars 5 gm, Protein 20 gm

Mexican-Style Grits

Mary Sommerfeld • Lancaster, PA

Makes 10–12 servings (Ideal slow cooker size: 4-quart)

1½ cups instant grits

4 ozs. fat-free cheddar cheese, cubed

½ tsp. garlic powder

2 4-oz. cans diced chilies

2 Tbsp. light, soft tub margarine

1. Prepare grits according to package directions.

2. Stir in cheese, garlic powder, and chilies, until cheese is melted.

3. Stir in margarine. Pour into greased slow cooker.

4. Cover. Cook on High 2–3 hours, or on Low 4–6 hours.

Exchange List Values: Starch 1.0

Basic Nutritional Values: Calories 91 (Calories from Fat 9), Total Fat 1 gm (Saturated Fat 0.1 gm, Polyunsat Fat 0.3 gm, Monounsat Fat 0.5 gm, Cholesterol 1 mg), Sodium 167 mg, Total Carbohydrate 16 gm, Dietary Fiber 2 gm, Sugars 0 gm, Protein 5 gm

Creamy Old-Fashioned Oatmeal

Mary Wheatley • Mashpee, MA

Makes 5 servings (Ideal slow cooker size: 3-quart)

1⅓ cups dry old-fashioned rolled oats

2½ cups plus 1 Tbsp. water

dash salt

1. Mix together cereal, water, and salt in slow cooker.

2. Cook on Low 6 hours.

Exchange List Values: Starch 1.0

Basic Nutritional Values: Calories 83 (Calories from Fat 12), Total Fat 1 gm (Saturated Fat 0.3 gm, Polyunsat Fat 0.5 gm, Monounsat Fat 0.4 gm, Cholesterol 0 mg), Sodium 1 mg, Total Carbohydrate 14 gm, Dietary Fiber 2 gm, Sugars 0 gm, Protein 3 gm

VARIATION: Before cooking, stir in a few chopped dates or raisins for each serving, if you wish.

Cathy Boshart • Lebanon, PA

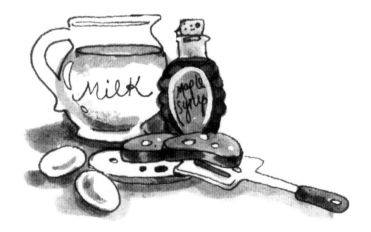

Apple Oatmeal

Frances B. Musser • Newmanstown, PA

Makes 4–5 servings (Ideal slow cooker size: 3-quart)

2 cups fat-free milk

1 Tbsp. honey

1 Tbsp. light, soft tub margarine

1/4 tsp. salt

1/2 tsp. cinnamon

1 cup dry old-fashioned oats

1 cup chopped apples

1/2 cup chopped walnuts

1 Tbsp. brown sugar

brown sugar substitute to equal 1/2 Tbsp.

1. Mix together all ingredients in greased slow cooker.

2. Cover. Cook on Low 5–6 hours.

3. Serve with milk or ice cream.

Exchange List Values: Carbohydrate 2.0, Fat 1.5

Basic Nutritional Values: Calories 220 (Calories from Fat 89), Total Fat 10 gm (Saturated Fat 1.1 gm, Polyunsat Fat 6.3 gm, Monounsat Fat 1.9 gm, Cholesterol 2 mg), Sodium 180 mg, Total Carbohydrate 28 gm, Dietary Fiber 3 gm, Sugars 15 gm, Protein 8 gm

VARIATION: Add 1/2 cup light or dark raisins to mixture.

Jeanette Oberholtzer • Manheim, PA

Peanut Butter Granola

Dawn Ranck • Harrisonburg, VA

Recipe photo appears in color section.

Makes 26 servings (Ideal slow cooker size: 5-quart)

6 cups dry oatmeal

1/2 cup wheat germ

1/4 cup toasted coconut

1/4 cup sunflower seeds

1/2 cup raisins

8 Tbsp. light, soft tub margarine

3/4 cup peanut butter

1/2 cup brown sugar

brown sugar substitute to equal 4 Tbsp.

1. Combine oatmeal, wheat germ, coconut, sunflower seeds, and raisins in large slow cooker.

2. Melt together margarine, peanut butter, brown sugar, and sugar substitute. Pour over oatmeal in cooker. Mix well.

3. Cover. Cook on Low 1 1/2 hours, stirring every 15 minutes.

4. Allow to cool in cooker, stirring every 30 minutes or so, or spread onto cookie sheet. When thoroughly cooled, break into chunks and store in airtight container.

Exchange List Values: Starch 0.5, Carbohydrate 1.0, Fat 1.5

Basic Nutritional Values: Calories 179 (Calories from Fat 73), Total Fat 8 gm (Saturated Fat 1.5 gm, Polyunsat Fat 2.8 gm, Monounsat Fat 3.3 gm, Cholesterol 0 mg), Sodium 70 mg, Total Carbohydrate 22 gm, Dietary Fiber 3 gm, Sugars 7 gm, Protein 6 gm

Breakfast Apple Cobbler

Anona M. Teel • Banga, PA

**Makes 6–8 servings
(Ideal slow cooker size: 4-quart)**

8 medium apples, cored, peeled, sliced

2 Tbsp. sugar

sugar substitute to equal 1 Tbsp.

dash cinnamon

juice of 1 lemon

2 Tbsp. light, soft tub margarine, melted

2 cups granola

1. Combine ingredients in slow cooker.

2. Cover. Cook on Low 7–9 hours (while you sleep!), or on High 2–3 hours (after you're up in the morning).

Exchange List Values: Starch 1.5, Fruit 1.5, Fat 1.0

Basic Nutritional Values: Calories 221 (Calories from Fat 57), Total Fat 6 gm (Saturated Fat 2.1 gm, Polyunsat Fat 1.9 gm, Monounsat Fat 1.7 gm, Cholesterol 0 mg), Sodium 102 mg, Total Carbohydrate 42 gm, Dietary Fiber 4 gm, Sugars 29 gm, Protein 2 gm

Dulce Leche (Sweet Milk)

Dorothy Horst • Tiskilwa, IL

Makes 38 (1 Tbsp.) servings (Ideal slow cooker size: 3–4-quart)

2 14-oz. cans fat-free sweetened condensed milk

1. Place unopened cans of milk in slow cooker. Fill cooker with warm water so that it comes above the cans by 1½"–2".

2. Cover cooker. Cook on High 2 hours.

3. Cool unopened cans.

4. When opened, the contents should be thick and spreadable. Use as a filling between 2 cookies or crackers.

Exchange List Values: Carbohydrate 1.0

Basic Nutritional Values: Calories 58 (Calories from Fat 0), Total Fat 0 gm (Saturated Fat 0 gm, Polyunsat Fat 0.1 gm, Monounsat Fat 0.5 gm, Cholesterol 0 mg), Sodium 21 mg, Total Carbohydrate 13 gm, Dietary Fiber 0 gm, Sugars 13 gm, Protein 2 gm

When on a tour in Argentina, we were served this at breakfast-time as a spread on toast or thick slices of bread. We were also presented with a container of prepared Dulce Leche as a parting gift to take home. This dish also sometimes appears on Mexican menus.

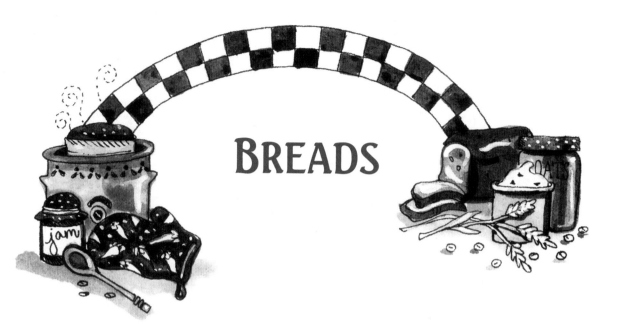

BREADS

Healthy Whole Wheat Bread

Esther Becker • Gordonville, PA

Makes 16 servings (Ideal slow cooker size: 5–6-quart)

2 cups warm reconstituted fat-free powdered milk (²/₃ cup powder to 1¹/₃ cups water)

2 Tbsp. canola oil

¼ cup honey or brown sugar

¾ tsp. salt

1 pkg. active dry yeast

2½ cups whole wheat flour

1¼ cups white flour

1. Mix together milk, oil, honey or brown sugar, salt, yeast, and half the flour in electric mixer bowl. Beat with mixer for 2 minutes. Add remaining flour. Mix well.

2. Place dough in well-greased bread or cake pan that will fit into your cooker. Cover with greased tinfoil. Let stand for 5 minutes. Place in slow cooker.

3. Cover cooker and bake on High 2½–3 hours. Remove pan and uncover. Let stand 5 minutes. Serve warm.

Exchange List Values: Starch 1.0, Fat 0.5

Basic Nutritional Values: Calories 142 (Calories from Fat 20), Total Fat 2 gm (Saturated Fat 0.1 gm, Polyunsat Fat 0.7 gm, Monounsat Fat 1.1 gm, Cholesterol 1 mg), Sodium 126 mg, Total Carbohydrate 27 gm, Dietary Fiber 3 gm, Sugars 6 gm, Protein 5 gm

Boston Brown Bread

Jean Butzer • Batavia, NY

Makes 21 servings (3 loaves) (Ideal slow cooker size: 6-quart)

3 16-oz. vegetable cans, cleaned and emptied

1/2 cup rye flour

1/2 cup yellow cornmeal

1/2 cup whole wheat flour

3 Tbsp. sugar

1 tsp. baking soda

3/4 tsp. salt

1/2 cup chopped walnuts

1/2 cup raisins

1 cup low-fat buttermilk*

1/3 cup molasses

1. Spray insides of vegetable cans, and one side of 3 6"-square pieces of foil, with nonstick cooking spray. Set aside.

2. Combine rye flour, cornmeal, whole wheat flour, sugar, baking soda, and salt in a large bowl.

3. Stir in walnuts and raisins.

4. Whisk together buttermilk and molasses. Add to dry ingredients. Stir until well mixed. Spoon into prepared cans.

5. Place one piece of foil, greased side down, on top of each can. Secure foil with rubber bands or cotton string. Place upright in slow cooker.

6. Pour boiling water into slow cooker to come halfway up sides of cans. (Make sure foil tops do not touch boiling water.)

7. Cover cooker. Cook on Low 4 hours, or until skewer inserted in center of bread comes out clean.

8. To remove bread, lay cans on their sides. Roll and tap gently on all sides until bread releases. Cool completely on wire racks.

9. Serve with butter or cream cheese and bowls of soup.

Exchange List Values: Carbohydrate 1.0, Fat 0.5

Basic Nutritional Values: Calories 85 (Calories from Fat 20), Total Fat 2 gm (Saturated Fat 0.2 gm, Polyunsat Fat 1.4 gm, Monounsat Fat 0.3 gm, Cholesterol 0 mg), Sodium 158 mg, Total Carbohydrate 16 gm, Dietary Fiber 2 gm, Sugars 8 gm, Protein 2 gm

*To substitute for buttermilk, pour 1 Tbsp. lemon juice into 1-cup measure. Add enough milk to fill the cup. Let stand 5 minutes before mixing with molasses.

Make one meal today free of meat and cheese. Your heart will thank you.

Corn Bread from Scratch

Dorothy M. Van Deest • Memphis, TN

Makes 9 servings (Ideal slow cooker size: 6-quart)

1¼ cups flour

¾ cup yellow cornmeal

¼ cup sugar

4½ tsp. baking powder

½ tsp. salt

1 egg, slightly beaten

1 cup fat-free milk

¼ cup canola oil

1. In mixing bowl sift together flour, cornmeal, sugar, baking powder, and salt. Make a well in the center.

2. Pour egg, milk, and oil into well. Mix into the dry mixture until just moistened.

3. Pour mixture into a greased 2-quart mold that will fit into your cooker. Cover with a plate. Place on a trivet or rack in the bottom of slow cooker.

4. Cover. Cook on High 2–3 hours.

Exchange List Values: Starch 2.0, Fat 1.0

Basic Nutritional Values: Calories 200 (Calories from Fat 64), Total Fat 7 gm (Saturated Fat 0.7 gm, Polyunsat Fat 2.1 gm, Monounsat Fat 4.0 gm, Cholesterol 24 mg), Sodium 330 mg, Total Carbohydrate 29 gm, Dietary Fiber 1 gm, Sugars 7 gm, Protein 4 gm

Lemon Bread

Ruth Ann Gingrich • New Holland, PA

Makes 12 servings (Ideal slow cooker size: 4-quart)

¼ cup canola oil

6 Tbsp. sugar

sugar substitute to equal 3 Tbsp.

2 eggs, beaten

1⅔ cups flour

1⅔ tsp. baking powder

½ tsp. salt

½ cup fat-free milk

4 ozs. chopped walnuts

grated peel from 1 lemon

GLAZE:

¼ cup confectioners' sugar

juice of 1 lemon

1. Cream together oil, sugar, and sugar substitute. Add eggs. Mix well.

2. Sift together flour, baking powder, and salt. Add flour mixture and milk alternately to shortening mixture.

3. Stir in nuts and lemon peel.

4. Spoon batter into well-greased 2-lb. coffee can and cover with well-greased tinfoil. Place in cooker set on High for 2–2¼ hours, or until done. Remove bread from coffee can.

5. Mix together confectioners' sugar and lemon juice. Pour over loaf.

6. Serve plain or with cream cheese.

Exchange List Values: Starch 1.5, Fat 1.0

Basic Nutritional Values: Calories 176 (Calories from Fat 66), Total Fat 7 gm (Saturated Fat 0.9 gm, Polyunsat Fat 2.7 gm, Monounsat Fat 3.3 gm, Cholesterol 37 mg), Sodium 168 mg, Total Carbohydrate 24 gm, Dietary Fiber 1 gm, Sugars 10 gm, Protein 4 gm

Date and Nut Loaf

Jean Butzer • Batavia, NY

Recipe photo appears in color section.

Makes 20 servings (Ideal slow cooker size: 6-quart)

1½ cups boiling water

1½ cups chopped dates

¾ cup sugar

sugar substitute to equal ¼ cup

1 egg

2 tsp. baking soda

½ tsp. salt

1 tsp. vanilla

1 Tbsp. light, soft tub margarine, melted

2½ cups flour

1 cup walnuts, chopped

2 cups hot water

1. Pour 1½ cups boiling water over dates. Let stand 5–10 minutes.

2. Stir in sugar, sugar substitute, egg, baking soda, salt, vanilla, and margarine.

3. In separate bowl, combine flour and nuts. Stir into date mixture.

4. Pour into 2 greased 11½-oz. coffee cans or one 8-cup baking insert. If using coffee cans, cover with foil and tie. If using baking insert, cover with its lid. Place cans or insert on rack in slow cooker. (If you don't have a rack, use rubber jar rings instead.)

5. Pour hot water around cans, up to half their height.

6. Cover slow cooker tightly. Cook on High 3½–4 hours.

7. Remove cans or insert from cooker. Let bread stand in coffee cans or baking insert for 10 minutes. Turn out onto cooling rack. Slice. Spread with butter, cream cheese, or peanut butter, if you wish.

Exchange List Values: Carbohydrate 2.0, Fat 0.5

Basic Nutritional Values: Calories 168 (Calories from Fat 41), Total Fat 5 gm (Saturated Fat 0.5 gm, Polyunsat Fat 3.0 gm, Monounsat Fat 0.8 gm, Cholesterol 11 mg), Sodium 193 mg, Total Carbohydrate 30 gm, Dietary Fiber 2 gm, Sugars 17 gm, Protein 3 gm

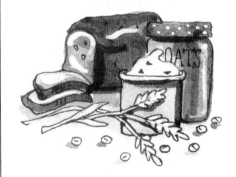

Broccoli Corn Bread

Winifred Ewy • Newton, KS

Makes 10 servings (Ideal slow cooker size: 3-4-quart)

3 Tbsp. light, soft tub margarine, melted

10-oz. pkg. chopped broccoli, cooked and drained

1 medium onion, chopped

8½-oz. box corn bread mix

1 egg, well beaten

3 egg whites

8 ozs. 1% fat cottage cheese

⅛ tsp. salt

1. Combine all ingredients. Mix well.

2. Pour into greased slow cooker. Cook on Low 6 hours, or until toothpick inserted in center comes out clean.

3. Serve like spoon bread, or invert the pot, remove bread, and cut into wedges.

Exchange List Values: Starch 1.0, Vegetable 1.0, Fat 0.5

Basic Nutritional Values: Calories 119 (Calories from Fat 34), Total Fat 4 gm (Saturated Fat 1.4 gm, Polyunsat Fat 0.6 gm, Monounsat Fat 1.4 gm, Cholesterol 22 mg), Sodium 370 mg, Total Carbohydrate 20 gm, Dietary Fiber 2 gm, Sugars 7 gm, Protein 7 gm

Banana Loaf

Sue Hamilton • Minooka, IL

Makes 10 servings (Ideal slow cooker size: 4-5-quart)

3 very ripe, medium bananas

¼ cup margarine, softened

2 eggs

1 tsp. vanilla

½ cup sugar

sugar substitute to equal ¼ cup

1 cup flour

1 tsp. baking soda

1. Combine all ingredients in an electric mixing bowl. Beat 2 minutes or until well blended. Pour into well-greased 2-lb. coffee can.

2. Place can in slow cooker. Cover can with 6 layers of paper towels between cooker lid and bread.

3. Cover cooker. Bake on High 2-2½ hours, or until toothpick inserted in center comes out clean. Cool 15 minutes before removing from can.

Exchange List Values: Carbohydrate 2.0, Fat 1.0

Basic Nutritional Values: Calories 177 (Calories from Fat 53), Total Fat 6 gm (Saturated Fat 1.3 gm, Polyunsat Fat 1.7 gm, Monounsat Fat 2.5 gm, Cholesterol 43 mg), Sodium 192 mg, Total Carbohydrate 29 gm, Dietary Fiber 1 gm, Sugars 16 gm, Protein 3 gm

Cheery Cherry Bread

Shirley Sears • Tiskilwa, IL

Recipe photo appears in color section.

Makes 10 servings (Ideal slow cooker size: 4–5-quart)

6-oz. jar maraschino cherries

1½ cups flour

1½ tsp. baking powder

¼ tsp. salt

2 eggs

6 Tbsp. sugar

sugar substitute to equal 3 Tbsp.

¾ cup coarsely chopped pecans

1. Drain cherries, reserving ⅓ cup syrup. Cut cherries in pieces. Set aside.

2. Combine flour, baking powder, and salt.

3. Beat eggs, sugar, and sugar substitute together until thickened.

4. Alternately add flour mixture and cherry syrup to egg mixture, mixing until well blended after each addition.

5. Fold in cherries and pecans. Spread in well-greased and floured baking insert or 2-lb. coffee can. If using baking insert, cover with its lid; if using a coffee can, cover with 6 layers of paper towels. Set in slow cooker.

6. Cover cooker. Cook on High 2–3 hours.

7. Remove from slow cooker. Let stand 10 minutes before removing from pan.

8. Cool before slicing.

Exchange List Values: Carbohydrate 2.0, Fat 1.5

Basic Nutritional Values: Calories 213 (Calories from Fat 70), Total Fat 8 gm (Saturated Fat 1.0 gm, Polyunsat Fat 2.1 gm, Monounsat Fat 4.3 gm, Cholesterol 43 mg), Sodium 126 mg, Total Carbohydrate 31 gm, Dietary Fiber 2 gm, Sugars 15 gm, Protein 4 gm

Gingerbread with Lemon Sauce

Jean Butzer • Batavia, NY /
Marie Shank • Harrisonburg, VA

Makes 16 servings (Ideal slow cooker size: 4–5-quart)

¼ cup margarine, softened

¼ cup sugar

sugar substitute to equal 2 Tbsp.

1 egg, lightly beaten

1 cup sorghum molasses

2½ cups flour

1½ tsp. baking soda

1 tsp. cinnamon

2 tsp. ground ginger

½ tsp. ground cloves

½ tsp. salt

1 cup hot coffee or hot water

½ cup confectioners' sugar

2 tsp. cornstarch

pinch salt

juice of 2 lemons

½ cup water

1 Tbsp. butter

confectioners' sugar for garnish

1. Cream together ¼ cup margarine, sugar, and sugar substitute.

2. Add egg. Mix well.

3. Add molasses. Mix well.

4. Sift together flour, baking soda, cinnamon, ginger, cloves, and salt. Stir into creamed mixture.

5. Add coffee or 1 cup water. Beat well.

6. There are two ways to bake the gingerbread:

a. If you have a baking insert, or a 2-lb. coffee can, grease and flour the inside of it. Pour in batter. Place in slow cooker. Pour water around insert or coffee can. Cover insert with its lid, or cover coffee can with 6–8 paper towels.

b. Cut waxed paper or parchment paper to fit bottom of slow cooker. Place in bottom of cooker. Spray paper and sides of cooker's interior with nonstick cooking spray. Pour batter into pre-heated slow cooker.

7. Cover cooker with its lid slightly ajar to allow excess moisture to escape. Cook on High 1¾–2 hours, or on Low 3–4 hours, or until edges are golden and knife inserted in center comes out clean.

8. If you used a baking insert or coffee can, remove from cooker. Cool on cake rack. Let stand 5 minutes before running knife around outer edge of cake and inverting onto serving plate. If you baked the gingerbread directly in the cooker, cut the cake into wedges after allowing it to cool for 30 minutes, and carefully lift the wedges out of the cooker onto serving plates.

9. In saucepan, mix together ½ cup confectioners' sugar, cornstarch, and salt. Add lemon juice and ½ cup water, stirring with each addition. Cook over medium heat until thick and bubbly, about 1 minute. Remove from heat. Stir in butter.

10. If gingerbread has been cooling on a rack, cut it into wedges. To serve, top with sauce and sprinkle with confectioners' sugar.

Exchange List Values: Carbohydrate 2.5, Fat 0.5

Basic Nutritional Values: Calories 198 (Calories from Fat 37), Total Fat 4 gm (Saturated Fat 1.1 gm, Polyunsat Fat 1.1 gm, Monounsat Fat 1.6 gm, Cholesterol 15 mg), Sodium 239 mg, Total Carbohydrate 38 gm, Dietary Fiber 1 gm, Sugars 23 gm, Protein 2 gm

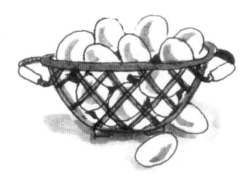

Old-Fashioned Gingerbread

Mary Ann Westerberg • Rosamond, CA

Recipe photo appears in color section.

Makes 16 servings (Ideal slow cooker size: 4-quart)

4 Tbsp. margarine, softened

4 Tbsp. sugar

sugar substitute to equal 2 Tbsp.

1 egg

1 cup light molasses

2½ cups flour

1½ tsp. baking soda

1 tsp. ground cinnamon

2 tsp. ground ginger

½ tsp. ground cloves

½ tsp. salt

1 cup hot water

warm applesauce, optional

whipped cream, optional

nutmeg, optional

1. Cream together margarine, sugar, and sugar substitute. Add egg and molasses. Mix well.

2. Stir in flour, baking soda, cinnamon, ginger, cloves, and salt. Mix well.

3. Add hot water. Beat well.

4. Pour batter into greased and floured 2-lb. coffee can.

5. Place can in cooker. Cover top of can with 6–8 paper towels. Cover cooker and bake on High 2½–3 hours.

6. Serve with applesauce, if desired. Top with whipped cream and sprinkle with nutmeg, if desired.

Exchange List Values: Carbohydrate 2.0, Fat 0.5

Basic Nutritional Values: Calories 168 (Calories from Fat 30), Total Fat 3 gm (Saturated Fat 0.7 gm, Polyunsat Fat 1.0 gm, Monounsat Fat 1.4 gm, Cholesterol 13 mg), Sodium 235 mg, Total Carbohydrate 32 gm, Dietary Fiber 1 gm, Sugars 16 gm, Protein 2 gm

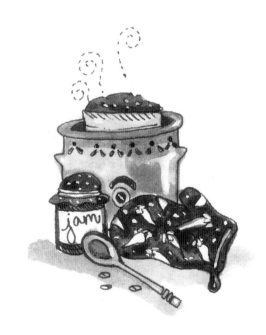

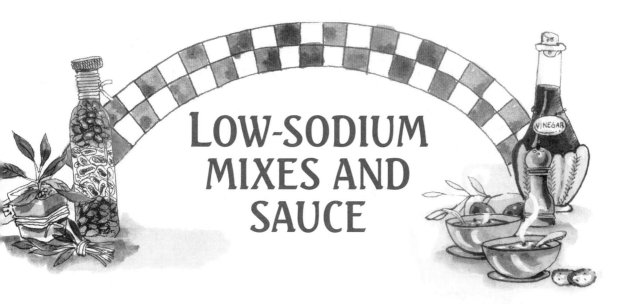

LOW-SODIUM MIXES AND SAUCE

Italian Seasoning Mix

Madelyn L. Wheeler • Zionsville, IN

Makes 13 (1 Tbsp.) servings

6 tsp. marjoram, dried

6 tsp. thyme leaves, dried

6 tsp. rosemary, dried

6 tsp. savory, ground

3 tsp. dry sage, ground

6 tsp. oregano leaves, dried

6 tsp. basil leaves, dried

Combine all ingredients.

Exchange List Values: Vegetable 2.0, Meat, lean 4.0

Basic Nutritional Values: Calories 8 (Calories from Fat 2), Total Fat 0 gm (Saturated Fat 0.1 gm, Polyunsat Fat 0.1 gm, Monounsat Fat 0 gm, Cholesterol 0 mg), Sodium 1 mg, Total Carbohydrate 2 gm, Dietary Fiber 1 gm, Sugars 0 gm, Protein 0 gm

This recipe should be made with dried leaves if available, rather than ground, except for the savory and sage.

Low-Sodium Taco Seasoning Mix

Madelyn L. Wheeler • Zionsville, IN

Makes 3 servings; serving size is ⅓ of recipe (about 7 tsp.)

6 tsp. chili powder

5 tsp. paprika

4½ tsp. cumin seed

3 tsp. onion powder

1 tsp. garlic powder

⅔ Tbsp. dry cornstarch

1. Combine all ingredients in bowl.

2. One-third of mix (about 7 tsp.) is equivalent to 1 pkg. (1.25 ozs.) purchased taco seasoning mix.

Exchange List Values: Carbohydrate 0.5

Basic Nutritional Values: Calories 56 (Calories from Fat 19), Total Fat 2 gm (Saturated Fat 0 gm, Polyunsat Fat 0.9 gm, Monounsat Fat 0.7 gm, Cholesterol 0 mg), Sodium 61 mg, Total Carbohydrate 10 gm, Dietary Fiber 3 gm, Sugars 3 gm, Protein 2 gm

Sodium-Free Onion Soup Mix

Madelyn L. Wheeler • Zionsville, IN

Makes 1 serving (equivalent to 1 pkg. purchased dry onion soup mix)

2⅔ Tbsp. dried onion, minced, flaked, or chopped

4 tsp. sodium-free beef instant bouillon powder

1 tsp. onion powder

¼ tsp. celery seed

Combine all ingredients.

Exchange List Values: Carbohydrate 1.5

Basic Nutritional Values: Calories 106 (Calories from Fat 2), Total Fat 0 gm (Saturated Fat 0 gm, Polyunsat Fat 0.1 gm, Monounsat Fat 0.1 gm, Cholesterol 0 mg), Sodium 5 mg, Total Carbohydrate 23 gm, Dietary Fiber 2 gm, Sugars 11 gm, Protein 2 gm

Phyllis's Homemade Barbecue Sauce

Phyllis Barrier • Little Rock, AR

Makes 16 (2 Tbsp.) servings

2 8-oz. cans no-salt-added tomato sauce

¼ cup cider vinegar

brown sugar substitute to equal 2 Tbsp.

½ cup fresh onions, minced

1 tsp. garlic powder

½ tsp. dry mustard powder

6 tsp. chili powder

⅛ tsp. Tabasco sauce

½ tsp. black pepper

6 tsp. Worcestershire sauce

1 tsp. paprika

1 tsp. liquid smoke

¼ tsp. salt

Mix all ingredients together and cook in microwave until minced onion is tender and sauce has thickened.

Exchange List Values: Carbohydrate 0.5

Basic Nutritional Values: Calories 24 (Calories from Fat 2), Total Fat 0 gm (Saturated Fat 0 gm, Polyunsat Fat 0.1 gm, Monounsat Fat 0 gm, Cholesterol 0 mg), Sodium 81 mg, Total Carbohydrate 5 gm, Dietary Fiber 1 gm, Sugars 5 gm, Protein 0 gm

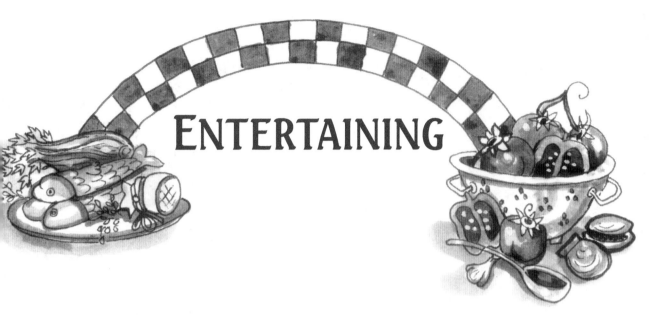

ENTERTAINING

Home-Style Beef Cubes

Dorothy Horst • Tiskilwa, IL

Makes 8–10 servings (Ideal slow cooker size: 6-quart)

1/2 cup flour

1 tsp. salt

1/8 tsp. pepper

4 lbs. top or bottom round beef cubes

1/2 cup chopped shallots or green onions

2 4-oz. cans sliced mushrooms, drained, or
    1/2 lb. fresh mushrooms, sliced

14 1/2-oz. can lower-sodium beef broth

1 tsp. Worcestershire sauce

2 tsp. ketchup

1/4 cup water

3 Tbsp. flour

1. Combine 1/2 cup flour, salt, and pepper. Toss beef in flour mixture to coat. Place in slow cooker.

2. Add shallots or onions and mushrooms.

3. Combine broth, Worcestershire sauce, and ketchup. Pour into slow cooker. Mix well.

4. Cover. Cook on Low 7–12 hours.

5. One hour before serving, make a smooth paste of water and 3 Tbsp. flour. Stir into slow cooker. Cover and cook until broth thickens.

6. Serve over hot noodles.

Exchange List Values: Starch 0.5, Vegetable 0.5, Meat, lean 5.5

Basic Nutritional Values: Calories 298 (Calories from Fat 79); Total Fat 9 gm (Saturated Fat 3 gm, Polyunsat Fat 0.5 gm, Monounsat Fat 4 gm, Cholesterol 118 mg), Sodium 491 mg, Total Carbohydrate 9 gm, Dietary Fiber 0.5 gm, Sugars 1 gm, Protein 43 gm

MENU IDEA

Home-Style Beef Cubes

Hot buttered noodles

Tossed salad with oil and vinegar dressing

    To make dressing, combine:

    1/2 cup red wine vinegar

    1/2 cup olive oil

    1 tsp. salt

    1 tsp. sugar

Melt-in-Your-Mouth Mexican Meat Dish

Marlene Bogard • Newton, KS

Makes 10 servings (Ideal slow cooker size: 6-quart)

4-lb. boneless round roast

½ tsp. salt

1 tsp. pepper

2 Tbsp. oil

1 onion, chopped

1 tsp. chili powder

1 tsp. garlic powder

1¼ cups diced fresh green chili peppers

½ cup chipotle salsa

¼ cup hot pepper sauce

water

1. Season roast with salt and pepper. Sear on all sides in oil in skillet. Place in slow cooker.

2. Mix together remaining ingredients, except water, and spoon over meat. Pour in water down along the side of the cooker (so as not to wash off the topping) until roast is one-third covered.

3. Cover. Cook on High 6 hours. Reduce to Low 2–4 hours, until meat falls apart.

4. Thicken sauce with flour if you like.

5. This highly seasoned meat is perfect for shredded beef Mexican tacos or burritos.

Exchange List Values: Vegetable 0.5, Meat, medium fat 4, Fat 1.5

Basic Nutritional Values: Calories 334 (Calories from Fat 186), Total Fat 21 gm (Saturated Fat 8 gm, Polyunsat Fat 2 gm, Monounsat Fat 8 gm, Cholesterol 92 mg), Sodium 380 mg, Total Carbohydrate 3 gm, Dietary Fiber 1 gm, Sugars 2 gm, Protein 32 gm

Hosting Idea

Get two slow cookers going—one with this beef dish and one with the same recipe, but using chicken as the meat. Host a Mexican fiesta and let guests build their own combinations. Prepare bowls of olives, cheese (either shredded or cubed), chopped tomatoes, shredded lettuce, a variety of beans, and guacamole as go-alongs.

Fruited Beef Tagine

Naomi E. Fast • Hesston, KS

Makes 8 servings (Ideal slow cooker size: 5-quart)

2-lb. boneless top round beef, cut into 2" cubes

1 Tbsp. oil

4 cups sliced onions

2 tsp. ground coriander

1½ tsp. ground cinnamon

¾ tsp. ground ginger

14½-oz. can lower-sodium beef broth, plus enough water to equal 2 cups

16 ozs. pitted prunes

salt to taste

fresh ground pepper to taste

juice of 1 lemon

1. Brown beef cubes in oil in skillet. Place beef in slow cooker. Reserve drippings.

2. Saute onions in drippings until lightly browned, adding more oil if needed. Add to slow cooker.

3. Add remaining ingredients, except lemon juice.

4. Simmer on Low 5–6 hours, adding lemon juice during last 10 minutes.

Exchange List Values: Fruit 2.0, Vegetable 1.0, Meat, lean 4.0, Fat 1.0

Basic Nutritional Values: Calories 367 (Calories from Fat 104), Total Fat 2 gm (Saturated Fat 4 gm, Polyunsat Fat 1 gm, Monounsat Fat 5 gm, Cholesterol 47 mg), Sodium 205 mg, Total Carbohydrate 41 gm, Dietary Fiber 6 gm, Sugars 3 gm, Protein 28 gm

VARIATIONS:

1. Mix in a few very thin slices of lemon peel to add flavor and eye appeal.
2. You can substitute lamb cubes for the beef.

MENU IDEA

Fruited Beef Tagine

Tossed green salad

Whole wheat couscous

Mango sorbet

Saucy Italian Roast

Sharon Miller • Holmesville, OH

Makes 10 servings (Ideal slow cooker size: 5-quart)

3–3½-lb. boneless rump roast

½ tsp. salt

½ tsp. garlic powder

¼ tsp. pepper

4½-oz. jar mushroom pieces, drained

1 medium onion, diced

14-oz. jar spaghetti sauce

¼-½ cup lower-sodium beef broth

1 lb. hot cooked pasta

1. Cut roast in half.

2. Combine salt, garlic powder, and pepper. Rub over both halves of the roast. Place in slow cooker.

3. Top with mushrooms and onions.

4. Combine spaghetti sauce and broth. Pour over roast.

5. Cover. Cook on Low 8–9 hours.

6. Slice roast. Serve in sauce over pasta.

Exchange List Values: Starch 2.0, Meat, lean 3.0

Basic Nutritional Values: Calories 400 (Calories from Fat 89), Total Fat 10 gm (Saturated Fat 3 gm, Polyunsat Fat 1 gm, Monounsat Fat 4 gm, Cholesterol 79 mg), Sodium 402 mg, Total Carbohydrate 39 gm, Dietary Fiber 2 gm, Sugars 2 gm, Protein 36 gm

MENU IDEA

Saucy Italian Roast

Caesar salad with low-fat dressing

Zesty Pears, page 274

Best Ever Beef Stew

Barbara Walker • Sturgis, SD

Makes 6 servings (Ideal slow cooker size: 4-quart)

2 cups water

1 pkg. beef stew mix

2 lbs. boneless bottom round beef, cubed

3 lbs. fresh new potatoes

1 cup sliced celery

10–12 small white onions, peeled

1–1½ cups sliced carrots

8 ozs. fresh mushrooms

1. Combine water and beef stew mix in slow cooker.

2. Layer meat in slow cooker.

3. Add remaining ingredients.

4. Cover. Cook on High 6–7 hours.

Exchange List Values: Starch 2.0, Vegetable 1.0, Meat, lean 3.0

Basic Nutritional Values: Calories 418 (Calories from Fat 89), Total Fat 10 gm (Saturated Fat 3.5 gm, Polyunsat Fat 0.5 gm, Monounsat Fat 4 gm, Cholesterol 92 mg), Sodium 743 mg, Total Carbohydrate 39 gm, Dietary Fiber 5 gm, Sugars 3 gm, Protein 41 gm

MENU IDEA

Best Ever Beef Stew

Spinach salad with low-fat French dressing

Fruit kebabs

Sunday Roast Beef

Beverly Flatt-Getz • Warriors Mark, PA

Makes 8 servings (Ideal slow cooker size: 4–5-quart)

4 potatoes, peeled and quartered

½ cup peeled small onions

1 cup carrot chunks

3-lb. beef chuck roast

1 Tbsp. olive oil

1 pkg. George Washington seasoning

½ tsp. onion salt

½ tsp. minced garlic

½ tsp. garlic salt

1 cup water

few drops Worcestershire sauce

1 Tbsp. cornstarch

½ cup cold water

1. Place potatoes, onions, and carrots in bottom of slow cooker.

2. Sear beef in olive oil in skillet. Add to vegetables in slow cooker.

3. Sprinkle with seasonings.

4. Pour water around roast.

5. Cover. Cook on Low 8–10 hours.

6. Remove meat and vegetables from juice. Season juice with Worcestershire sauce.

7. Dissolve cornstarch in cold water. Add to slow cooker. Cook on High, until thick and bubbly.

Exchange List Values: Starch 1.0, Vegetable 0.5, Meat, lean 5.0, Fat 0.5

Basic Nutritional Values: Calories 327 (Calories from Fat 80), Total Fat 9 gm (Saturated Fat 3 gm, Polyunsat Fat 0.5 gm, Monounsat Fat 4 gm, Cholesterol 75 mg), Sodium 371 mg, Total Carbohydrate 20 gm, Dietary Fiber 2 gm, Sugars 2 gm, Protein 39 gm

MENU IDEA

Sunday Roast Beef

Creamed onions or creamed peas and onions

Dinner rolls with butter

Hot apple pie with vanilla ice cream and cinnamon sauce

Italian Beef Stew

Kathy Hertzler • Lancaster, PA

Makes 6 servings (Ideal slow cooker size: 4-quart)

2 Tbsp. flour

2 tsp. chopped fresh thyme

½ tsp. salt

¼–½ tsp. freshly ground pepper

2 lbs. boneless top round, cubed

3 Tbsp. olive oil

1 onion, chopped

1 cup tomato sauce

1 cup beef stock

1 cup red wine

3 cloves garlic, minced

2 Tbsp. tomato paste

2 cups frozen peas, thawed but not cooked

1 tsp. sugar

1. Spoon flour into small dish. Season with thyme, salt, and pepper. Add beef cubes and coat evenly.

2. Heat oil in slow cooker on High. Add floured beef and brown on all sides.

3. Stir in remaining ingredients except peas and sugar.

4. Cover. Cook on Low 6 hours.

5. Add peas and sugar. Cook an additional 30 minutes, or until beef is tender and peas are warm.

Exchange List Values: Starch 0.5, Vegetable 1.0, Meat, lean 5.0, Fat 1.5

Basic Nutritional Values: Calories 390 (Calories from Fat 126), Total Fat 14 gm (Saturated Fat 4 gm, Polyunsat Fat 1 gm, Monounsat Fat 8 gm, Cholesterol 98 mg), Sodium 554 mg, Total Carbohydrate 17 gm, Dietary Fiber 3 gm, Sugars 7 gm, Protein 39 gm

MENU IDEA

Italian Beef Stew

Mashed potatoes

Iceberg wedge with low-fat Thousand Island dressing

Biscotti

Beef Pot Roast

Nancy Wagner Graves • Manhattan, KS

Makes 8 servings (Ideal slow cooker size: 5-quart)

3–4-lb. beef chuck roast

1 clove garlic, cut in half

salt to taste

pepper to taste

1 carrot, chopped

1 rib celery, chopped

1 small onion, sliced

¾ cup light sour cream

3 Tbsp. flour

½ cup dry white wine

1. Rub roast with garlic. Season with salt and pepper. Place in slow cooker.

2. Add carrots, celery, and onion.

3. Combine sour cream, flour, and wine. Pour into slow cooker.

4. Cover. Cook on Low 6–7 hours.

Exchange List Values: Vegetable 0.5, Meat, lean 5.0, Fat 0.5

Basic Nutritional Values: Calories 288 (Calories from Fat 87), Total Fat 10 gm (Saturated Fat 4 gm, Polyunsat Fat 0.5 gm, Monounsat Fat 4 gm, Cholesterol 83 mg), Sodium 192 mg, Total Carbohydrate 6 gm, Dietary Fiber 0.5 gm, Sugars 1 gm, Protein 39 gm

MENU IDEA

Beef Pot Roast

Herbed Potatoes, page 252

Steamed broccoli

Peach pie

Slow Cooker Beef with Mushrooms

Grace W. Yoder • Harrisonburg, VA

Makes 6 servings (Ideal slow cooker size: 4-quart)

2 medium onions, thinly sliced

½ lb. mushrooms, sliced, or 2 4-oz. cans sliced mushrooms, drained

2¼-lb. beef flank, or round steak

salt to taste

pepper to taste

1 Tbsp. Worcestershire sauce

1 Tbsp. oil

paprika to taste

1. Place sliced onions and mushrooms in slow cooker.

2. Score top of meat about ½" deep in diamond pattern.

3. Season with salt and pepper. Rub in Worcestershire sauce and oil. Sprinkle top with paprika.

4. Place meat on top of onions.

5. Cover. Cook on Low 7–8 hours.

6. To serve, cut beef across grain in thin slices. Top with mushrooms and onions.

Exchange List Values: Vegetable 1.0, Meat, lean 5.0, Fat 1.5

Basic Nutritional Values: Calories 328 (Calories from Fat 148), Total Fat 16 gm (Saturated Fat 0 gm, Polyunsat Fat 1 gm, Monounsat Fat 7 gm, Cholesterol 70 mg), Sodium 145 mg, Total Carbohydrate 5 gm, Dietary Fiber 1 gm, Sugars 2 gm, Protein 37 gm

MENU IDEA

Slow Cooker Beef with Mushrooms

Orange Glazed Carrots, page 230

Dinner rolls

Cantaloupe wedges

Barbecued Chuck Steak

Rhonda Burgoon • Collingswood, NJ

Makes 4 servings (Ideal slow cooker size: 4-quart)

1½-lb. boneless chuck steak, 1½" thick

1 clove garlic, minced

¼ cup wine vinegar

1 Tbsp. brown sugar

1 tsp. paprika

2 Tbsp. Worcestershire sauce

⅓ cup ketchup

¼ tsp. salt

1 tsp. prepared mustard

¼ tsp. black pepper

1. Cut beef on diagonal across the grain into 1"-thick slices. Place in slow cooker.

2. Combine remaining ingredients. Pour over meat. Stir to mix.

3. Cover. Cook on Low 3–5 hours.

Exchange List Values: Starch 0.5, Meat, lean 4.0

Basic Nutritional Values: Calories 239 (Calories from Fat 59), Total Fat 7 gm (Saturated Fat 2 gm, Polyunsat Fat 6.5 gm, Monounsat Fat 3.5 gm, Cholesterol 92 mg), Sodium 634 mg, Total Carbohydrate 1 gm, Dietary Fiber 0 gm, Sugars 9 gm, Protein 33 gm

MENU IDEA

Barbecued Chuck Steak

Brown rice

Steamed green beans

Chocolate Pudding Cake, page 288

Corned Beef and Cabbage with Potatoes and Carrots

Rosaria Strachan • Fairfield, CT

Makes 7 servings (Ideal slow cooker size: 5-quart)

3–4 carrots, sliced

3–4 potatoes, cubed

1 onion, sliced

2½–3½-lb. lean corned beef brisket

10–12 peppercorns

4–6 cabbage wedges

1. Place carrots, potatoes, and onions in bottom of slow cooker.

2. Place beef over vegetables.

3. Cover with water.

4. Add peppercorns.

5. Cover. Cook on Low 8–10 hours, or on High 5–6 hours.

6. Add cabbage. Cook on High 2–3 hours more.

7. Cut up meat and serve on large platter with mustard or horseradish as a condiment. Pass vegetables with meat or in their own serving dish.

Exchange List Values: Starch 0.5, Vegetable 2.0, Meat, lean 5.0, Fat 1.0

Basic Nutritional Values: Calories 341 (Calories from Fat 109), Total Fat 12 gm (Saturated Fat 4 gm, Polyunsat Fat 0.5 gm, Monounsat Fat 6 gm, Cholesterol 100 mg), Sodium 165 mg, Total Carbohydrate 21 gm, Dietary Fiber 4 gm, Sugars 6 gm, Protein 37 gm

MENU IDEA

Crudités with hummus

Corned Beef and Cabbage with Potatoes and Carrots

Seven Layer Bars, page 289

Meat Loaf

Colleen Heatwole • Burton, MI

Makes 8 servings (Ideal slow cooker size: 4-quart)

2 lbs. 95%-lean ground beef

2 eggs

²/₃ cup quick oats

1 pkg. dry onion soup mix

¹/₂–1 tsp. liquid smoke

1 tsp. ground mustard

¹/₂ cup ketchup, divided

1. Combine ground beef, eggs, dry oats, dry soup mix, liquid smoke, ground mustard, and all but 2 Tbsp. ketchup. Shape into loaf and place in slow cooker.

2. Top with remaining ketchup.

3. Cover. Cook on Low 8–10 hours, or on High 4–6 hours.

Exchange List Values: Starch 0.5, Meat, lean 3.5

Basic Nutritional Values: Calories 227 (Calories from Fat 69), Total Fat 8 gm (Saturated Fat 3 gm, Polyunsat Fat 0.5 gm, Monounsat Fat 3 gm, Cholesterol 123 mg), Sodium 568 mg, Total Carbohydrate 11 gm, Dietary Fiber 1 gm, Sugars 4 gm, Protein 27 gm

MENU IDEA

Meat Loaf
Baked potatoes
Zucchini Special, page 232
Ice cream with fresh berries

Comfort Meat Loaf

Trudy Kutter • Corfu, NY

Recipe photo appears in color section.

Makes 6 servings (Ideal slow cooker size: 4-quart)

2 eggs, beaten

¹/₂ cup milk

²/₃ cup bread crumbs

2 Tbsp. grated, or finely chopped, onion

³/₄ tsp. salt

¹/₂ tsp. sage

1¹/₂ lbs. 95%-lean ground beef

2–3 Tbsp. tomato sauce, or ketchup

1. Combine everything but tomato sauce. Shape into 6" round loaf and place in cooker.

2. Cover. Cook on Low 6 hours.

3. Spoon tomato sauce over meat loaf.

4. Cover. Cook on High 30 minutes.

Exchange List Values: Starch 0.5, Meat, lean 3.5, Fat 0.5

Basic Nutritional Values: Calories 245 (Calories from Fat 78), Total Fat 9 gm (Saturated Fat 4 gm, Polyunsat Fat 0.5 gm, Monounsat Fat 3 gm, Cholesterol 143 mg), Sodium 520 mg, Total Carbohydrate 11 gm, Dietary Fiber 1 gm, Sugars 2 gm, Protein 29 gm

MENU IDEA

Comfort Meat Loaf
Baked French fries
Steamed green beans
Chocolate Pudding Cake, page 288

Arlene's BBQ Meatballs

Arlene Groff • Lewistown, PA

Makes 12 servings (Ideal slow cooker size: 5-quart)

2-lbs. 95%-lean ground beef

2 eggs

1 small onion, chopped

¼ cup 1% milk

1½ cups crushed crackers (equal to 1 packaged column of saltines)

1 tsp. prepared mustard

1 tsp. salt

½ tsp. pepper

oil

1½ cups tomato juice

⅓ cup vinegar

1 Tbsp. soy sauce

1 Tbsp. Worcestershire sauce

½ cup brown sugar

brown sugar substitute to equal ¼ cup

2 Tbsp. cornstarch

1 tsp. prepared mustard

1. Combine beef, eggs, onion, milk, crackers, 1 tsp. mustard, salt, and pepper. Form into small balls. Brown in oil in skillet. Place in slow cooker.

2. Combine remaining ingredients. Pour over meatballs.

3. Cover. Cook on High 2 hours. Stir well. Cook an additional 2 hours.

Exchange List Values: Starch 1.0, Vegetable 1.5, Meat, lean 2.0

Basic Nutritional Values: Calories 213 (Calories from Fat 59), Total Fat 7 gm (Saturated Fat 2 gm, Polyunsat Fat 1 gm, Monounsat Fat 3 gm, Cholesterol 82 mg), Sodium 558 mg, Total Carbohydrate 19 gm, Dietary Fiber 1 gm, Sugars 10 gm, Protein 19 gm

MENU IDEA

Arlene's BBQ Meatballs

Whole wheat hoagie rolls

Cole slaw

Fruit kebabs with vanilla yogurt

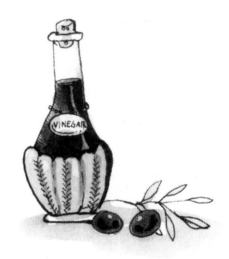

Applesauce Meatballs

Mary E. Wheatley • Mashpee, MA

Makes 6 servings (Ideal slow cooker size: 4-quart)

¾ lb. 95%-lean ground beef

¼ lb. ground pork (16% fat), if available

1 egg

¾ cup soft bread crumbs

½ cup unsweetened applesauce

¾ tsp. salt

¼ tsp. pepper

oil

¼ cup ketchup

¼ cup water

1. Combine beef, pork, egg, bread crumbs, applesauce, salt, and pepper. Form into 1½" balls.

2. Brown in oil in batches in skillet. Transfer meat to slow cooker, reserving drippings.

3. Combine ketchup and water and pour into skillet. Stir up browned drippings and mix well. Spoon over meatballs.

4. Cover. Cook on Low 4–6 hours.

5. Serve with steamed rice and green salad.

Exchange List Values: Meat, lean 2.0, Meat, medium fat 0.5, Fat 0.5

Basic Nutritional Values: Calories 178 (Calories from Fat 76), Total Fat 8 gm (Saturated Fat 3 gm, Polyunsat Fat 0 gm, Monounsat Fat 0 gm, Cholesterol 83 mg), Sodium 503 mg, Total Carbohydrate 8 gm, Dietary Fiber 2 gm, Sugars 4 gm, Protein 17 gm

MENU IDEA

Applesauce Meatballs

Steamed rice

Green salad with low-fat balsamic vinegar

Chocolate Peanut Butter Cake, page 284

Dawn's Spaghetti and Meat Sauce

Dawn Day • Westminster, CA

Makes 6–8 servings (Ideal slow cooker size: 4-quart)

1 lb. 95%-lean ground beef

1 Tbsp. canola oil, if needed

½ lb. mushrooms, sliced

1 medium onion, chopped

3 cloves garlic, minced

½ tsp. dried oregano

½ tsp. salt

¼ cup grated Parmesan, or Romano, cheese

6-oz. can tomato paste

2 15-oz. cans tomato sauce

14.5-oz. can no-salt-added diced tomatoes

1. Brown ground beef in skillet, in oil if needed. Reserve drippings and transfer meat to slow cooker.

2. Saute mushrooms, onion, and garlic in drippings until onions are transparent. Add to slow cooker.

3. Add remaining ingredients to cooker. Mix well.

4. Cover. Cook on Low 6 hours.

Exchange List Values: Vegetable 2.5, Meat, lean 2.0, Fat 0.5

Basic Nutritional Values: Calories 180 (Calories from Fat 55), Total Fat 6 gm (Saturated Fat 2 gm, Polyunsat Fat 1 gm, Monounsat Fat 2 gm, Cholesterol 39 mg), Sodium 831 mg, Total Carbohydrate 5 gm, Dietary Fiber 3 gm, Sugars 10 gm, Protein 17 gm

Note: This recipe freezes well.

MENU IDEA

Dawn's Spaghetti and Meat Sauce
Whole grain spaghetti
Green salad with oil and vinegar

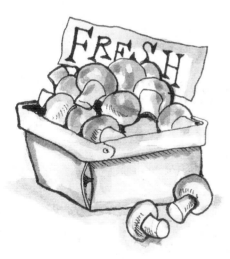

Slow Cooker Lasagna

Crystal Brunk • Singers Glen, VA

Makes 8 servings (Ideal slow cooker size: 6-quart)

1 lb. 95%-lean ground beef, browned

4-5 cups lower-in-sodium spaghetti sauce, depending upon how firm or how juicy you want the finished lasagna

1 egg

24-oz. container 2% cottage cheese

8–10 lasagna noodles, uncooked

2–3 cups shredded mozzarella cheese

1. Combine ground beef and spaghetti sauce.

2. Combine egg and cottage cheese.

3. Layer half of the ground beef mixture, the dry noodles, the cottage cheese mixture, and the mozzarella cheese in the slow cooker. Repeat layers.

4. Cover. Cook on High 4–5 hours, or on Low 6–8 hours.

Exchange List Values: Starch 2.0, Meat, lean 3.0, Meat, medium fat 1.0, Fat 0.5

Basic Nutritional Values: Calories 346 (Calories from Fat 110), Total Fat 12 gm (Saturated Fat 4 gm, Polyunsat Fat 2 gm, Monounsat Fat 4 gm, Cholesterol 73 mg), Sodium 546 mg, Total Carbohydrate 23 gm, Dietary Fiber 2 gm, Sugars 9 gm, Protein 34 gm

MENU IDEA

Slow Cooker Lasagna
Peas
Garlic bread

Pork Roast
with Sauerkraut

Betty K. Drescher • Quakertown, PA

Recipe photo appears in color section.

Makes 10 servings (Ideal slow cooker size: 6-quart)

3-4-lb. lean boneless pork roast, trimmed of fat

32-oz. bag sauerkraut

2 apples, peeled and sliced

1 medium onion, sliced thin

14½-oz. can Italian tomatoes, drained and smashed

1. Place roast in slow cooker.

2. Add sauerkraut.

3. Layer apples and onion over roast.

4. Top with tomatoes.

5. Cover. Cook on Low 7–9 hours, or until meat is tender.

Exchange List Values: Fruit 0.5, Vegetable 1.0, Meat, lean 4.0

Basic Nutritional Values: Calories 227 (Calories from Fat 50), Total Fat 6 gm (Saturated Fat 1.4 gm, Polyunsat Fat 0.9 gm, Monounsat Fat 3.3 gm, Cholesterol 86 mg), Sodium 701 mg, Total Carbohydrate 11 gm, Dietary Fiber 3 gm, Sugars 6.5 gm, Protein 31 gm

VARIATION: If you like a brothy dish, add 1 cup water along with sauerkraut in Step 2.

MENU IDEA

Pork Roast with Sauerkraut

Steamed brown and wild rice blend

Baked Acorn Squash, page 234

Pork Chop Casserole

Nancy Wagner Graves • Manhattan, KS

Makes 4-6 servings (Ideal slow cooker size: 5-quart)

6 (1½ lb.) boneless, center loin pork chops

salt to taste

pepper to taste

oil

2 medium potatoes, peeled and sliced

1 large onion, sliced

1 large green pepper, sliced

½ tsp. dried oregano

16-oz. can crushed tomatoes

1. Season pork chops with salt and pepper. Brown in oil in skillet. Transfer to slow cooker.

2. Add remaining ingredients in order listed.

3. Cover. Cook on Low 8–10 hours, or on High 3–4 hours.

Exchange List Values: Starch 0.5, Vegetable 1.5, Meat, lean 3.0

Basic Nutritional Values: Calories 241 (Calories from Fat 57), Total Fat 6 gm (Saturated Fat 2 gm, Polyunsat Fat 0.8 gm, Monounsat Fat 2.7 gm, Cholesterol 63 mg), Sodium 161 mg, Total Carbohydrate 20 gm, Dietary Fiber 4 gm, Sugars 2.5 gm, Protein 26 gm

MENU IDEA

Pork Chop Casserole

Whole grain noodles

Tossed salad with low-fat honey mustard dressing

Mandarin oranges

Barbecued Pork Chops

LaVerne A. Olson • Lititz, PA

Makes 8 servings (Ideal slow cooker size: 5-quart)

8 (1½ lb.) boneless, center loin pork chops, lightly browned in skillet

½ cup ketchup

½ tsp. salt

1 tsp. celery seed

½ tsp. ground nutmeg

⅓ cup vinegar

½ cup water

1 bay leaf

1. Place pork chops in slow cooker.

2. Combine remaining ingredients. Pour over chops.

3. Cover. Cook on Low 2–3 hours, or until chops are tender.

4. Remove bay leaf before serving.

Exchange List Values: Meat, lean 2.5

Basic Nutritional Values: Calories 139 (Calories from Fat 42), Total Fat 5 gm (Saturated Fat 1.6 gm, Polyunsat Fat 0.5 gm, Monounsat Fat 2 gm, Cholesterol 47 mg), Sodium 357 mg, Total Carbohydrate 6 gm, Dietary Fiber 0 gm, Sugars 5 gm, Protein 17 gm

MENU IDEA

Barbecued Pork Chops

Baked sweet potatoes

Sauteed zucchini and onion

Corn bread

Autumn Pork Chops

Leesa Lesenski • Whately, MA

Makes 6 servings (Ideal slow cooker size: 5-quart)

6 boneless pork chops

2 cups apple juice

½ tsp. ground cinnamon

1. Place pork chops in slow cooker.

2. Cover with apple juice.

3. Sprinkle with cinnamon.

4. Cover. Cook on Low 10 hours.

Exchange List Values: Fruit 0.5, Meat, lean 2.0

Basic Nutritional Values: Calories 141 (Calories from Fat 37), Total Fat 4 gm (Saturated Fat 1.4 gm, Polyunsat Fat 0.5 gm, Monounsat Fat 1.8 gm, Cholesterol 42 mg), Sodium 39 mg, Total Carbohydrate 10 gm, Dietary Fiber 0 gm, Sugars 9 gm, Protein 15 gm

MENU IDEA

Autumn Pork Chops

Rice or potatoes

Applesauce

Italian Sausage

Lauren Eberhard • Seneca, IL

Makes 15 servings (Ideal slow cooker size: 6-quart)

3½ lbs. Italian sausage in casing

4 large green peppers, sliced

3 large onions, sliced

1–2 cloves garlic, minced

28-oz. can no-salt-added tomato puree

14-oz. can no-salt-added tomato sauce

12-oz. can no-salt-added tomato paste

1 Tbsp. dried oregano

1 Tbsp. dried basil

½ tsp. garlic powder

¼ tsp. salt

2 tsp. sugar

1. Cut sausage into 4" or 5" pieces and brown on all sides in batches in skillet.

2. Saute peppers, onions, and garlic in drippings.

3. Combine tomato puree, sauce, and paste in bowl. Add seasonings and sugar.

4. Layer half of sausage, onions, and peppers in 6-qt. slow cooker, or in 2 4-qt. cookers. Cover with half the tomato mixture. Repeat layers.

5. Cover. Cook on High 1 hour, and Low 5–6 hours.

Exchange List Values: Vegetable 3.0, Meat, lean 2.0

Basic Nutritional Values: Calories 192 (Calories from Fat 35), Total Fat 4 gm (Saturated Fat 1.3 gm, Polyunsat Fat 0.1 gm, Monounsat Fat 0 gm, Cholesterol 35 mg), Sodium 787 mg, Total Carbohydrate 24 gm, Dietary Fiber 4 gm, Sugars 12 gm, Protein 19 gm

MENU IDEA

Antipasto salad

Italian Sausage

Whole grain penne

Tiramisu

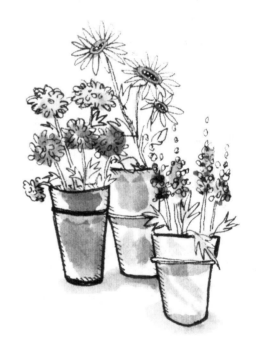

One-Pot Easy Chicken

Jean Robinson • Cinnaminson, NJ

Makes 8 servings (Ideal slow cooker size: 6-quart)

6–8 potatoes, quartered

1–2 large onions, sliced

3–5 carrots, cubed

4-lb. chicken, skin removed (quarters or legs and thighs work well)

1 small onion, chopped

1 tsp. black pepper

1 Tbsp. whole cloves

1 Tbsp. garlic salt

1 Tbsp. chopped fresh oregano

1 tsp. dried rosemary

½ cup lemon juice, or chicken broth

1. Layer potatoes, sliced onions, and carrots in bottom of slow cooker.

2. Rinse and pat chicken dry. In bowl, mix together chopped onions, pepper, cloves, and garlic salt. Dredge chicken in seasonings. Place in cooker over vegetables. Spoon any remaining seasonings over chicken.

3. Sprinkle with oregano and rosemary. Pour lemon juice over chicken.

4. Cover. Cook on Low 6 hours.

Exchange List Values: Starch 1.5, Vegetable 1.0, Meat, lean 3.5

Basic Nutritional Values: Calories 314 (Calories from Fat 47), Total Fat 5 gm (Saturated Fat 1.3 gm, Polyunsat Fat 1.3 gm, Monounsat Fat 1.6 gm, Cholesterol 105 mg), Sodium 468 mg, Total Carbohydrate 37 gm, Dietary Fiber 5 gm, Sugars 4 gm, Protein 30 gm

MENU IDEA
One-Pot Easy Chicken
Celery and carrot sticks
Green beans
Sugar-free Jello salad

This is a lifesaver when the grandchildren come for a weekend. I get to play with them, and dinner is timed and ready when we are.

Delicious Chicken with Curried Cream Sauce

Jennifer J. Gehman • Harrisburg, PA

Makes 4–6 servings (Ideal slow cooker size: 5-quart)

4–6 boneless, skinless chicken breasts, or legs and thighs

oil

salt to taste

pepper to taste

10¾-oz. can reduced-sodium cream of chicken soup

½ cup mayonnaise

1–2 Tbsp. curry powder

½ tsp. salt

⅛ tsp. pepper

1 lb. fresh, or 15-oz. can, asparagus spears

½–1 cup shredded reduced-fat cheddar cheese

1. Brown chicken on all sides in skillet in oil. Season with salt and pepper. Place in slow cooker.

2. Combine soup, mayonnaise, curry powder, salt, and pepper. Pour over chicken.

3. Cover. Cook on High 3 hours, or on Low 5 hours.

4. If using fresh asparagus, steam lightly until just tender. If using canned asparagus, heat. Drain asparagus and place in bottom of serving dish.

5. Cover asparagus with chicken. Sprinkle with cheese.

6. Serve with egg noodles or white rice. Add another cooked vegetable, along with fruit salad, applesauce, or mandarin oranges, as side dishes.

Exchange List Values: Starch 0.5, Vegetable 0.5, Meat, lean 2.0, Meat, medium fat 0.5

Basic Nutritional Values: Calories 179 (Calories from Fat 50), Total Fat 6 gm (Saturated Fat 2.2 gm, Polyunsat Fat 0.6 gm, Monounsat Fat 0.9 gm, Cholesterol 62 mg), Sodium 592 mg, Total Carbohydrate 11 gm, Dietary Fiber 2.5 gm, Sugars 3.4 gm, Protein 22 gm

MENU IDEA

Delicious Chicken with Curried Cream Sauce

Steamed brown rice

Sugar-free vanilla pudding with fresh berries

Garlic Lime Chicken

Loretta Krahn • Mt. Lake, MN

Makes 5 servings (Ideal slow cooker size: 4-quart)

5 skinless chicken breast halves

1/2 cup low-sodium soy sauce

1/4–1/3 cup lime juice, according to your taste preference

1 Tbsp. low- sodium Worcestershire sauce

2 cloves garlic, minced, or 1 tsp. garlic powder

1/2 tsp. dry mustard

1/2 tsp. ground pepper

1. Place chicken in slow cooker.

2. Combine remaining ingredients and pour over chicken.

3. Cover. Cook on High 4–6 hours, or on Low 6–8 hours.

Exchange List Values: Meat, lean 3.0

Basic Nutritional Values: Calories 154 (Calories from Fat 29), Total Fat 3 gm (Saturated Fat 0.7 gm, Polyunsat Fat 0.5 gm, Monounsat Fat 0.9 gm, Cholesterol 76 mg), Sodium 714 mg, Total Carbohydrate 4 gm, Dietary Fiber 0.3 gm, Sugars 1 gm, Protein 26 gm

MENU IDEA

Garlic Lime Chicken

Scalloped Corn, page 243

Carrot and celery sticks with low-fat ranch dressing dip

Orange sugar-free Jello with whipped cream

Herbed Chicken

Laverne A. Olson • Lititz, PA

Makes 8 servings (Ideal slow cooker size: 4-quart)

4 whole skinless chicken breasts, halved

10 3/4-oz. can reduced-sodium cream of mushroom, or chicken, soup

1/4 cup low-sodium soy sauce

1/4 cup olive oil

1/4 cup wine vinegar

3/4 cup water

1/2 tsp. minced garlic

1 tsp. ground ginger

1/2 tsp. dried oregano

1 Tbsp. brown sugar

1. Place chicken in slow cooker.

2. Combine remaining ingredients. Pour over chicken.

3. Cover. Cook on Low 2–2 1/2 hours. Uncover and cook 15 minutes more. Serve with rice.

Exchange List Values: Meat, lean 3.0, Fat 0.5

Basic Nutritional Values: Calories 182 (Calories from Fat 55), Total Fat 6 gm (Saturated Fat 1.3 gm, Polyunsat Fat 1.4 gm, Monounsat Fat 2.4 gm, Cholesterol 76 mg), Sodium 412 mg, Total Carbohydrate 4 gm, Dietary Fiber 0.2 gm, Sugars 2.5 gm, Protein 26 gm

MENU IDEA

Herbed Chicken

Whole wheat couscous

Steamed asparagus

Chocolate pudding

A favorite with the whole family, even grandchildren. The gravy is delicious.

Chicken Stew with Peppers and Pineapples

Judi Manos • West Islip, NY

Makes 4 servings (Ideal slow cooker size: 4-quart)

1 lb. boneless, skinless chicken breasts, cut in 1½" cubes

4 medium carrots, sliced into 1" pieces

½ cup lower-sodium chicken broth

2 Tbsp. gingerroot, chopped

1 Tbsp. brown sugar

2 Tbsp. soy sauce

½ tsp. ground allspice

½ tsp. red pepper sauce

8-oz. can pineapple chunks, drained (reserve juice)

1 Tbsp. cornstarch

1 medium sweet green pepper, cut in 1" pieces

1. Combine chicken, carrots, chicken broth, gingerroot, sugar, soy sauce, allspice, and red pepper sauce in slow cooker.

2. Cover. Cook on Low 7–8 hours, or on High 3–4 hours.

3. Combine pineapple juice and cornstarch until smooth. Stir into chicken mixture. Add pineapple and green pepper.

4. Cover. Cook on High 15 minutes, or until slightly thickened.

Exchange List Values: Fruit 0.5, Vegetable 1.0, Meat, lean 3.0

Basic Nutritional Values: Calories 222 (Calories from Fat 29), Total Fat 3 gm (Saturated Fat 0.7 gm, Polyunsat Fat 0.6 gm, Monounsat Fat 0.9 gm, Cholesterol 73 mg), Sodium 340 mg, Total Carbohydrate 23 gm, Dietary Fiber 3 gm, Sugars 15 gm, Protein 26 gm

VARIATION: Add 1 cut-up fresh tomato 30 minutes before end of cooking time.

> **MENU IDEA**
> Chicken Stew with Peppers and Pineapples
> Whole wheat couscous
> Dump Cake, page 281

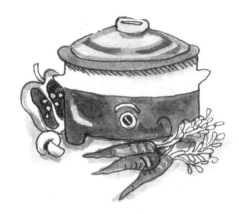

Janie's Chicken a la King

Lafaye M. Musser • Denver, PA

Makes 4 servings (Ideal slow cooker size: 4-quart)

10¾-oz. can reduced-sodium
 cream of chicken soup

3 Tbsp. flour

¼ tsp. salt

¼ tsp. pepper

dash cayenne pepper

1 lb. boneless, skinless chicken breast,
 uncooked and cut in pieces

1 rib celery, chopped

½ cup chopped green pepper

¼ cup chopped onions

9-oz. bag frozen peas, thawed

1. Combine soup, flour, salt, pepper, and
 cayenne pepper in slow cooker.

2. Stir in chicken, celery, green pepper,
 and onion.

3. Cover. Cook on Low 7–8 hours.

4. Stir in peas.

5. Cover. Cook 30 minutes longer.

**Exchange List Values: Starch 1.0,
Vegetable 0.5, Meat, lean 3.0**

Basic Nutritional Values: Calories 254 (Calories
from Fat 39), Total Fat 4 gm (Saturated Fat 1 gm,
Polyunsat Fat 0.9 gm, Monounsat Fat 1.2 gm,
Cholesterol 77 mg), Sodium 633 mg, Total
Carbohydrate 23 gm, Dietary Fiber 4 gm, Sugars
4.6 gm, Protein 30 gm

> MENU IDEA
>
> Almond Tea, page 315
> Janie's Chicken a la King
> Pastry cups or toast
> Quartered oranges
> Fortune cookies

Turkey Loaf and Potatoes

Lizzie Weaver • Ephrata, PA

Makes 7 servings (Ideal slow cooker size: 5-quart)

2 lbs. 93%-lean ground turkey

1½ cups soft bread crumbs, or oatmeal

2 eggs, slightly beaten

1 small onion, chopped

¼ tsp. salt

1 tsp. dry mustard

¼ cup ketchup

¼ cup evaporated milk

4 medium-sized potatoes, quartered

1. Combine all ingredients except potatoes.
 Form into loaf to fit in slow cooker.

2. Tear 4 strips of aluminum foil, each
 18" x 2". Position them in the slow cooker,
 spoke-fashion, with the ends sticking out
 over the edges of the cooker to act as
 handles. Place loaf down in the cooker,
 centered over the foil strips.

3. Place potatoes around meat.

4. Cover. Cook on High 4–5 hours, or until
 potatoes are soft.

**Exchange List Values: Starch 1.0, Meat,
lean 3.5**

Basic Nutritional Values: Calories 328 (Calories
from Fat 96), Total Fat 11 gm (Saturated Fat 3.3 gm,
Polyunsat Fat 0.4 gm, Monounsat Fat 0.7 gm,
Cholesterol 138 mg), Sodium 372 mg, Total
Carbohydrate 28 gm, Dietary Fiber 3 gm, Sugars
5 gm, Protein 31 gm

> MENU IDEA
>
> Turkey Loaf and Potatoes
> Steamed broccoli and cauliflower
> Cole slaw

Slow and Easy Macaroni and Cheese

Janice Muller • Derwood, MD

Makes 14 servings (Ideal slow cooker size: 4-quart)

1 lb. dry macaroni

$\frac{1}{2}$ cup light, soft tub margarine

2 eggs

12-oz. can fat-free evaporated milk

10$\frac{3}{4}$-oz. can cheddar cheese soup

1 cup skim milk

4 cups shredded reduced-fat cheddar cheese, divided

$\frac{1}{8}$ tsp. paprika

1. Cook macaroni until al dente. Drain and pour hot macaroni into slow cooker.

2. Add margarine to macaroni. Stir until melted.

3. Combine eggs, evaporated milk, soup, and milk. Add 3 cups cheese. Pour over macaroni and mix well.

4. Cover. Cook on Low 4 hours. Sprinkle with remaining cheese. Cook 15 minutes, until cheese melts.

5. Sprinkle with paprika before serving.

Exchange List Values: Starch 1.5, Milk, fat-free 0.5, Meat, medium fat 1.0, Fat 1.0

Basic Nutritional Values: Calories 270 (Calories from Fat 91), Total Fat 10 gm (Saturated Fat 4.7 gm, Polyunsat Fat 2 gm, Monounsat Fat 1.4 gm, Cholesterol 50 mg), Sodium 409 mg, Total Carbohydrate 31 gm, Dietary Fiber 1 gm, Sugars 6 gm, Protein 14 gm

VARIATION: Add 12-oz. can drained tuna to Step 3.

MENU IDEA

Slow and Easy Macaroni and Cheese
Chopped vegetable salad
Sugar-free pistachio pudding

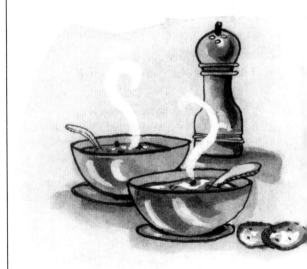

Dawn's Special Beans

Dawn Day • Westminster, CA

Makes 14 servings (Ideal slow cooker size: 4-quart)

16-oz. can kidney beans

16-oz. can small white beans

16-oz. can butter beans

16-oz. can small red beans

1 cup chopped onions

2 tsp. dry mustard

½ tsp. hickory-smoke flavoring

½ cup dark brown sugar

½ cup honey

1 cup low-sodium barbecue sauce

2 Tbsp. apple cider vinegar

1. Combine all ingredients in slow cooker.

2. Cover. Cook on Low 6 hours.

3. Serve with hot dogs, hamburgers, and any other picnic food. These beans are also great for a potluck.

Exchange List Values: Starch 1.0, Carbohydrate 1.0

Basic Nutritional Values: Calories 152 (Calories from Fat 3), Total Fat 0.4 gm (Saturated Fat 0 gm, Polyunsat Fat 0 gm, Monounsat Fat 0 gm, Cholesterol 0 mg), Sodium 329 mg, Total Carbohydrate 34 gm, Dietary Fiber 6 gm, Sugars 14 gm, Protein 7 gm

Note: If you like soupy beans, do not drain the beans before adding them to the cooker. If you prefer a drier outcome, drain all beans before pouring into cooker.

MENU IDEA

Grilled hot dogs

Dawn's Special Beans

Tomato, cucumber, and olives tossed in low-fat Italian dressing

Strawberry sorbet

Tex-Mex Black Bean Soup

Sue Tjon • Austin, TX

Makes 6 servings (Ideal slow cooker size: 4-quart)

1 lb. dry black beans

2 10-oz. cans Rotel tomatoes

1 medium onion, chopped

1 medium green bell pepper, chopped

1 Tbsp. minced garlic

14½-oz. can chicken, or vegetable, broth

water

Cajun seasoning to taste

1. Cover beans with water and soak for 8 hours, or overnight. Drain well. Place beans in slow cooker.

2. Add tomatoes, onions, pepper, garlic, and chicken or vegetable broth. Add water just to cover beans. Add Cajun seasoning.

3. Cover. Cook on High 8 hours. Mash some of the beans before serving for a thicker consistency.

Exchange List Values: Starch 2.5, Vegetable 1.0

Basic Nutritional Values: Calories 218 (Calories from Fat 3), Total Fat 0.3 gm (Saturated Fat 0 gm, Polyunsat Fat 0 gm, Monounsat Fat 0 gm, Cholesterol 0 mg), Sodium 266 mg, Total Carbohydrate 40 gm, Dietary Fiber 6 gm, Sugars 7.5 gm, Protein 12 gm

Note: Leftovers freeze well.

MENU IDEA

Tex-Mex Black Bean Soup

Steamed rice

Romaine lettuce with low-fat creamy Italian dressing

Cherry Delight, page 286

Many-Bean Soup

Trudy Kutter • Corfu, NY

Makes 12 servings (Ideal slow cooker size: 5-quart)

20-oz. pkg. dried 15-bean soup mix, or 2¼ cups dried beans

5 14½-oz. cans lower-sodium chicken or vegetable broth

2 cups chopped carrots

1½ cups chopped celery

1 cup chopped onions

2 Tbsp. tomato paste

1 tsp. Italian seasoning

½ tsp. pepper

14½-oz. can diced tomatoes

1. Combine all ingredients except tomatoes in slow cooker.

2. Cover. Cook on Low 8–10 hours, or until beans are tender.

3. Stir in tomatoes.

4. Cover. Cook on High 10–20 minutes, or until soup is heated through.

Exchange List Values: Starch 1.5, Vegetable 1.0

Basic Nutritional Values: Calories 200 (Calories from Fat 18), Total Fat 2 gm (Saturated Fat 0.3 gm, Polyunsat Fat 0.2 gm, Monounsat Fat 0.2 gm, Cholesterol 0 mg), Sodium 183 mg, Total Carbohydrate 33 gm, Dietary Fiber 4 gm, Sugars 4 gm, Protein 13 gm

MENU IDEA

Many-Bean Soup

12-grain bread

Tossed salad with low-fat ranch dressing

Baked apples

Slow Cooker Bean Soup

Betty B. Dennison • Grove City, PA

Makes 12 servings (Ideal slow cooker size: 6-quart)

3 15-oz. cans pinto beans, undrained

3 15-oz. cans Great Northern beans, undrained

4 cups lower-sodium chicken or vegetable broth

3 potatoes, peeled and chopped

4 carrots, sliced

2 ribs celery, sliced

1 large onion, chopped

1 green pepper, chopped

1 sweet red pepper, chopped, optional

2 cloves garlic, minced

½ tsp. salt, or to taste

¼ tsp. pepper, or to taste

1 bay leaf, optional

½ tsp. liquid barbecue smoke, optional

1. Empty beans into 6-qt. slow cooker, or divide ingredients between 2 4- or 5-qt. cookers.

2. Cover. Cook on Low while preparing vegetables.

3. Cook broth and vegetables in stockpot until vegetables are tender-crisp. Transfer to slow cooker.

4. Add remaining ingredients and mix well.

5. Cover. Cook on Low 4–5 hours.

6. Serve with tossed salad and Italian bread or corn bread.

Exchange List Values: Starch 2.5, Vegetable 1.0

Basic Nutritional Values: Calories 243 (Calories from Fat 13), Total Fat 1.5 gm (Saturated Fat 0 gm, Polyunsat Fat 1 gm, Monounsat Fat 0 gm, Cholesterol 0 mg), Sodium 463 mg, Total Carbohydrate 45 gm, Dietary Fiber 13 gm, Sugars 5 gm, Protein 15 gm

Notes:

1. You can add the broth and vegetables to the cooker without cooking them in advance. Simply extend the slow cooker cooking time to 8 hours on Low.

2. This is a stress-free recipe when you're expecting guests but you're not sure of their arrival time. Slow Cooker Bean Soup can burble on Low heat for longer than its appointed cooking time without being damaged.

3. Make a tossed salad and have the dressing ready to go. Add dressing to salad as your guests make their way to the table.

MENU IDEA

Tossed salad
Slow Cooker Bean Soup
Corn bread
Low-fat cheesecake

Garbanzo Souper

Willard E. Roth • Elkhart, IN

Makes 8 servings (Ideal slow cooker size: 6-quart)

1 lb. dry garbanzo beans

4 ozs. raw baby carrots, cut in halves

1 large onion, diced

3 ribs celery, cut in 1" pieces

1 large green pepper, diced

½ tsp. dried basil

½ tsp. dried oregano

½ tsp. dried rosemary

½ tsp. dried thyme

2 28-oz. cans lower-sodium vegetable broth

1 broth can of water

8-oz. can no-salt-added tomato sauce

8 ozs. prepared hummus

½ tsp. sea salt

1. Soak beans overnight. Drain. Place in bottom of slow cooker.

2. Add carrots, onion, celery, and green pepper.

3. Sprinkle with basil, oregano, rosemary, and thyme.

4. Cover with broth and water.

5. Cover. Cook on High 6 hours.

6. Half an hour before serving, stir in tomato sauce, hummus, and salt. Cook until hot.

Exchange List Values: Starch 2.5, Vegetable 1.0, Fat 0.5

Basic Nutritional Values: Calories 292 (Calories from Fat 54), Total Fat 6 gm (Saturated Fat 0.5 gm, Polyunsat Fat 1 gm, Monounsat Fat 1 gm, Cholesterol 0 mg), Sodium 362 mg, Total Carbohydrate 47 gm, Dietary Fiber 14 gm, Sugars 12 gm, Protein 15 gm

A fine meal for vegetarians on St. Patrick's Day!

MENU IDEA

Garbanzo Souper
Irish soda bread
Lemon curd

Hearty Bean and Vegetable Soup

Jewel Showalter • Landisville, PA

Makes 10 servings (Ideal slow cooker size: 6-quart)

2 medium onions, sliced

2 cloves garlic, minced

2 Tbsp. olive oil

8 cups lower-sodium chicken, or vegetable, broth

1 small head cabbage, chopped

2 large red potatoes, chopped

2 cups chopped celery

2 cups chopped carrots

4 cups corn

2 tsp. dried basil

1 tsp. dried marjoram

$\frac{1}{4}$ tsp. dried oregano

$\frac{1}{2}$ tsp. salt

$\frac{1}{2}$ tsp. pepper

2 15-oz. cans navy beans, rinsed and drained

1. **Saute onions and garlic in oil. Transfer to large slow cooker.**

2. **Add remaining ingredients, mixing together well.**

3. **Cover. Cook on Low 6–8 hours.**

Exchange List Values: Starch 2.0, Vegetable 1.5, Fat 0.5

Basic Nutritional Values: Calories 242 (Calories from Fat 45), Total Fat 5 gm (Saturated Fat 0.5 gm, Polyunsat Fat 1 gm, Monounsat Fat 3 gm, Cholesterol 0 mg), Sodium 481 mg, Total Carbohydrate 42 gm, Dietary Fiber 8 gm, Sugars 8 gm, Protein 12 gm

VARIATION: Add 2–3 cups cooked and cut-up chicken 30 minutes before serving, if you wish.

MENU IDEA
Hearty Bean and Vegetable Soup
Homemade bread
Cheese cubes and crackers
Fruit
Cookies

I discovered this recipe after my husband's heart attack. It's a great, nutritious soup using only a little fat.

Polish Sausage Bean Soup

Janie Steele • Moore, OK

Makes 10 servings (Ideal slow cooker size: 6-quart)

1-lb. pkg. dried Great Northern beans

28-oz. can whole tomatoes

2 8-oz. cans no-salt-added tomato sauce

2 large onions, chopped

3 cloves garlic, minced

¼–½ tsp. pepper, according to your taste preference

3 ribs celery, sliced

1 bell pepper, sliced

1 large ham bone, or ham hock

1–2 lbs. lean smoked sausage links, sliced

1. Cover beans with water and soak for 8 hours. Rinse and drain.

2. Place beans in 6-qt. cooker and cover with water.

3. Combine all other ingredients, except sausage, in large bowl. Stir into beans in slow cooker.

4. Cover. Cook on High 1–1½ hours. Reduce to Low. Cook 7 hours.

5. Remove ham bone or hock and debone. Stir ham pieces back into soup.

6. Add sausage links.

7. Cover. Cook on Low 1 hour.

Exchange List Values: Starch 2.0, Vegetable 2.0, Meat, lean 0.5

Basic Nutritional Values: Calories 271 (Calories from Fat 27), Total Fat 3 gm (Saturated Fat 1 gm, Polyunsat Fat 0.5 gm, Monounsat Fat 1 gm, Cholesterol 16 mg), Sodium 564 mg, Total Carbohydrate 45 gm, Dietary Fiber 12 gm, Sugars 7 gm, Protein 17 gm

Note: For enhanced flavor, brown sausage before adding to soup.

MENU IDEA

Polish Sausage Bean Soup
Cucumber and sour cream salad
Deluxe Tapioca Pudding, page 267

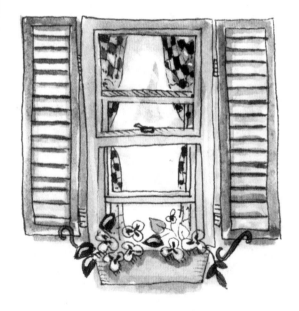

Party Bean Soup

Jo Haberkamp • Fairbank, IA

Makes 9 servings (Ideal slow cooker size: 5-quart)

1 cup dry navy beans

1 qt. water

1 lb. lower-sodium, lean smoked or plain
   ham hocks

1 cup chopped onions

½ cup chopped celery

1 clove garlic, minced

8-oz. can tomatoes, cut up

2 14½-oz. cans lower-sodium chicken broth

⅛ tsp. salt

⅛ tsp. pepper

1 cup (4 ozs.) shredded reduced-fat cheddar
   cheese

1 Tbsp. dried parsley flakes

1. Place beans and water in slow cooker.

2. Cover. Cook on Low for 12 hours.

3. Add ham hocks, onions, celery, garlic,
   tomatoes, chicken broth, salt, and pepper.

4. Cover. Cook on Low 8–10 hours.

5. Add cheese and parsley. Stir until cheese
   is melted.

**Exchange List Values: Starch 1.0,
Vegetable 0.5, Meat, medium fat 0.5**

Basic Nutritional Values: Calories 215 (Calories
from Fat 58), Total Fat 6 gm (Saturated Fat 3 gm,
Polyunsat Fat 0.7 gm, Monounsat Fat 1.6 gm,
Cholesterol 36 mg), Sodium 677 gm, Total
Carbohydrate 19 gm, Dietary Fiber 6 gm, Sugars
3 gm, Protein 21 gm

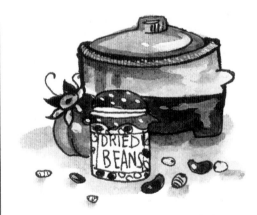

Hosting Idea

Buy 10–18 different kinds of dried beans. Mix them
together in a large bag or jar. Scoop them into small
bags (8 ozs. is a good size). Top each with a dried
bay leaf to discourage bugs, tie them shut, and
present them to the friends who have just eaten
from your buffet table.

A bag full of these dried beans is also a welcome
and interesting addition to a gift basket.

—Alix Nancy Botsford

Green Bean and Potato Soup

Bernita Boyts • Shawnee Mission, KS

Makes 6 servings (Ideal slow cooker size: 6-quart)

1 medium onion, chopped

2 carrots, sliced

2 ribs celery, sliced

1 Tbsp. olive oil

5 medium potatoes, cubed

10-oz. pkg. frozen green beans

2 14½-oz. cans chicken broth

2 broth cans water

⅓ lb. link sausage, sliced, or bulk sausage, browned

2 Tbsp. chopped fresh parsley (or 2 tsp. dried)

1-2 Tbsp. chopped fresh oregano (or ½ Tbsp. dried)

1 tsp. Italian spice

salt to taste

pepper to taste

1. Saute onion, carrots, and celery in oil in skillet until tender.

2. Combine all ingredients in slow cooker.

3. Cover. Cook on High 1–2 hours, and then on Low 6–8 hours.

4. Serve with freshly baked bread or corn bread.

Exchange List Values: Starch 2.0, Vegetable 1.5, Meat, lean 0.5, Fat 0.5

Basic Nutritional Values: Calories 242 (Calories from Fat 37), Total Fat 4 gm (Saturated Fat 1 gm, Polyunsat Fat 0.5 gm, Monounsat Fat 2 gm, Cholesterol 8 mg), Sodium 640 mg, Total Carbohydrate 40 gm, Dietary Fiber 6 gm, Sugars 6 gm, Protein 11 gm

VARIATION: If you like it hot, add ground red pepper or hot sauce just before serving.

MENU IDEA

Red Pepper Cheese Dip, page 291

Green Bean and Potato Soup

Lemon Bread, page 327

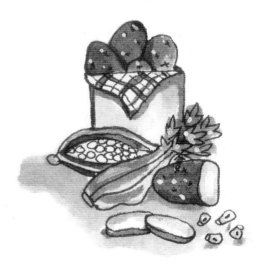

Grandma's Barley Soup

Andrea O'neil • Fairfield, CT

Makes 12 servings (Ideal slow cooker size: 5-quart)

2 lean smoked ham hocks

4 carrots, sliced

4 potatoes, cubed

1 cup dried lima beans

1 cup no-salt-added tomato paste

1½–2 cups cooked barley

salt, if needed

1. Combine all ingredients in slow cooker, except salt.

2. Cover with water.

3. Cover. Simmer on Low 6–8 hours.

4. Debone ham hocks and return cut-up meat to soup.

5. Taste before serving. Add salt, if needed.

Exchange List Values: Starch 2.0, Vegetable 1.0

Basic Nutritional Values: Calories 221 (Calories from Fat 23), Total Fat 2.5 gm (Saturated Fat 0.8 gm, Polyunsat Fat 0.5 gm, Monounsat Fat 1 gm, Cholesterol 18 mg), Sodium 374 gm, Total Carbohydrate 37 gm, Dietary Fiber 8 gm, Sugars 5.6 gm, Protein 14 gm

Note: If you want to reduce the amount of meat you eat, this dish is flavorful using only 1 ham hock.

MENU IDEA

Grandma's Barley Soup

Corn bread

Cole slaw

Raisin Nut-Stuffed Apples, page 268

Broccoli, Potato, and Cheese Soup

Ruth Shank • Gridley, IL

Makes 6 servings (Ideal slow cooker size: 5-quart)

2 cups cubed, or diced, potatoes

3 Tbsp. chopped onion

10-oz. pkg. frozen broccoli cuts, thawed

2 Tbsp. light, soft tub margarine, melted

1 Tbsp. flour

2 cups cubed Velveeta Light cheese

½ tsp. salt

5½ cups skim milk

1. Cook potatoes and onion in boiling water in saucepan until potatoes are crisp-tender. Drain. Place in slow cooker.

2. Add remaining ingredients. Stir together.

3. Cover. Cook on Low 4 hours.

Exchange List Values: Starch 0.5, Vegetable 0.5, Milk, reduced fat 1.0, Meat, lean 1.0, Fat 1.0

Basic Nutritional Values: Calories 260 (Calories from Fat 87), Total Fat 10 gm (Saturated Fat 5 gm, Polyunsat Fat 1 gm, Monounsat Fat 2 gm, Cholesterol 32 mg), Sodium 674 mg, Total Carbohydrate 26 gm, Dietary Fiber 2 gm, Sugars 15 gm, Protein 16 gm

MENU IDEA

Broccoli, Potato, and Cheese Soup

Apple salad

Whole grain rolls

Crockery Cocoa, page 317

Au Gratin Green Beans

Donna Lantgen • Rapid City, SD

Makes 8 servings (Ideal slow cooker size: 4-quart)

2 16-oz. cans green beans, drained

¼ cup diced onions

½ cup cubed Velveeta cheese

¼ cup evaporated milk

1 tsp. flour

½ tsp. salt

dash pepper

1. Combine all ingredients in slow cooker.

2. Cover. Cook on Low 4 hours.

3. Garnish with sliced almonds at serving time, if you wish.

Exchange List Values: Vegetable 0.5

Basic Nutritional Values: Calories 54 (Calories from Fat 21), Total Fat 2 gm (Saturated Fat 1.5 gm, Polyunsat Fat 0 gm, Monounsat Fat 0 gm, Cholesterol 8 mg), Sodium 422 mg, Total Carbohydrate 5 gm, Dietary Fiber 2 gm, Sugars 2 gm, Protein 3 gm

MENU IDEA

Perfect Pork Chops, page 64

Au Gratin Green Beans

Baked sweet potatoes

Lemon sorbet

Green Bean Casserole

Darla Sathre • Baxter, MN

Makes 10 servings (Ideal slow cooker size: 4-quart)

2 16-oz. bags frozen French-style green beans, drained

2 10¾-oz. cans reduced-sodium cream of mushroom soup

6-oz. can French-fried onion rings

2 cups shredded reduced-fat cheddar cheese

2 tsp. dried basil

5-oz. can evaporated skim milk

1. In greased slow cooker, layer half of each ingredient, except milk, in order given. Repeat. Pour milk over all.

2. Cover. Cook on Low 6–10 hours.

Exchange List Values: Starch 1.0, Fat 2.0

Basic Nutritional Values: Calories 263 (Calories from Fat 146), Total Fat 16 gm (Saturated Fat 5 gm, Polyunsat Fat 0 gm, Monounsat Fat 0 gm, Cholesterol 14 mg), Sodium 640 mg, Total Carbohydrate 19 gm, Dietary Fiber 3 gm, Sugars 5 gm, Protein 10 gm

MENU IDEA

Roast turkey with stuffing

Green Bean Casserole

Sweet Potatoes and Apples, page 258

Pumpkin pie

Scalloped Corn and Celery

Darla Sathre • Baxter, MN

Makes 8 servings (Ideal slow cooker size: 4-quart)

2 16-oz. cans whole-kernel corn, drained

2 16-oz. cans no-salt-added cream-style corn

2 cups chopped celery

40 saltine crackers, crushed

$\frac{1}{8}$–$\frac{1}{4}$ tsp. pepper

2 Tbsp. soft tub margarine or trans fat-free spread

12-oz. can evaporated skim milk

1. Layer in greased slow cooker, half of whole-kernel corn, cream-style corn, celery, crackers, pepper, and butter. Repeat. Pour milk over all.

2. Cover. Cook on Low 8–12 hours.

Exchange List Values: Starch 2.0, Fat 0.5

Basic Nutritional Values: Calories 212 (Calories from Fat 41), Total Fat 5 gm (Saturated Fat 2 gm, Polyunsat Fat 1 gm, Monounsat Fat 1 gm, Cholesterol 6 mg), Sodium 373 mg, Total Carbohydrate 35 gm, Dietary Fiber 3 gm, Sugars 11 gm, Protein 6 gm

MENU IDEA

Garlic Lime Chicken, page 351

Scalloped Corn and Celery

Carrot and celery sticks with ranch dressing dip

Sugar-free orange jello with whipped cream

Broccoli Casserole

Dorothy Van Deest • Memphis, TN

Makes 6 servings (Ideal slow cooker size: 4-quart)

10-oz. pkg. frozen chopped broccoli

6 eggs, beaten

24-oz. carton small-curd 1% cottage cheese

6 Tbsp. flour

6 ozs. mild cheese of your choice, diced

3 Tbsp. soft tub margarine, melted

2 green onions, chopped

1. Place frozen broccoli in colander. Run cold water over it until it thaws. Separate into pieces. Drain well.

2. Combine remaining ingredients in large bowl and mix until well blended. Stir in broccoli. Pour into greased slow cooker.

3. Cover. Cook on High 1 hour. Stir well, then resume cooking on Low 2–4 hours.

Exchange List Values: Starch 0.5, Vegetable 0.5, Meat, lean 1.5, Meat, medium fat 0.5, Fat 2.0

Basic Nutritional Values: Calories 333 (Calories from Fat 164), Total Fat 18 gm (Saturated Fat 8 gm, Polyunsat Fat 2 gm, Monounsat Fat 3 gm, Cholesterol 180 mg), Sodium 691 mg, Total Carbohydrate 16 gm, Dietary Fiber 2 gm, Sugars 6 gm, Protein 23 gm

MENU IDEA

Hot Crab Dip, page 297

Baked ham

Broccoli Casserole

Carrot salad

Flourless chocolate cake

Refrigerator Mashed Potatoes

Deborah Swartz • Grottoes, VA

Makes 10 servings (Ideal slow cooker size: 6-quart)

5 lbs. potatoes

8-oz. pkg. cream cheese, softened

1 cup light sour cream

1 tsp. salt

¼ tsp. pepper

¼ cup crisp bacon, crumbled

2 Tbsp. butter

1. Cook and mash potatoes.

2. Add remaining ingredients except butter. Put in slow cooker. Dot with butter.

3. Cover. Cook on Low 2 hours.

Exchange List Values: Starch 1.5, Meat, high fat 0.5, Fat 1.0

Basic Nutritional Values: Calories 226 (Calories from Fat 86), Total Fat 10 gm (Saturated Fat 4.5 gm, Polyunsat Fat 1 gm, Monounsat Fat 2.5 gm, Cholesterol 23 mg), Sodium 454 mg, Total Carbohydrate 26 gm, Dietary Fiber 3 gm, Sugars 3 gm, Protein 8 gm

VARIATIONS:

1. These potatoes can be made several days ahead and refrigerated. Cook refrigerated potatoes on Low 5 hours.

2. If you wish, sprinkle 1 cup cheddar cheese over top of potatoes during their last half hour in the slow cooker.

3. Substitute chopped ham for the bacon.

4. Add 2 Tbsp. chopped fresh chives to Step 2.

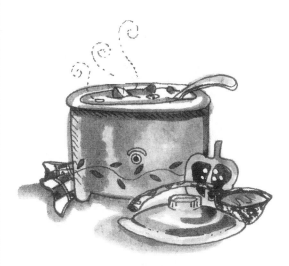

Hosting Idea

My mom always prepared mashed potatoes for any get-togethers at my grandmother's house. She made them ahead of time, put them in her slow cooker, and transported them, turning on the cooker when we arrived. The potatoes were always hot, steamy, and wonderful whenever we got around to eating.

—Lucille Amos

Sunday Dinner Potatoes

Ruth Ann Penner • Hillsboro, KS

Makes 8 servings (Ideal slow cooker size: 4-quart)

4 cups cooked, sliced potatoes

1/3 cup soft tub margarine

1/4 cup flour

2 cups 2% milk

1 tsp. salt

pepper to taste

1 tsp. onion powder

1. Place potatoes in slow cooker.

2. Melt margarine in small skillet. Add flour and stir. Slowly add milk, stirring constantly.

3. Add salt, pepper, and onion powder. When smooth and thickened, pour over potatoes.

4. Cover. Cook on High 2–3 hours, or Low 4–5 hours.

Exchange List Values: Starch 1.0, Fat 1.0

Basic Nutritional Values: Calories 167 (Calories from Fat 66), Total Fat 7 gm (Saturated Fat 2 gm, Polyunsat Fat 2 gm, Monounsat Fat 3 gm, Cholesterol 5 mg), Sodium 383 mg, Total Carbohydrate 22 gm, Dietary Fiber 2 gm, Sugars 4 gm, Protein 4 gm

MENU IDEA

Horseradish Beef, page 33

Sunday Dinner Potatoes

Steamed green beans

Macaroons

Company Potatoes

Deborah Swartz • Grottoes, VA /
Julia A. Fisher • New Carlisle, OH

Makes 6–8 servings (Ideal slow cooker size: 4-quart)

6 medium-sized potatoes, cooked, cooled, and shredded

2 cups shredded reduced-fat cheddar cheese

1/3 cup finely chopped onions

1/4 cup soft tub margarine, melted

1 tsp. salt

1/4 tsp. pepper

1 1/2–2 cups light sour cream

butter

1. Combine potatoes, cheese, onions, margarine, salt, pepper, and sour cream in slow cooker. Dot with butter.

2. Cover. Cook on Low 4 hours.

Exchange List Values: Starch 1.0, Meat, medium fat 1.0, Fat 1.5

Basic Nutritional Values: Calories 236 (Calories from Fat 103), Total Fat 11 gm (Saturated Fat 5.5 gm, Polyunsat Fat 1 gm, Monounsat Fat 2 gm, Cholesterol 25 mg), Sodium 472 mg, Total Carbohydrate 24 gm, Dietary Fiber 2 gm, Sugars 4 gm, Protein 0 gm

VARIATIONS:

1. Use garlic salt instead of regular salt.

2. Add 1/2 tsp. chopped parsley to Step 1.

3. Use 1 cup milk and 1 cup sour cream instead of 2 cups sour cream.

Kim Stoltzfus • New Holland, PA

MENU IDEA

Pork roast

Company Potatoes

Sauteed red onion and spinach

Slow Cooker Tapioca, page 267

Cheese Scalloped Potatoes

Mary Jane Musser • Manheim, PA /
Miriam Nolt • New Holland, PA

Makes 10 servings (Ideal slow cooker size: 4-quart)

6–8 good-sized potatoes

3 Tbsp. soft tub margarine

2 Tbsp. flour

3 cups 2% milk

2 Tbsp. chopped onion

1 tsp. salt

1/8 tsp. pepper

1 tsp. parsley

1 1/2 cups diced reduced-fat mild cheese

1. Cook potatoes in saucepan until tender. Peel and refrigerate. When thoroughly cooled, shred.

2. Melt margarine in saucepan. Stir in flour. Gradually add milk, stirring constantly, until smooth and thickened.

3. Stir in onions, seasonings, and cheese, a half cup at a time. Continue stirring over heat until cheese melts.

4. Combine potatoes and sauce in slow cooker.

5. Cover. Cook on Low 4 hours.

Exchange List Values: Starch 1.0, Fat 1.0

Basic Nutritional Values: Calories 182 (Calories from Fat 68), Total Fat 8 gm (Saturated Fat 3 gm, Polyunsat Fat 1 gm, Monounsat Fat 2.5 gm, Cholesterol 6 mg), Sodium 400 mg, Total Carbohydrate 21 gm, Dietary Fiber 1 gm, Sugars 4 gm, Protein 9 gm

Note: Cook and shred the potatoes the day before serving them. That will relieve the pressure on the day you're having guests.

MENU IDEA

Barbecued chicken
Cheese Scalloped Potatoes
Broccoli salad
Sugar-free jello squares

Hash Brown Potato Casserole

Michelle Strite • Goshen, IN

Makes 10 servings (Ideal slow cooker size: 4-quart)

26-oz. pkg. frozen shredded hash browns

3 Tbsp. canola oil

2 cups chopped ham, optional

2 10 3/4-oz. cans cream of potato soup

1/2 cup grated Parmesan cheese

8-oz. container light sour cream

1 cup fat-free half-and-half

4 ozs. shredded cheddar cheese

1. Brown hash browns in oil in skillet. Transfer to slow cooker.

2. Add remaining ingredients and stir well.

3. Cover. Cook on Low 3 hours.

Exchange List Values: Starch 1.0, Fat 1.0

Basic Nutritional Values: Calories 210 (Calories from Fat 86), Total Fat 10 gm (Saturated Fat 4 gm, Polyunsat Fat 1 gm, Monounsat Fat 3 gm, Cholesterol 15 mg), Sodium 591 mg, Total Carbohydrate 23 gm, Dietary Fiber 1 gm, Sugars 3 gm, Protein 9 gm

MENU IDEA

Ham Balls, page 80
Hash Brown Potato Casserole
Apple Crisp, page 271, or Cranberry Baked Apples, page 269, or Fruit and Nut Baked Apples, pages 270

Mushroom Stuffing

Laverne Stoner • Scottdale, PA

Makes 8 cups stuffing (Ideal slow cooker size: 6-quart)

1 cup finely chopped onions

1 cup finely chopped celery

1/3 cup soft tub margarine

8-oz. can sliced mushrooms, drained

1/4 cup chopped parsley

1 1/2–2 tsp. poultry seasoning

1/4 tsp. salt

1/8 tsp. pepper

12 cups toasted bread cubes*

2 eggs, well beaten

1 1/2 cups reduced-sodium chicken broth

1. Saute onion and celery in margarine in skillet until cooked. Stir in mushrooms and parsley.

2. Combine seasonings and sprinkle over bread cubes.

3. Gently add remaining ingredients. Spoon lightly into slow cooker.

4. Cover. Cook on High 1 hour, then reduce to Low and cook 1–2 hours.

*Toast 18–22 slices of bread for 15 minutes at 300°.

Exchange List Values: Starch 2.0, Vegetable 0.5, Fat 1.0

Basic Nutritional Values: Calories 289 (Calories from Fat 102), Total Fat 11 gm (Saturated Fat 4 gm, Polyunsat Fat 3.5 gm, Monounsat Fat 5 gm, Cholesterol 54 mg), Sodium 635 mg, Total Carbohydrate 38 gm, Dietary Fiber 2 gm, Sugars 4 gm, Protein 9 gm

Note: This is not as much a time-saver as it is a space-saver. If your oven is full, make your stuffing in your slow cooker.

MENU IDEA
Roast chicken
Mushroom Stuffing
Green beans almondine
Apple pie

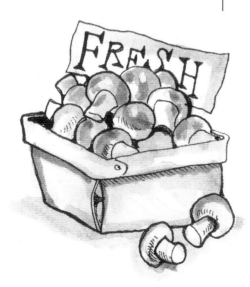

Herbed Stuffing

Allison Ingels • Maynard, IA

Makes 10–12 servings (Ideal slow cooker size: 6-quart)

12–13 cups dry bread cubes (equal to a 20-oz. loaf of bread)

¼ cup dried parsley

2 eggs, beaten

giblets, cooked and chopped (reserve broth)

1 tsp. salt

¼ tsp. pepper

½ tsp. sage

1½ tsp. poultry seasoning

2 low-sodium chicken bouillon cubes

3½ cups turkey broth (from cooking giblets)

2 cups finely chopped celery

1 cup finely chopped onion

½ cup soft tub margarine

1. Combine bread cubes and parsley in slow cooker.

2. Add eggs, giblets, and seasonings.

3. Dissolve bouillon in turkey broth. Add to cooker.

4. Saute celery and onion in margarine in skillet. Stir into bread mixture.

5. Cover. Cook on High 1 hour, and then on Low 2 hours, stirring occasionally.

Exchange List Values: Starch 2.0, Vegetable 0.5, Meat, lean 2.0, Fat 1.5

Basic Nutritional Values: Calories 317 (Calories from Fat 118), Total Fat 13 gm (Saturated Fat 2.5 gm, Polyunsat Fat 4 gm, Monounsat Fat 6 gm, Cholesterol 222 mg), Sodium 630 mg, Total Carbohydrate 30 gm, Dietary Fiber 2 gm, Sugars 3 gm, Protein 19 gm

Note: A convenient way to free up oven space—or keep your kitchen cool.

MENU IDEA

Easy and Delicious Turkey Breast, page 110
Herbed Stuffing
Mashed sweet potatoes
Caramelized pearl onions
Apple-cranberry pie

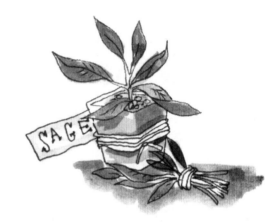

A Week of Menus

If you're trying to stick to a daily meal plan with a specific number of calories, here is help. Each day in this Week of Menus is designed with 3 meals and 2 snacks, for a total of about 1,500 calories.

One or two recipes each day come from this *Fix-It and Forget-It Diabetic Cookbook,* making it easy to eat healthfully, despite busy lives and chaotic schedules.

You'll quickly see the Exchange Value for each part of the meal, as well as the nutritional breakdown of each food. In addition, the total number of nutrients for each day's menu is given, and then compared to healthy, nutritional goals. You'll soon see how easy it is to eat well.

Sunday

Food Item	Amount to Serve	Exchanges	Cal	Carb (gm)	Prot (gm)	Fat (gm)	Sod (mg)
BREAKFAST							
Breakfast Skillet (p 321), lower fat, sat fat	1 serving	1½ Starch; ½ Milk, fat-free; 2 Meat, lean	251	29	20	7	941
Fresh fruit mix	¾ cup	1 Fruit	61	15	1	0	4
			312	**44**	**21**	**8**	**945**
LUNCH							
Pita bread, whole wheat	1 pita	2 Starch	140	30	5	1	130
Ham, boneless, extra-lean, lower-sodium, roasted	1 oz.	1 Meat, very lean	30	1	5	1	230
Cheese, Monterey Jack, reduced fat	1 oz.	1 Meat, med fat	81	0	9	5	222
Tomato, cucumber, onion mix, raw	1 cup	1 Vegetable	30	7	1	0	9
Orange, fresh	1 orange	1 Fruit	62	15	1	0	0
			342	**53**	**22**	**7**	**592**
AFTERNOON SNACK							
Yogurt, non-fat, vanilla	1 container (6 ozs.)	1 Milk, fat-free	90	16	6	0	95
			90	**16**	**6**	**0**	**95**
DINNER							
Savory Slow Cooker Chicken (p 84—lower sodium)	1 serving	2 Vegetable; 3 Meat, lean	230	11	30	7	427
Potato, mashed	½ cup	1 Starch	85	19	2	0	12
Roll, multi-grain	1 roll, medium	1½ Starch	125	23	3	2	244
Margarine, light, soft tub	1 Tbsp.	1 Fat	40	0	0	4	90
Watermelon, fresh	1¼ cups	1 Fruit	61	14	1	1	4
			541	**67**	**36**	**15**	**777**
EVENING SNACK							
Milk, fat-free (non-fat, skim)	1 cup	1 Milk, fat-free	83	12	8	0	108
Wheaties	¾ cup	1 Starch	80	18	2	1	163
			163	**30**	**11**	**1**	**271**

Sunday—Totals for the Day

Nutrient	Quantity	DRI Comparison (- = Under)	% of Day's Calories	Goals
Calories	1,449			1,450 to 1,550
Fat	31 gm		19%	0 to 30%
Saturated fat	11 gm		7%	0 to 10%
Polyunsat fat	6 gm		3%	
Monounsat fat	11 gm		7%	More than 10%
Cholesterol	310 mg			Less than 300 mg
Sodium	2,680 mg			0 to 2,400 mg
Carbohydrate	210 gm		56%	150 to 230 gm
Dietary fiber	20 gm			More than 17 gm
Sugars	93 gm			Less than 150 gm
Protein	95 gm	45	25%	12 to 20%
Calcium	1,088 mg	-112		More than 1,200 mg
Carb (Breakfast)	44 gm			
Carb (AM Snack)	0 gm			
Carb (Lunch)	53 gm			
Carb (PM Snack)	16 gm			
Carb (Dinner)	67 gm			
Carb (EV Snack)	30 gm			
Glycemic index	41			
Starch	97 gm			
Phosphorus	1,602 mg	902		More than 700 mg
Potassium	2,806 mg			

Monday

Food Item	Amount to Serve	Exchanges	Cal	Carb (gm)	Prot (gm)	Fat (g)	Sod (mg)
BREAKFAST							
Bagel, plain	½ large (4" dia)	2 Starch	155	30	6	1	302
Cream cheese, reduced fat (Neufchatel)	1½ Tbsp.	1 Fat	54	1	2	5	92
Milk, fat-free (non-fat, skim)	1 cup	1 Milk, fat-free	83	12	8	0	108
Orange juice, fresh	½ cup	1 Fruit	56	13	1	0	1
			348	**56**	**17**	**6**	**502**
LUNCH							
Southwestern Bean Soup with Cornmeal Dumplings (p 163)	1 serving	2 Starch; 2 Vegetable	197	39	9	1	367
Nuts, mixed	6 nuts	1 Fat	37	1	1	3	26
Fresh fruit mix	¾ cup	1 Fruit	61	15	1	0	4
Cheese, cheddar, reduced fat	2 ozs.	2 Meat, med fat	115	1	14	12	480
			410	**56**	**25**	**17**	**877**
AFTERNOON SNACK							
Crackers, whole wheat, reduced fat (Triscuits)	5 Triscuits	1 Starch	80	15	2	2	110
Sunflower seeds, dry roasted	1 Tbsp.	1 Fat	47	2	2	4	0
			127	**17**	**3**	**6**	**110**
DINNER							
Snapper, cooked	4 ozs.	4 Meat, very lean	145	0	30	2	65
Beans, green, fresh, cooked	1 cup	2 Vegetable	44	10	2	0	4
Potato, baked with skin	6 ozs.	2 Starch	158	36	4	0	17
Margarine, light, soft tub	1 Tbsp.	1 Fat	40	0	0	4	90
Pear, fresh	½ pear	1 Fruit	62	16	0	0	0
			449	**62**	**37**	**7**	**176**
EVENING SNACK							
Yogurt, non-fat, vanilla	1 container (6 ozs.)	1 Milk, fat-free	90	16	6	0	95
Walnuts, English	4 halves	1 Fat	52	1	1	5	0
			142	**17**	**7**	**6**	**95**

Monday—Totals for the Day

Nutrient	Quantity	DRI Comparison (- = Under)	% of Day's Calories	Goals
Calories	1,476			1,450 to 1,550
Fat	42 gm		24%	0 to 30%
Saturated fat	14 gm		8%	0 to 10%
Polyunsat fat	12 gm		7%	
Monounsat fat	12 gm		7%	More than 10%
Cholesterol	117 mg			Less than 300 mg
Sodium	1,760 mg			0 to 2,400 mg
Carbohydrate	208 gm		53%	150 to 230 gm
Dietary fiber	26 gm			More than 18 gm
Sugars	76 gm			Less than 150 gm
Protein	90 gm	40	23%	12 to 20%
Calcium	1,117 mg	-83		More than 1,200 mg
Carb (Breakfast)	56 gm			
Carb (AM Snack)	0 gm			
Carb (Lunch)	56 gm			
Carb (PM Snack)	17 gm			
Carb (Dinner)	62 gm			
Carb (EV Snack)	17 gm			
Glycemic index	46			
Starch	104 gm			
Phosphorus	1,672 mg	972		More than 700 mg
Potassium	3,855 mg			

Tuesday

Food Item	Amount to Serve	Exchanges	Cal	Carb (gm)	Prot (gm)	Fat (gm)	Sod (mg)
BREAKFAST							
Wheat bread, toasted	2 slices	2 Starch	130	24	5	2	265
Margarine, light, soft tub	1 Tbsp.	1 Fat	40	0	0	4	90
Jelly/preserves, low or reduced sugar	2 tsp.	Free food	16	4	0	0	0
Fresh fruit mix	¾ cup	1 Fruit	61	15	1	0	4
Milk, fat-free (non-fat, skim)	1 cup	1 Milk, fat-free	83	12	8	0	108
			330	**55**	**14**	**7**	**467**
MORNING SNACK							
Cranberries, dried	3 Tbsp.	1 Fruit	66	16	0	1	0
Walnuts, English	4 halves	1 Fat	52	1	1	5	0
			119	**17**	**1**	**6**	**0**
LUNCH							
Cottage cheese, low-fat, 1% milkfat	½ cup	2 Meat, very lean	81	3	14	1	459
Crackers, whole wheat, reduced fat (Triscuits)	10 Triscuits	2 Starch	160	30	4	4	220
Grapes, fresh seedless, small	17 grapes	1 Fruit	60	15	1	0	2
Tomato, raw	3 slices, medium	—	13	3	0	0	5
			314	**51**	**19**	**6**	**686**
AFTERNOON SNACK							
Milk, fat-free (non-fat, skim)	1 cup	1 Milk, fat-free	83	12	8	0	108
Popcorn, popped, no salt/fat added	3 cups	1 Starch	92	19	3	1	1
			175	**31**	**11**	**1**	**109**
DINNER							
Turkey and Sweet Potato Casserole (p 115)	1 serving	2 Starch; 1 Vegetable; 4 Meat, very lean	318	35	37	3	473
Salad greens mix	2 cups	1 Vegetable	15	3	1	0	15

Food Item	Amount to Serve	Exchanges	Cal	Carb (gm)	Prot (gm)	Fat (gm)	Sod (mg)
Salad dressing, Italian, fat-free	1 Tbsp.	Free food	7	2	0	0	155
Cantaloupe, fresh	1 cup	1 Fruit	56	13	1	0	14
			397	**53**	**40**	**3**	**657**

EVENING SNACK

Food Item	Amount to Serve	Exchanges	Cal	Carb (gm)	Prot (gm)	Fat (gm)	Sod (mg)
Crackers, graham	3 crackers	1 Starch	89	16	1	2	127
Peanut butter, smooth/crunchy	1 Tbsp.	1 Meat, high fat	96	3	4	8	80
			185	**19**	**5**	**10**	**207**

Tuesday—Totals for the Day

Nutrient	Quantity	DRI Comparison (- = Under)	% of Day's Calories	Goals
Calories	1,520			1,450 to 1,550
Fat	34 gm		19%	0 to 30%
Saturated fat	7 gm		4%	0 to 10%
Polyunsat fat	12 gm		7%	
Monounsat fat	12 gm		7%	More than 10%
Cholesterol	107 mg			Less than 300 mg
Sodium	2,126 mg			0 to 2,400 mg
Carbohydrate	226 gm		58%	150 to 230 gm
Dietary fiber	24 gm			More than 18 gm
Sugars	102 gm			Less than 150 gm
Protein	90 gm	40	23%	12 to 20%
Calcium	755 mg	-445		More than 1,200 mg
Carb (Breakfast)	55 gm			
Carb (AM Snack)	17 gm			
Carb (Lunch)	51 gm			
Carb (PM Snack)	31 gm			
Carb (Dinner)	53 gm			
Carb (EV Snack)	19 gm			
Glycemic index	37			
Starch	81 gm			
Phosphorus	1,309 mg	609		More than 700 mg
Potassium	2,755 mg			

Wednesday

Food Item	Amount to Serve	Exchanges	Cal	Carb (gm)	Prot (gm)	Fat (gm)	Sod (mg)
BREAKFAST							
Oatmeal, cooked	1 cup	2 Starch	145	25	6	2	2
Raisins, dark, seedless	2 Tbsp.	1 Fruit	54	14	1	0	2
Almonds, dry roasted	6 almonds	1 Fat	48	2	2	4	0
Milk, fat-free (non-fat, skim)	1 cup	1 Milk, fat-free	83	12	8	0	108
			330	**53**	**17**	**7**	**112**
MORNING SNACK							
Snack Mix (p 303)	1 serving	1 Starch; 1 Fat	110	14	2	5	278
			110	**14**	**2**	**5**	**278**
LUNCH							
Bread, whole wheat	2 slices	2 Starch	138	26	5	2	295
Tuna salad, fresh	½ cup	½ Carbohydrate; 2 Meat, lean; 1 Fat	192	10	16	9	412
Lettuce, leaf	2 leaves	—	2	0	0	0	1
Tomato, raw	3 slices, medium	—	13	3	0	0	5
Apple, with peel	1 small (2½" dia)	1 Fruit	55	15	0	0	1
			399	**53**	**23**	**11**	**715**
DINNER							
Beef, chuck, lean only (extras from Saturday)	4 ozs.	4 Meat, lean	245	0	37	9	75
Hot German Potato Salad (p 255)	1 serving	2 Starch	149	30	4	2	397
Cabbage, red, cooked, shredded	1 cup	2 Vegetable	44	10	2	0	12
Applesauce, unsweetened	½ cup	1 Fruit	52	14	0	0	2
			490	**54**	**44**	**11**	**486**

Food Item	Amount to Serve	Exchanges	Cal	Carb (gm)	Prot (gm)	Fat (gm)	Sod (mg)
EVENING SNACK							
Gingersnap cookies, regular	3 cookies	1 Carbohydrate	87	16	1	2	137
Milk, fat-free (non-fat, skim)	1 cup	1 Milk, fat-free	83	12	8	0	108
			170	**28**	**9**	**2**	**245**

Wednesday—Totals for the Day

Nutrient	Quantity	DRI Comparison (- = Under)	% of Day's Calories	Goals
Calories	1,499			1,450 to 1,550
Fat	36 gm		22%	0 to 30%
Saturated fat	9 gm		5%	0 to 10%
Polyunsat fat	9 gm		5%	
Monounsat fat	16 gm		10%	More than 10%
Cholesterol	141 mg			Less than 300 mg
Sodium	1,836 mg			0 to 2,400 mg
Carbohydrate	203 gm		53%	150 to 230 gm
Dietary fiber	23 gm			More than 18 gm
Sugars	83 gm			Less than 150 gm
Protein	96 gm	46	25%	12 to 20%
Calcium	719 mg	-481		More than 1,200 mg
Carb (Breakfast)	53 gm			
Carb (AM Snack)	14 gm			
Carb (Lunch)	53 gm			
Carb (PM Snack)	0 gm			
Carb (Dinner)	54 gm			
Carb (EV Snack)	28 gm			
Glycemic index	46			
Starch	83 gm			
Phosphorus	1,463 mg	763		More than 700 mg
Potassium	3,093 mg			

Thursday

Food Item	Amount to Serve	Exchanges	Cal	Carb (gm)	Prot (gm)	Fat (gm)	Sod (mg)
BREAKFAST							
Egg, scrambled with	1 egg	1 Meat, med fat	75	1	6	5	63
pepper, green bell, raw	⅛ cup, sliced	⅛ Vegetable	2	1	0	0	0
onions, fresh	⅛ cup	⅛ Vegetable	7	2	0	0	1
Salsa	¼ cup	Free food	15	3	1	0	168
English muffin, whole wheat	1 muffin	2 Starch	126	25	5	1	220
Margarine, light, soft tub	1 Tbsp.	1 Fat	40	0	0	4	90
Orange juice, fresh	½ cup	1 Fruit	56	13	1	0	1
			322	**44**	**14**	**11**	**543**
MORNING SNACK							
Milk, fat-free (non-fat, skim)	1 cup	1 Milk, fat-free	83	12	8	0	108
			83	**12**	**8**	**0**	**108**
LUNCH							
Pirate Stew (p 181), lower sodium	1 serving	2 Starch; 1 Vegetable; 2 Meat, lean; ½ Fat	310	38	22	8	611
Papaya, fresh	1 cup	1 Fruit	55	14	1	0	4
			365	**52**	**23**	**8**	**615**
AFTERNOON SNACK							
Snack Mix (p 303)	1 serving (extras from a previous day)	1 Starch; 1 Fat	110	14	2	5	278
			110	**14**	**2**	**5**	**278**
DINNER							
Salmon, fresh, broiled or baked	3 ozs.	3 Meat, lean	183	0	23	9	56
Vegetables, mixed (with corn), frozen cooked	1 cup	1 Starch	80	18	4	0	80
Roll, multi-grain	1 roll, medium	1½ Starch	125	23	3	2	244
Margarine, light, soft tub	1 Tbsp.	1 Fat	40	0	0	4	90

Food Item	Amount to Serve	Exchanges	Cal	Carb (gm)	Prot (gm)	Fat (gm)	Sod (mg)
Salad greens mix	2 cups	1 Vegetable	15	3	1	0	15
Salad dressing, Italian, fat-free	2 Tbsp.	Free food	15	3	0	0	310
Banana, fresh	1 extra small	1 Fruit	75	19	1	0	1
			533	**66**	**32**	**17**	**796**

EVENING SNACK

Food Item	Amount to Serve	Exchanges	Cal	Carb (gm)	Prot (gm)	Fat (gm)	Sod (mg)
Yogurt, non-fat, vanilla	1 container (6 ozs.)	1 Milk, fat-free	90	16	6	0	95
			90	**16**	**6**	**0**	**95**

Thursday—Totals for the Day

Nutrient	Quantity	DRI Comparison (- = Under)	% of Day's Calories	Goals
Calories	1,503			1,450 to 1,550
Fat	42 gm		25%	0 to 30%
Saturated fat	10 gm		6%	0 to 10%
Polyunsat fat	8 gm		5%	
Monounsat fat	19 gm		11%	More than 10%
Cholesterol	341 mg			Less than 300 mg
Sodium	2,435 mg			0 to 2,400 mg
Carbohydrate	204 gm		53%	150 to 230 gm
Dietary fiber	24 gm			More than 18 gm
Sugars	86 gm			Less than 150 gm
Protein	85 gm	35	22%	12 to 20%
Calcium	858 mg	-342		More than 1,200 mg
Carb (Breakfast)	44 gm			
Carb (AM Snack)	12 gm			
Carb (Lunch)	52 gm			
Carb (PM Snack)	14 gm			
Carb (Dinner)	66 gm			
Carb (EV Snack)	16 gm			
Glycemic index	48			
Starch	92 gm			
Phosphorus	1,548 mg	848		More than 700 mg
Potassium	3,874 mg			

Friday

Food Item	Amount to Serve	Exchanges	Cal	Carb (gm)	Prot (gm)	Fat (gm)	Sod (mg)
BREAKFAST							
Mexican-Style Grits (p 322), lower fat	2 servings	2 Starch	182	32	9	2	334
Fresh fruit mix	¾ cup	1 Fruit	61	15	1	0	4
Milk, fat-free (non-fat, skim)	1 cup	1 Milk, fat-free	83	12	8	0	108
			326	**59**	**18**	**3**	**445**
LUNCH							
Soy patty, chicken flavor	1 patty	1 Starch; 1 Meat, med fat	150	12	13	6	470
Pita bread, whole wheat	½ pita	1 Starch	70	15	3	1	65
Tomato, cucumber, onion mix, raw	1 cup	1 Vegetable	30	7	1	0	9
Lettuce, leaf	2 leaves	—	2	0	0	0	1
Salad dressing, ranch, light	1 Tbsp.	1 Fat	40	2	0	4	140
Plum, fresh	2 plums	1 Fruit	73	17	1	1	0
			367	**53**	**19**	**10**	**686**
AFTERNOON SNACK							
Yogurt, non-fat, vanilla	1 container (6 ozs.)	1 Milk, fat-free	90	16	6	0	95
			90	**16**	**6**	**0**	**95**
DINNER							
Mjeddrah (p 214)	1 serving	2 Starch; ½ Fat	173	29	9	3	196
Meatless burger, soy-based	2½ cup	1 Carbohydrate; 2 Meat, very lean	140	14	22	1	440
Raisins, dark, seedless	2 Tbsp.	1 Fruit	54	14	1	0	2
Cashews, unsalted	1 Tbsp.	1 Fat	52	3	1	4	1
Carrots, fresh cooked	1 cup	2 Vegetable	70	16	2	0	102
			488	**76**	**34**	**9**	**742**

Food Item	Amount to Serve	Exchanges	Cal	Carb (gm)	Prot (gm)	Fat (gm)	Sod (mg)
EVENING SNACK							
Tortilla chips, baked (low-fat)	¾ oz	1 Starch	83	18	2	1	150
Hummus	⅓ cup	1 Starch; 1 Fat	137	12	7	8	313
			219	**30**	**9**	**9**	**463**

Friday—Totals for the Day

Nutrient	Quantity	DRI Comparison (- = Under)	% of Day's Calories	Goals
Calories	1,491			1,450 to 1,550
Fat	30 gm		18%	0 to 30%
Saturated fat	5 gm		3%	0 to 10%
Polyunsat fat	10 gm		6%	
Monounsat fat	11 gm		7%	More than 10%
Cholesterol	12 mg			Less than 300 mg
Sodium	2,431 mg			0 to 2,400 mg
Carbohydrate	233 gm		60%	150 to 230 gm
Dietary fiber	38 gm			More than 18 gm
Sugars	78 gm			Less than 150 gm
Protein	86 gm	36	22%	12 to 20%
Calcium	841 mg	-359		More than 1,200 mg
Carb (Breakfast)	59 gm			
Carb (AM Snack)	0 gm			
Carb (Lunch)	53 gm			
Carb (PM Snack)	16 gm			
Carb (Dinner)	76 gm			
Carb (EV Snack)	30 gm			
Glycemic index	35			
Starch	117 gm			
Phosphorus	1,823 mg	1,123		More than 700 mg
Potassium	2,422 mg			

Saturday

Food Item	Amount to Serve	Exchanges	Cal	Carb(gm)	Prot(gm)	Fat(gm)	Sod(mg)
BREAKFAST							
Milk, fat-free (non-fat, skim)	1 cup	1 Milk, fat-free	83	12	8	0	108
Kashi, puffed cereal	1 cup	1 Starch	70	13	3	1	2
Apricots, dried	8 halves	1 Fruit	67	18	1	0	3
Almonds, dry roasted	6 almonds	1 Fat	48	2	2	4	0
Wheat bread, toasted	1 slice	1 Starch	65	12	2	1	132
			333	**56**	**17**	**6**	**245**
MORNING SNACK							
Banana, fresh	1 extra small	1 Fruit	75	19	1	0	1
			75	**19**	**1**	**0**	**1**
LUNCH							
Slow Cooker Minestrone (p 169)—lower sodium	1 serving	1 Starch; 2 Vegetable; 1 Meat, lean	183	21	17	4	413
Crackers, whole wheat, reduced fat (Triscuit)	5 Triscuits	1 Starch	80	15	2	2	110
Apple, with peel	1 small (2½" dia)	1 Fruit	55	15	0	0	1
			318	**51**	**19**	**6**	**524**
AFTERNOON SNACK							
Popcorn, popped, no salt/fat added	3 cups	1 Starch	92	19	3	1	1
Nuts, mixed	6 nuts	1 Fat	37	1	1	3	26
			129	**20**	**4**	**4**	**27**
DINNER							
Pot Roast (p 7)	1 serving	1 Starch; 1 Vegetable; 3 Meat, lean	219	14	26	6	361
Roll, multi-grain	1 roll, medium	1½ Starch	125	23	3	2	244
Margarine, light, soft tub	1 Tbsp.	1 Fat	40	0	0	4	90
Salad greens mix	2 cups	1 Vegetable	15	3	1	0	15

Food Item	Amount to Serve	Exchanges	Cal	Carb (gm)	Prot (gm)	Fat (gm)	Sod (mg)
Salad dressing, Italian, fat-free	1 Tbsp.	Free food	7	2	0	0	155
Fresh fruit mix	¾ cup	1 Fruit	61	15	1	0	4
			468	**57**	**31**	**13**	**869**

EVENING SNACK

Milk, fat-free (non-fat, skim)	1 cup	1 Milk, fat-free	83	12	8	0	108
Oatmeal, cooked	½ cup	1 Starch	73	13	3	1	1
			156	**25**	**11**	**1**	**10**

Saturday—Totals for the Day

Nutrient	Quantity	DRI Comparison (- = Under)	% of Day's Calories	Goals
Calories	1,479			1,450 to 1,550
Fat	31 gm		18%	0 to 30%
Saturated fat	8 gm		4%	0 to 10%
Polyunsat fat	7 gm		4%	
Monounsat fat	14 gm		8%	More than 10%
Cholesterol	126 mg			Less than 300 mg
Sodium	1,775 mg			0 to 2,400 mg
Carbohydrate	228 gm		60%	150 to 230 gm
Dietary fiber	30 gm			More than 17 gm
Sugars	94 gm			Less than 150 gm
Protein	82 gm	32	22%	12 to 20%
Calcium	726 mg	-474		More than 1,200 mg
Carb (Breakfast)	56 gm			
Carb (AM Snack)	19 gm			
Carb (Lunch)	51 gm			
Carb (PM Snack)	20 gm			
Carb (Dinner)	57 gm			
Carb (EV Snack)	25 gm			
Glycemic index	42			
Starch	83 gm			
Phosphorus	1,339 mg	639		More than 700 mg
Potassium	3,197 mg			

Averages for the Week

Nutrient	Quantity	DRI Comparison (- = Under)	% of Day's Calories	Goals
Calories	1,488			1,450 to 1,550
Fat	36 gm		21%	0 to 30%
Saturated fat	9 gm		5%	0 to 10%
Polyunsat fat	9 gm		5%	
Monounsat fat	14 gm		8%	More than 10%
Cholesterol	165 mg			Less than 300 mg
Sodium	2,149 mg			0 to 2,400 mg
Carbohydrate	216 gm		56%	150 to 230 gm
Dietary fiber	26 gm			More than 18 gm
Sugars	88 gm			Less than 150 gm
Protein	89 gm	39	23%	12 to 20%
Calcium	872 mg	-328		More than 1,200 mg
Carb (Breakfast)	52 gm			
Carb (AM Snack)	9 gm			
Carb (Lunch)	53 gm			
Carb (PM Snack)	16 gm			
Carb (Dinner)	62 gm			
Carb (EV Snack)	24 gm			
Glycemic index	42			
Starch	94 gm			
Phosphorus	1,537 mg	837		More than 700 mg
Potassium	3,143 mg			

10 Most Asked Questions about Diabetes

1. Can people with diabetes eat sugar?

Yes, they can. Sugar is just another carbohydrate to the body. All carbohydrates, whether they come from dessert, breads, or carrots, raise blood sugar. An equal serving of brownie and of baked potato raise your blood sugar the same amount. If you know that a rise in blood sugar is coming, it is wise to focus on the size of the serving.

The question of "how much sugar is too much?" has to be answered by each one of us. No one who wants to be healthy eats a lot of sugar.

2. Do people with diabetes have to eat a special diet?

No, they should eat the same foods that are healthy for everyone—whole grains, vegetables, fruit, and small portions of lean meat. Like everyone else, people with diabetes should eat breakfast, lunch, and dinner and not put off eating until dinnertime. By then, you are ravenous and will eat too much. This sends the blood sugar levels soaring in people with diabetes, and doesn't allow them to feel hungry for breakfast the next morning. Some people (with or without diabetes) do best when they eat five or six tiny meals or snacks a day.

3. What is diabetes?

Let's begin with insulin. It is a hormone that is produced in the pancreas, which is an organ located near your stomach. When you eat food, it is digested and broken down into glucose, a sugar. In this form it can travel around to feed all the cells in your body by way of the bloodstream. But the glucose cannot get into your cells unless insulin is there to open the door. Without insulin, the glucose stays in the bloodstream. And each time you eat, more glucose goes into your bloodstream. High levels of blood glucose or blood sugar is the sign that you have diabetes.

In type 1 diabetes, the body cannot produce insulin at all. Something has caused the body to destroy the cells in the pancreas that make insulin. People with type 1 diabetes must have insulin injections or use an insulin pump to stay alive.

In type 2 diabetes, the body is either not making enough insulin or not using it well. People can help their bodies use the insulin more effectively by losing weight and being active every day. Some people have to take diabetes pills or insulin to get their blood sugar levels back to normal.

4. What causes diabetes?

To start with, you need to have the gene for diabetes. Then there has to be something that triggers the gene. For many people who develop type 2 diabetes, the trigger is being over-weight and sedentary. For others, it might be a stress on the body such as pregnancy or a serious accident requiring surgery.

For a child with type 1 diabetes, a virus may have confused the immune system into identifying the beta cells in the pancreas as part of the virus, and so the immune system destroyed the beta cells and stopped the production of insulin.

5. How many people have diabetes in the United States?

About 18 million people have diabetes in the United States, but 8 million of those don't know it. There are 1 million new cases of diabetes diagnosed every year. The most distressing of these are the growing number of teens and older children who are developing type 2 diabetes—which usually occurs much later in life.

6. Why don't people know that they have diabetes?

The people who develop type 1 diabetes know because it comes on quickly and the symptoms are serious. But it affects only about 10 percent of the people with diabetes.

Type 2 accounts for the other 90 percent. Because it doesn't hurt and the symptoms come on gradually, people have usually had type 2 diabetes for 7 to 10 years when they get diagnosed.

7. Is there a cure for diabetes?

Not yet. Some people with type 2 diabetes may seem to have cured it by losing weight and getting regular daily exercise, because their blood sugar returns to normal levels and stays there. This may continue for years, but eventually the pancreas just wears out, and they will need medication to manage their blood sugar levels.

A small number of people with type 1 diabetes who have had a successful pancreas or islet cell transplant no longer have diabetes because their bodies are producing insulin again. However, they have to take powerful immunosuppressant drugs for the rest of their lives to prevent their bodies from rejecting the transplant.

8. Is there a type of diabetes that only happens when a woman is pregnant?

Yes, it is called gestational diabetes. After the baby is born, the woman no longer has diabetes, but she needs to take care to be active and to maintain a healthy weight or she might develop type 2 diabetes later on in life. During the last two months of her pregnancy, she will need to follow a meal plan to keep her blood sugar in normal ranges, or her baby may grow too big, causing problems for her and the baby during the birth process.

9. Does diabetes hurt?

High blood sugar can make you feel tired and irritable, but it comes on so gradually that you may not realize what is happening. It can blur your vision. That's on the outside. On the inside, constantly high blood sugar levels are silently damaging your blood vessels and nerves and can cause problems everywhere from your eyes to your feet, and especially to your heart. If diabetes starts hurting, damage has already been done.

10. Is there any way to avoid the damage that diabetes can do to the body?

Yes. We now know how to manage blood sugar levels, and persons with diabetes can learn what to do to keep healthy. Working with dietitians to develop a meal plan of foods that they like helps them get the nutrients their bodies need and not eat too much carbohydrate at any one meal or snack. Checking their blood sugar, in the morning or two hours after a meal, for example, with a small glucose meter gives them and their health care providers information about how high their blood sugar is going and when, and about the effect of any diabetes medication they are taking. A daily 30- to 45-minute walk is another simple but powerful way to lower blood sugar and to be healthier all over.

Learning to bring blood sugar levels back to normal every day is the key to preventing diabetes from doing any damage. We have extensive research to show that this is true. People can even prevent diabetes from developing at all by taking the same steps of eating healthy meals and getting daily exercise. These are also the tools that can reverse some of the damage that might have already been done.

Recommended Reading List

(ADA is the American Diabetes Association.)

Diabetes Burnout: What to Do When You Can't Take It Anymore, William H. Polonsky, PhD, CDE; ADA,1999, 348 pages. Also available on audiocassette.

Diabetes Meal Planning Made Easy, 4th ed., Hope S. Warshaw, MMSc, RD, CDE, BC-ADM; ADA, 2010, 362 pages.

Dr. Gavin's Health Guide for African Americans, James R. Gavin, MD, PhD, with Sherrye Landrum; Small Steps Press, 2004, 278 pages.

A Field Guide to Type 1 Diabetes, ADA, 2002, 210 pages.

A Field Guide to Type 2 Diabetes: The Essential Resource from the Diabetes Experts, ADA, 2004, 295 pages.

Help! My Underwear Is Shrinking! Jo Ann Hattner, MPH, RD; Ann Coulston, MS, RD; and E. Michael Goodkind; ADA, 2003, 140 pages.

Mastering Your Diabetes (Before Diabetes Masters You), Janette Kirkham, RN, CDE, ECT; ADA, 2003, 132 pages.

The Official Pocket Guide to Diabetic Exchanges: Choose Your Foods, 3rd ed., ADA, 2011, 72 pages.

What to Do When You Have Type 2 Diabetes, ADA, 2002, 64 pages.

Index

An asterisk (*) indicates that photos are shown in the insert pages.

About the Author

Phyllis Pellman Good is a *New York Times* bestselling author whose books have sold nearly 10 million copies.

Good is the author of the nationally acclaimed *Fix-It and Forget-It* slow cooker cookbooks, several of which have appeared on the *New York Times* bestseller list, as well as the bestseller lists of *USA Today, Publishers Weekly,* and *Book Sense.*

The series includes *Fix-It and Forget-It Cookbook* (Revised and Updated); *700 Great Slow Cooker Recipes; Fix-It and Forget-It Lightly: Healthy, Low-Fat Recipes for Your Slow Cooker; Fix-It and Forget-It 5-Ingredient Favorites: Comforting Slow-Cooker Recipes;* and *Fix-It and Forget-It Christmas Cookbook: 600 Slow Cooker Holiday Recipes.*

Phyllis Pellman Good is Executive Editor at Good Books. (Good Books has published hundreds of titles by more than 135 authors.) She received her BA and MA in English from New York University. She and her husband, Merle, live in Lancaster, Pennsylvania. They are the parents of two young-adult daughters.

For a complete listing of books by Phyllis Pellman Good, as well as excerpts and reviews, visit www.Fix-ItandForget-It.com or www.GoodBooks.com.

American Diabetes Association
Cure · Care · Commitment

The American Diabetes Association is the nation's leading voluntary health organization supporting diabetes research, information, and advocacy. Its mission is to prevent and cure diabetes and to improve the lives of all people affected by diabetes. The American Diabetes Association is the leading publisher of comprehensive diabetes information. Its huge library of practical and authoritative books for people with diabetes covers every aspect of self-care-cooking and nutrition, fitness, weight control, medications, complications, emotional issues, and general self-care.

To order ADA books, call 1-800-232-6733.

Or go to the web bookstore at store.diabetes.org (no www is needed).

For more information about diabetes, call 1-800-342-2383.